APPROACHES TO THE MIND

MOVEMENT OF THE PSYCHIATRIC SCHOOLS FROM SECTS TOWARD SCIENCE

APPROACHES TO THE MIND

MOVEMENT OF THE PSYCHIATRIC SCHOOLS FROM SECTS TOWARD SCIENCE

·

Leston L. Havens, M.D.

Professor of Psychiatry at the
Massachusetts Mental Health Center,
Harvard Medical School, Boston

·

LITTLE, BROWN AND COMPANY
BOSTON

Library of Congress catalog card No. 73-1419

ISBN 0-316-35045

Published in Great Britain by
Churchill/Livingstone, Edinburgh and London

Printed in the United States of America

— Who wields a poem huger than the grave?
for only Whom shall time no refuge keep
though all the weird worlds must be opened?
) Love

                        e. e. cummings

                To

            Susan

        Christopher, Jeffrey,

        Jennifer, and Sarah

PREFACE

The purpose of this book is to help psychiatry move from the sectarianism that grips it toward science and a more effective practice. Today the different psychiatric schools institutionalize themselves to protect and teach their theories and methods. A lack of general medical validity makes everyone defensive while at the same time each school needs the others for special treatment situations and occasionally for referrals! Although any large collapse of the present situation awaits such overwhelmingly effective discoveries as those that broke the nineteenth century medical sects, for example the discovery of infectious agents, the present-day fragmentation and disputatiousness not only confuse practice but also obscure the extraordinary advances that have been made. One of my contentions in the book is that these advances concern *methods* of investigating human nature more than they do theories of human nature. The schools have developed distinct techniques for approaching troubled human beings; these techniques secure quite different types of information; the techniques and types of information are both the basis of the sectarianism and one means by which it may be overcome.

Psychiatry developed, first, from the application of objective-descriptive method and, during the first half of this century, from psychoanalytic method. Now new methods of social and existential psychiatry promise further advances. And there are undoubtedly many more methods waiting to be discovered.

The emphasis of this book is on methods and facts, seldom on theories. The nature of psychiatric information and concerns encourages theorizing. The result is that psychiatric theories lie around us like fogs. It is time, in Emerson's sharp language, "to pierce this rotten diction and fasten words again to visible things."

I have had splendid teachers over a long course of schooling, including psychoanalytic schooling, which is perhaps the most complex amalgam of treatment and training known. To Henry Wermer I owe the retrieval of a love of writing and practice that had first animated my movement into medicine. John Murray brought to our work a rich experience, courage, wisdom, and a clear, wonderfully cheerful mind. I spent my residency years, and much of the period since, at the Massachusetts Mental Health Center (the old Boston Psychopathic Hospital). Its recent professors and superintendents, Jack Ewalt and Harry Solomon, have made that institution representative of the best in the field, and have thereby struck against the prevailing sectarianism. There I have had teachers of the hand, heart, and head. Jack Ewalt is an administrative genius, who makes independent work possible. For a generation of medical students and residents, Elvin Semrad has been

Boston's leading teacher of the heart. Few psychiatric thinkers have surpassed Ives Hendrick in his clear use of the head.

Eleanor deRubeis, Molly Brittan, and Judith McLeod have provided wonderful secretarial help. Susan Payne gave invaluable library assistance, and Judith McLeod and Bea Limentani, saving editorial advice.

L. L. H.

CONTENTS

PREFACE   vii

Introduction   1
THE FOUR MAJOR SCHOOLS   4
THE LARGER SCENE   7

Part I. The Schools   11

1. Objective-Descriptive Psychiatry   13
EMIL KRAEPELIN   13
PIERRE JANET   34

2. Beginnings of Psychoanalysis   63
CHARCOT   63
BREUER AND FREUD   80

3. Freud and Psychoanalysis   93
   CONFLICT AND DISSOCIATION   95
   THE DORA CASE: REVERSAL OF AFFECTS AND
      DISPLACEMENT   104
   WISH AND FANTASY   116
   INFANTILE ELEMENTS   118

4. Existential Psychiatry   123
   JASPERS   124
   MINKOWSKI   133
   BINSWANGER   147
   ROLE OF EMOTION IN TREATMENT   156

5. Interpersonal (Social) Psychiatry   167
   ADOLF MEYER   171
   HARRY STACK SULLIVAN   183
   SOCIAL UNDERSTANDING OF HYSTERIA   199
   SOCIOLOGICAL PSYCHIATRY   206

Part II. Main Currents of Psychiatric
     Development   215

6. Temporal Development   219
   EVOLUTION IN PSYCHIATRY   226
   CONTRIBUTIONS OF THE SCHOOLS   228

7. Causes   235
   BURTON   235
   BENJAMIN RUSH   238
   PROCESSES   241
   FIRST CAUSE   247
   POINTS OF INTERVENTION   248

8. Relationship to the Patients   251
   GROWTH OF UNDERSTANDING   252
   COMING INTO RELATIONSHIP   257

9. Psychiatric Ideals   263
CHANGING IDEALS   264
UNITY OF IDEALS   269
DIVERGENT IDEALS   270

Part III. Toward a Pluralistic Psychiatry   275

10. Technology of the Schools   277
OBJECTIVE-DESCRIPTIVE PSYCHIATRY   278
PSYCHOANALYSIS   287
EXISTENTIAL METHOD   296
INTERPERSONAL PSYCHIATRY   305

11. Dilemmas and Solutions   313
AN ILLUSTRATION: DEALING WITH ANGER   315
THERAPISTS' DECISIONS   321
PLURALISM IN PSYCHIATRY   328

Notes   331

INDEX   365

APPROACHES
TO THE MIND

MOVEMENT OF THE
PSYCHIATRIC SCHOOLS
FROM SECTS TOWARD SCIENCE

INTRODUCTION

*Ludwig Richter relates in his reminiscences
how once, when he was in Tivoli as a
young man, he and three friends set out to
paint part of the landscape, all four firmly
resolved not to deviate from nature by a
hair's-breadth; and although the subject
was the same, and each quite creditably
reproduced what his eyes had seen, the result was four totally different pictures, as
different from each other as the personalities of the four painters. Whence the nar-
rator drew the conclusion that there is no
such thing as objective vision, and that
form and colour are always apprehended
differently according to temperament.*

Heinrich Wölfflin

I T I S N O T an idle matter to question whether we can apprehend human nature only according to our temperaments
or whether there is indeed an objective psychiatry. With
the split of psychiatry into schools, each teaches its own facts,
methods, and ideas, convinced it is *the* psychiatry. Students
shop among the schools, and the public asks psychiatrists and
psychologists what *kind* they are. Every year new varieties come
and go like fashion styles.

One reason for this flux is the wide range of psychiatric
data. The patient's social life, fantasies, physiology or chemistry, our reactions to him, the present, past, and future—all
this and much more feed facts of possible relevance to psychiatric understanding. Beginners in psychiatry sometimes play

the game of presenting one case to several seniors. The first teacher picks up depressive themes, a second oedipal ones, and a third the way incident after incident points to passive homosexual or narcissistic traits. If the issue is classic diagnosis, a few paranoid features may be underlined by one observer or catatonic signs by another, and either allowed to dominate the naming. There are usually enough disagreements to confound scientists and send the frightened back to chemistry.

The question is asked, "Does psychotherapy help and, if so, with what?" No two therapists agree on how *health* should be measured; even its definition is disputed. Acute psychoses seem to existential psychiatrists an improvement over many premorbid adaptations, but not so to community psychiatrists. Psychoanalysts may increase symptoms while they struggle to change underlying personality problems; behaviorists reduce symptoms but then are accused of ignoring what lies behind them. There is a great babble of voices but little talking back and forth.

We know, moreover, that every observation results from some method, some way of looking at or talking to the patient and family. Existentialism, psychoanalysis, interpersonalism, behaviorism, descriptive psychiatry—each school uses its own methods and thus is one source of the variety of facts. I visit your home but then have no time to hear you recount your fantasies; I listen to your fantasies and then cannot ask the questions that would expose your mentation or insight. I "encounter" you as a person but then cannot observe you objectively. Since no one psychiatric school makes use of an all-inclusive method, beginning students, who have to start somewhere, feel themselves prisoners of a point of view.

The traditional medical quest for diseases, special processes, and pathognomonic signs seems at odds with the humanistic interest in whole lives, inner states, and relationships with others. There are attempts at measurement, objectivity, instrumentation, and, simultaneously, a search for metaphors, analogies, empathy, inward sharing, the breaking down of boundaries, and the derogation of objectivity. The new psychiatrist quickly learns, not to bring together, but to set aside; not to unify, but to specialize. Humanists tend to become psychotherapists, inclining toward sectarian groupings and a tight grip on old ideas. Scientists enter the laboratory to explore more and more specialized techniques and areas of knowledge. There is a great hunger to emulate physics or chemistry along with an abrupt turning away from an earlier adulation of Freud's intuitive and speculative gifts. Everyone is in favor of research, and the continuing discovery of fresh physical methods and measurements provides endless possibilities of application to psychiatric problems; yet framing relevant questions proves a slippery business. Clinicians pooh-pooh the experimenters, and the latter condescend to the clinicians. An occasional individual tries to be both and satisfies no one. Bit by bit, each side becomes alienated from the other. The old ideal of a working relationship between clinic and laboratory, so critical to the development of general medicine, remains to be realized.

There is as much fragmentation among the clinicians themselves. Objective psychiatrists follow the old medical authoritative model—"The doctor knows best." Psychoanalysts are objective, too, but more passive and neutral. Existentialists eschew objectivity. What they want is "felt encounters," intimacy; nothing, one wrote, happens until the doctor is touched by the patient. Moreover, when therapists work with groups or families rather than individuals, the same school quarrels are repeated for the group situations. It is as if there were a school for every temperament and no "man for all seasons."

Many of us entered psychiatry and psychology seeking a bridge between science and the arts, a unity of knowledge and experience (something achieved by Leonardo and perhaps

Freud), certainly not their fragmentation. We wanted to carry all our life's experience, as well as the intuitions and colors of art, over into science and the practice of therapy. We wanted to be as much whole persons in our professional lives as elsewhere, to have each part serve every other part, whether personal, social, or professional. Interest in psychopathology often began in college with the exposure to Freud, Nietzsche, Dostoevski, James, Kretschmer, Reich, Laing, or others. There was at first the conviction of understanding a great deal through essentially literary methods and then the creeping suspicion that one had penetrated to possibilities, not facts. Here entered, if it was not present already, a yearning for experimental methods, for the sharp instruments and decisions of the laboratory which medical education soon poured out abundantly. Only then did psychiatry seem to bridge the two worlds.

For other than personal reasons we need an inclusive psychiatry, a truly general psychopathology, and professionals technically apt, tough-minded, and at the same time intuitively and humanistically free. The patient wants to get the treatment he needs, not the one treatment the doctor dispenses. Today we have therapists who give drugs and electric treatments or deconditioning or psychoanalysis or family therapy, no matter who rings the bell, like mad surgeons with one operation for everyone.

THE FOUR MAJOR SCHOOLS

"In growing sciences," Newton wrote, "examples teach more than precepts." The foundation of this book is case material from the principal investigators. It is necessary to grasp the empirical basis of psychiatry first, then the methods by which the various observations are made, and only cautiously the grand ideas through which psychopathology is too often approached. The central questions concern what has been discovered and what methods were used to make the discoveries. Psychiatry has evolved a powerful group of methods—we can say technologies—that govern the relationships of therapists and investigators with their patients and subjects in each of the major schools.

Careful description of the patient seen as an object for description gave the outlines of the major conditions. Kraepelin was the principal figure in establishing the structure of diagnosis still in worldwide use 75 years later. Furthermore, this objective manipulative medical position (Chapter 1) continues, not only in description and diagnosis, but in a typical treatment attitude: The doctor knows best and prescribes for the patient, whether it be chemicals, advice, or, most recently, conditioning and deconditioning treatments. The efforts of biological psychiatry fall mainly here, though a little into psychoanalysis too.

Similarly psychoanalysis (Chapters 2 and 3) began as an investigative method, although not concerned with the description of patients, but with collecting their mental content and their verbal productions. Here another objective approach was established, one that came to emphasize passivity and neutrality on the observer's part, instead of action and authority, together with a particular position of doctor and patient, specific instructions, and the like, all quite different from those of objective-descriptive psychiatry. This method was from the outset both investigative and therapeutic; the very act of discovery was claimed to be therapeutic.

A little later existential psychiatry (Chapter 3) emerged, partly out of and partly in revolt against both objective-descriptive and psychoanalytic psychiatry. The principal figures were Jaspers, Minkowski, and Binswanger. They evolved a clinical method still little understood. In fact, the description of it here may be more my creation than theirs!

Almost simultaneously, social or interpersonal psychiatry

(Chapter 4) appeared, thanks largely to Meyer and Sullivan. This was the first and only American school. Again, its methods have not been well described, only illustrated. Often elements of interpersonal, existential, and psychoanalytic psychiatry have been thrown together, as recently done by Szasz, Laing, and Greenson, to everyone's confusion. Although each of the great schools has developed its own version of group and family work, social psychiatry contributed most and indeed is often equated with "group process." The material of social psychiatry is social reality. This proves to be just as far outside consciousness as are many biological and intrapsychic events.

There can be no separation of facts and methods. Each fact is secured by a particular limited method, and each method is scientific only insofar as it secures consistent facts. These points should not be overlooked if one hopes to grasp the whole universe of mental phenomena with a few methods and facts. Psychoanalysis, for example, attempts to write a "general psychology" on the basis of the associative method and its special facts of mental content. This is no better or worse than the attempt to write a "general psychiatry" on the basis of symptoms, signs, and courses as they emerge in occasional face-to-face interviews between doctor and patient. No clinic presents better examples of megalomania.

Today there are four major psychiatries. Because each represents a significant attitude toward life and people and is strongly attractive to certain temperaments, the person who means to master psychiatry has to withstand strong exclusive pulls in one direction or another. Further, the psychiatrist or psychologist does not want to be merely eclectic, that is, borrowing whatever pleases him from various sources. He wants to be *pluralistic*, able to use all the methods and make the critical observations himself, and to be capable of grasping when and with whom each method should be applied. We can then speak of an inclusive or pluralistic psychiatry. Thus, having painted our portrait from more than one angle, we may be closer to objectivity.

THE LARGER SCENE

As Jaspers wrote more than two decades ago, "The new element in the situation [of psychopathology] is the general uncommittedness and the breadth of approach possible today"—a statement even more applicable at the present time. The final six chapters of this book therefore present the great schools and their contributions in general lines of development and then contrast and partly reconcile technologies. On this basis one can claim that investigators have been building a single psychiatry, no matter how diverse their ideas and methods.

For example, in early psychiatry many occurrences were *causally* related to mental disease. Some approaches were dropped, especially the astrological and demonological; schools were created on the basis of prejudices in favor of one set of factors or another; a general tendency emerged to think in terms of heredity, predisposition, character, stress, and immediate mechanisms of symptom formation, in that order. At the time of every fresh discovery, causal significance was attached to it, so that for brief periods all mental disorders were thought to result from homosexuality, thyroid abnormalities, psychic stress, and so on. Naturally everyone hoped for simple inclusive solutions. Instead, causes were gradually ordered into *sequences of events and interacting factors,* among which decisive elements are rare. The absence of reliable means to weigh the relative impacts of different factors prevented critical experimentation and allowed for continued speculation. Of course, therapeutic tests have been applied; the investigator, intervening at the point he thinks decisive, records a happy result and then claims first place for his causal factor. However, too often everything works, or nothing, and critical investigators go away empty-handed.

Also, a remarkable series of changes can be traced in the *relationship to patients*. At first, patients were distant objects, to be avoided, imprisoned, shackled, even killed, or on the other hand reverenced, sanctified, even deified, but in both extremes, placed apart. All psychiatric development depends on moving beyond this point, approaching the patient and losing fear of him if one is to learn more about him. Many sacred or forbidden areas must be entered; sex, the family, even the attitudes of the doctors themselves. A great hue and cry followed these investigations, just as it did grave-robbing and dissection. Much of the progress seems part of social and political developments. Important advances accompanied the French and American revolutions, and today liberal, democratic, or communistic ideals can be seen reflected in the psychiatric goal of throwing off the outer garments of achievement, cast, or class, to find the "person himself"; everything short of the person himself gets treated as a defense. In psychoanalysis the development is from considering patients as objects productive of mental content to considering them as alliance-forming colleagues, exploring the unconscious with the doctor. It is psychoanalysis that makes the most successful effort of any psychiatric school to describe the great leap from ourselves to others, how we go from self and family outward, and what steps and processes lie between being self-centered and investing in others.

The word *alienation* meant at one time mental derangement; hence the term *alienist* for the profession. However, the patients were not the only ones to turn away, and it is indeed difficult to know who took the first step away, the patient or those around him. In any case, there is a gradual movement toward the patient, and with it, an effort to describe the degrees and stages of relatedness, partly in parallel with a changing medical relatedness that reflects psychiatry's developing methods.

Each one of these technical developments is part of the general developments in science, literature, and art. Parallels to psychiatry's changes can be found in the expanding representation of reality in Western literature (as described by Auerbach in *Mimesis*), differences in artistic perception (for example, Wölfflin's categories), the development of physics from the classical position (as described in Einstein and Enfield's account), the erosion of the concept of discrete objects in favor of experiential and transactional processes (as suggested by Bergson and Whitehead), and many others. Further, to give psychiatry its due, with the appearance of Charcot, Freud, Sullivan, Jung, and the existential psychiatrists, literature and art begin to reflect psychiatry!

I

THE SCHOOLS

1

OBJECTIVE-DESCRIPTIVE PSYCHIATRY [1]

EMIL KRAEPELIN *

EMIL KRAEPELIN fell upon a psychiatric world exhausted with arranging and reordering symptoms along psychological lines largely without medical significance. He sought in psychological phenomena the key to *disease* states. Although an experimental psychologist and student of Wundt [2] and a lifelong investigator of what is today called psychopharmacology, he had little interest in psychological facts for themselves; he did not, for example, follow psychological facts to psychological processes, as Janet was to do. Nor was he a serious student of brain processes for themselves. His

* Leston L. Havens, "Emil Kraepelin," *Journal of Nervous and Mental Disease* 141:16, 1965. Copyright © 1965, The Williams & Wilkins Co. Reproduced, as revised, by permission.

overriding interest was disease and disease processes in the pathological tradition of Virchow; it was to the discovery and elucidation of diseases that the greatest part of his work was directed. He brought to the task enormous energy, a long life, and the gift of marshaling large numbers of facts about a few, powerful ideas.

The most important of these was the disease concept itself. Incidence and distribution, anatomy, pathogenesis, etiology, symptoms and signs, differential diagnosis, course and outcome, prognosis, treatment, and prevention comprise its parts; complete knowledge of a disease implies knowledge of all these. The goal of medicine has been to place any bodily or mental disturbance in one such sequence, and this was Kraepelin's goal for psychiatry. His pursuit of it, more than any other one thing, explains his enduring influence.

The *Psychiatrie,* first a *Compendium,* then a *Short Textbook,* and finally, in the Fifth Edition, *A Textbook,* carried the bulk of his observations and ideas [3]. It began modestly with distinctions along traditional clinical lines and with relatively little attention to organic states. Over the next three editions the material increased; more toxic and infectious states were included and gradually pushed to the front of the book. Several conditions, including "general neuroses," previously handled separately, were brought together, and there were tentative efforts at classification by cause. The climax of these developments, with their emphasis on clinical concepts, the formation of new groupings, and efforts toward a causal structure, was the Fifth Edition, in 1896. The overwhelming tradition of psychiatric diagnosis by the symptoms of first prominence, whether arrived at clinically or from psychological or neurological presuppositions, was abandoned, and known organic states were used as the models for disease types. The new classification was to be by etiology, that is, by knowledge of cause. Diseases of known cause were most truly diseases; it was to be hoped that to this standard other conditions would someday repair. In the meantime, they were given *provisional* etiologies. Thus cretinism—thyroid idiocy—led off metabolic diseases. To this were added dementia praecox, hypothesized to be metabolic, and general paresis, an infectious process which Kraepelin then thought was metabolic. The final grouping, of manic-depressive psychosis, paranoia, neurotic conditions, and a few others, was more or less thrown together in desperation on a *constitutional* basis, as had so often been done in the past; these were diseases of inherited nature, the old French degeneracy concept.

In the last three editions of his text, Kraepelin placed dementia praecox and manic-depressive psychosis in separate categories of their own, without specification of cause. They were no longer one among metabolic or constitutional disorders, although these remained his hypotheses of first choice. Diseases of known cause, for example, infectious or toxic psychoses, still led the list. The largest categories were organic states, endogenous psychoses, and deviant personalities. In broad outline this remains the organization of the official American nosology and of most classificatory efforts since. (The principal change has been the insertion of a neurotic category between the psychoses and what are today called personality or character disorders; we will see how the neurotic category was developed by Janet.)

Where etiology was obscure, Kraepelin arranged the syndromes, largely handed on from nineteenth-century predecessors, by their signs, course, and outcome—other parts of the disease concept. His assumption of underlying *physical processes* encouraged the study of signs and symptoms over time, for a disease process implied longitudinal effects. Just before the writing of the Fifth Edition, Ziehen, Kraepelin's near-contemporary and rival, had reached the university pinnacle of German psychiatry and brought psychological formalism to a sterile perfection. The clinical material was arranged by academic categories: Were the phenomena primarily intellectual, volitional, or emotional; was the location of distortions outside the patient, in the mind, or in the body? As a medical man concerned with prognosis, Kraepelin escaped this symptom-splitting petty warfare of his time by collecting clinical signs under broad distinctions of *outcome,* distinctions which were useful clinically. The clinician, if not given something to do, was at least given something to *expect.* This was the second guiding idea. His location at Heidelberg made its application possible. The numbers of patients were manageable, and the district was accessible and well organized; he was able to follow patients for years after discharge. Every scientific revolution depends upon a fresh idea and method; Kraepelin's revolution depended on the disease concept and the method of case study his clinical situation made possible. Almost in the same year the Freudian revolution was also beginning, with its conviction that psychological events, however obscure, were understandable and with the methods of case study Freud's clinical situation made possible. Freud was to lead psychiatric attention to the earliest and most remote crannies of childhood experience; Kraepelin was to lead it to later courses and eventual outcome, at the other end of time. Both were also to produce *genetic* psychiatries, one a theory of psychological development, the other on the basis of physical genetics.

Kraepelin traveled clinically with an extraordinary small baggage of psychological ideas. Perhaps the most important is the concept of *volition.* In the first case that follows he describes an impediment to will; in the second case, a lost or indifferent will. It is important to have in mind that such phenomena as lack of responsiveness or delayed responsiveness need not call up this idea of will. Energy or life force or libido will do for other investigators. As a student of Wundt, however, Kraepelin would not reduce mental life to a hypothetical energy; it must be reduced to some product of introspection. Will is something we feel in ourselves; whatever empirical roots it has are introspective. You *feel* "willfull" or "willing"; also, the term is used when some obstruction to action is experienced. Similarly, we suspect Wundt's influence on Kraepelin's concern with the "disunities" of much pathological mental life; the concept of *dissociation* is a natural outgrowth of the dominant psychology of the nineteenth century, associationism. His attention to the phenomena of "splitting" is not great, however, and may owe as much to Bleuler as to Wundt. Nowhere in Karepelin's clinical work is his psychological background very obvious. He does not reduce clinical material to a few elements, for example, sensations, and build it up again as in the mental chemistry of Wundt's Leipzig school. Medical interests predominate. There is the same considerable gulf between laboratory and clinical ideas, as well as methods, that persists in psychiatry to this day.

Manic-Depressive Insanity

The first of his cases to be discussed is taken from the *Lectures on Clinical Psychiatry*, a collection of demonstrations before students. Each lecture contains a series of case examples, the general points interpolated between observations. A "clinical picture" is first presented, and then dissected, in the search for crucial features. The material is all pointed toward *diagnosis* and the closely related prognosis; the suspense lies in his gradual working forward through the clinical details to the apparently decisive signs. These are "signs" to a particular disease. The disease in turn suggests a prognosis which is tested against the clinical facts. With the arrival at diagnosis and prognosis the interest of each case is largely dissipated. We are then brought up to the present.

He takes us immediately to the psychological examination: what the physician observes standing before the patient. Even the patient's complaints (symptoms) are little heeded. First attention is to "objective" *signs*. Similarly, history is incidental and almost all history of the *course of the signs*. It is to the obvious manifestations of disease—to the disease rather than the host—that our concern is directed. His was an unsurpassed interest in what patients presented to an intensely curious, persistent, and objective academic physician in a hospital setting, with no special concern for developing a therapeutic or confidential relationship. Throughout, the *content* of the patient's communications and behaviors is of less interest than their form, the contour, pace, and unity of the stream of life.

The patient is brought into the lecture hall and Kraepelin begins his description.

The patient you see before you today is a merchant, 43 years old, who has been in our hospital almost uninterruptedly for about five years. He is strongly built, but badly nourished, and has a pale complexion, and an invalid expression of face. He comes in with short, wearied steps, sits down slowly, and remains sitting in a rather bent position, staring in front of him almost without moving. When questioned, he turns his head a little, and, after a certain pause, answers softly, and in monosyllables, but to the point. We get the impression that speaking gives him a great deal of trouble, his lips moving for a little while before the sound comes out. The patient is clear about time and place, knows the doctors, and says that he has been ill for more than five years, but cannot give any further explanation of this than that his spirits are affected. He says he has no apprehension. He gives short and perfectly relevant answers to questions about his circumstances and past life. He does exercises in arithmetic slowly but correctly, even when they are fairly hard. He writes his name on the blackboard, when asked to do so, with firm though hesitating strokes, after having got up awkwardly. No delusions, particularly ideas of sin, can be made out, the patient only declaring that he is in low spirits, without knowing of any cause for it, except that his illness has lasted so long, and worries him. He hopes, however, to get well again [4, p. 11].

We have to do here, he asserts, with *emotional depression* or "low spirits." Straightaway he sets about the differential diagnosis. These are not the low spirits of the *melancholy* patients he had discussed in an earlier lecture. The present patient is not apprehensive, does not gesticulate, lament, or even complain, as they did. Indeed, it is difficult to draw any response from him, whether the subject be of interest or indifference, or the questioning emphatic or gentle. The dominant impression he conveys is of being under some *constraint*. This is a broad inhibition and suggests to Kraepelin "some general obstacle to utterance of speech," in fact to "all action of will." If it were fear alone that constrained him, why should he be silent on matters of indifference? Comprehension of even complex trains of thought is intact, and the patient seems to *try* to comply with requests, but something retards him. Between the will and action there is an impediment. This, Kraepelin maintains, is by far the most prominent feature of the case.

He has found, in this constraint and in the absence of "apprehensive restlessness," his keys to diagnosis. We have already reached the climax of the presentation. The diagnosis is maniacal-depressive insanity [5], "an entirely different disease" from melancholia. The patient is in a depressed stage of "circular stupor," the older French term for one type of the same condition. And diagnosis implies prognosis.

This disease generally runs its course in a *series of isolated attacks*, which are not uniform, but present either states of depression of the kind described or characteristic states of excitement. . . . The isolated attacks are generally separated by longer or shorter intervals of freedom [4, p. 13].

The conclusion is promptly tested by reference to the patient's history. He first became depressed when he was 23 (that age or a little earlier would be typical) and entered a state of excitement the next year. Again, at age 26, 31, and 36 years, there were depressed and excited episodes. From these we are given the first bits of history that are not solely the history of the patient's signs. At age 26 and 31 his depression followed disappointments in love. In fact, "his relations held his depression to be the result of the melancholy experiences he had been through." Kraepelin places their view in sharp contrast to his own. Both disappointments *followed* periods of excitement, he states, during the first of which the patient had married "a person very much beneath him" and in the second fallen into the hands of an "adventuress." It is the illness which precipitates the apparently stressful experiences. For the first time Kraepelin has made assumptions of fact; both the predisposing excitements were "probable"; neither could be documented.

This is a point at which to pause, for in Kraepelin's handling of "psychic causes," what are today called traumata or stresses, we see his viewpoint stated most baldly. He was to write at a later time:

Profound changes have marked the development of our theory of the physical causes and bases of insanity. Though our attitude toward the influence of psychic forces on the development of mental disorders has changed but slightly, our assessment of their importance has fluctuated. While the old psychic school assigned them a dominant role, the somatic school tended to consider them unimportant. Popular opinion steadfastly championed the importance of psychic influences in the etiology of insanity, and even Griesinger held that they were generally more decisive than physical injuries. Today we have apparently arrived at a clearcut definition. We know that frequently so-called psychic causes—unhappy love, failure in business, overwork—are the product rather than the cause of the disease, that they are but the outward manifestations of a preexisting condition, and finally that their effects depend for the most part on the subject's *anlage* [6].

"The patient's father, as well as his two brothers, were drunkards, while his sister was ill in the same way as himself."

Here is the family history. There are as yet no intensive investigations of the home, school, jobs, or the personalities of parents. Nor are we asked to pause long over the melancholy facts he gives us. Kraepelin is the farthest thing from being a sentimental physician. Even in his less formal, less academic writings, from which his energetic activities in behalf of the patients become evident, there is no stepping down from his objective position. The transmission of parental sickness is assumed to be by physical inheritance. The tough-minded approach to inheritance would remain for several decades nonpsychological.

From the brief family history we are taken to the history of medical illnesses and then to the patient's state on admission to the hospital. At first he had suffered from diabetes insipidus. "A doctor advised him, presumably on this account, to take a little wine, as too much water was not good for him. The patient followed this advice, and about five and one-half years ago suddenly fell ill of delirium tremens, immediately followed by a state of excitement, gradually and continually growing worse, which only disappeared slowly after two years." Thus the episode before the present one was said to be ushered in by delirium tremens, the trembling hallucinatory delirium of heavy drinkers. (It was named and given one of its first descriptions by Thomas Sutton in 1813, who practiced on a section of the English coast through which much smuggled wine and liquor were passed and sampled [7]). We are not told whether this diagnosis was Kraepelin's or a predecessor's: In some cases mania and the "d.t.'s" may be difficult to distinguish, especially when the acute illness passes into a chronic mania. Only a few weeks separated the end of the manic period from the sudden onset of an "extraordinarily severe impediment of volition," which led to the present hospitalization.

The patient remained motionless in bed, would not eat, was wet and dirty in his habits, could hardly speak, and expressed apprehensive ideas. . . . In spite of the most careful nursing, his condition has improved only very slowly and immaterially in the course of the last three years. Yet we may expect that this attack also will end in recovery, like those which have preceded it, if only the patient can live through so severe a disturbance.

The follow-up is given in a footnote. Six months later the patient died, of acute tuberculosis, the common scourge of mental hospitals until recent times. There was no opportunity to test Kraepelin's further prediction that the patient would again fall ill of depression and excitement.

The case report closes with a discussion of the patient's "fluctuations of weight." "Violent revolutions in the province of general nutrition" mark this disorder, the attacks being accompanied by great falls of weight and recoveries by rises. A decided increase of weight "is the most reliable sign that the attack has passed its worst." Patients were to be weighed regularly and charts kept—further links with medicine. These measurable physical signs, in contrast to the more subjective psychic ones, were interpreted as additional evidence of a disease process. How much prominence they are given still allows the reader of textbooks and articles to guess the writers' basic assumptions.

Our first case is the example with which Kraepelin introduced his lectures on manic-depressive insanity. Presentations of manic and mixed types followed. The delineation of this syndrome, a recurrent, remitting disorder, prominently marked by elevation or depression, excitement or inhibition of mood, thought, and behavior, was his least debatable achievement. It provided the most reliable confluence of signs and course among the new entities he espoused; to an extent remarkable in psychiatry, manic or depressive signs and episodic courses do appear together. (The only serious rivals in the extent of clarity of clinical pictures and the dependability of their relationship to course are late-life depressions, paranoia, and perhaps senile dementia.) In addition, the clinical phenomena were easily conceptualized as *excitements* or *inhibitions* of the various psychological functions, the idea of a change in the *speed* of function giving a pleasing unity and simplicity to the whole conception. The conception itself was based on old observations to which details had been added through the nineteenth century. Kraepelin climaxed this development by characteristically painting a picture in words of broad, unmistakable meaning and locating signs and symptoms in a context of course and outcome. It was an important victory, to leave behind the terms *depression* and *mania* and specify a syndrome or disease.

Under manic-depressive psychosis he placed simple mania, circular, periodic forms, and a few others, each until then separately described, just as he collected under dementia praecox another group of syndromes. Mania might precede or succeed depression; there could be a free interval or none; mania or depression might be present without the other. The facts in common were relapse and recovery and, less clearly defined, affective coloring. Each previously separated type was treated as only a lead to the other characteristics of the group as a whole. The *differences* were regarded as superficial, particularly since similarity in outcome suggested a common underlying process.

Dementia Praecox

The next case illustrates the same method applied to Kraepelin's other new grouping of psychoses, dementia praecox. Again, the patient is brought in and at once described.

The merchant, aged 25, whom you see before you today, has made himself conspicuous by putting leaves and ferns into his buttonhole. He takes a seat with a certain amount of ceremony, and gives positive, concise, and generally relevant answers to our questions. We learn that he was admitted to the hospital a year ago, that he afterwards spent six weeks at home, and that he has now been here again for six months. The patient makes no explicit statements about the nature of the disturbances which appeared, but he admits, when he is asked about it, that he did not speak for some time, he does not know why. But he remembers most of the details of what he has been through. Although he knows where he is, he mistakes the people about him, calls us by wrong names, and takes us for merchants. While he is more or less indifferent at first, taking very little interest in us and looking around with a conceited expression, he gradually becomes rather excited, grows rude, irritable, and threatening, and breaks out into an incoherent flood of words, in which there is a quite senseless play on syllables— "Macbeth—mach'ins Bett," "Irr ich mich nicht—Klinik," "je suis— Jesus," and so on [4, p. 151].

He also intimates that he is the German Emperor and has been promised the Grand Duke's daughter in marriage. He is divertible, frequently breaking off his remarks and interspersing them "with curious snorting noises." "Often, more especially when he makes his jesting play on words, the patient bursts into a tittering laugh." Despite this, and his generally exalted mood, he does not seem excited. The description closes with a remark on his "deportment": it is pompous and affected.

While the emotional impact on us of the first case is likely to be sorrow or puzzlement, the effects of this one are something else. The ridiculous bizarre tone of the patient is conveyed immediately. We are inclined to smile at him or be angry or a little uncomfortable. He seems alien, hardly human. Indeed it is the "peculiar aberrations" of the patient's behavior which determine Kraepelin's diagnosis: the mannerisms, play on words, negativism, and emotional indifference, "while he is quite collected." "The patient does not consider himself ill, but stays here without making any resistance, does not worry at all, forms no plans for the future, and expresses no desires." The *common denominator* of these "peculiar aberrations" is difficult to establish, but "we know the picture well already as a form in which dementia praecox appears." He has brought us from a brief clinical description to this dread conclusion.

The dementia praecox concept was the boldest hypothesis Kraepelin gave the psychiatric world: the concept of *verblodungsprocesse,* or process of mental deterioration separate from the usual toxic and involutional psychoses. Mental deterioration, he argued, was not the occasional outcome of depression, mania, or hypochondriasis, as in the old vesania concept, but present from the start and a distinct clinical entity unto itself. Full remissions occurred, but they were the exceptions that proved the rule. *Syphilitic* dementia (general paresis or dementia paralytica), with its tortuous, deteriorating course and rich variety of psychological pictures, presented a suggestive model (just as *hysterical* phenomena served as the paradigms for many of Freud's explanatory principles). Kraepelin found the diagnosis, as well as the example, of syphilitic dementia appealing; there was a sharp drop in the number of such diagnoses at the Heidelberg Clinic after the introduction of the Wassermann test. (Later the number of dementia praecox diagnoses again fell, as time dealt kindly with originally harsh expectations [8].)

"The patient is said to belong to a healthy family. He was clever at school, always serious and conscientious, and served as a one-year's conscript" [4, p. 152]. Such are the family facts and past history. Very soon Meyer would direct the psychiatric world's attention to such "seriousness" and "conscientiousness" as qualities of medical interest, but Kraepelin takes us without pause to the first complaints and incapacity.

So far back as three years ago he complained of being shaky and excited, and no longer able to work as he had once done. Then, after he had been particularly active and enterprising for some time, marked depression of spirit set in fifteen months ago.

The patient became sleepless, and complained of pains in the back of his head. He felt stupid and unfit for work, took no pleasure in his business, played apathetically with his fingers, lay in bed all day, and thought that he had abused his principal's confidence and embezzled. In this way he came to the hospital. Here he showed a striking conjunction of emotional dullness with good comprehension and perfect lucidity [4, p. 152].

We recall the first case; a similar depression of spirits followed excitement and with no loss of comprehension or mental clearness. But in the present instance a group of bizarre characteristics appeared.

Very soon he sank into a stupor, became dumb, showed signs of automatic obedience, alternating with negativism, and masturbated very much. He was afraid that the French were coming, that the knife would be whetted and people made away with, heard threatening voices, felt electricity in bed, wished to die, and ate hardly anything. He was perfectly indifferent when he was visited. It was only quite slowly that he became a little more active, got out of bed, followed the doctor in his shirt, without speaking, or at the most murmured in a low tone to himself, or occasionally uttered irrelevant expressions, as to the meaning of which nothing could be learned from him [4, pp. 152 and 153].

On seeing a gold piece, "Louis d'or, Napoleon, Empress Eugenie, la France, Spain, thither will we go." He often spoke out of the window, and said he was talking to spirits or acting a play. His sleep was very much disturbed. The physical examination showed no abnormalities worth noticing, but great dermatography and mechanical excitability of the facialis. His weight had increased considerably [4, p. 153].

At first the diagnosis had been "maniacal-depressive insanity," and, even later, the patient's divertibility and quibbling suggested mania. Yet, "in maniacal cases it is only in the very worst states of excitement that the incoherence reaches as high a degree as it did here, where rationality was fully maintained and the excitement was comparatively slight." In addition, there were *catatonic* signs, negativism, mannerisms, automatic obedience, and confusion of speech. These, more than the delusional, hallucinatory, or affective phenomena, secured the diagnosis, even though the lecture title for the case is the *paranoidal* forms of dementia praecox. (Why has he put this among the *paranoidal* forms? Are the paranoidal or the catatonic features more prominent? Or is it the catatonic features in the paranoidal picture that shape the prognosis? The subjective or impressionistic nature of psychiatric diagnosis is nowhere more apparent. The clinician is asked to *weigh* details, subtly.) Surely Kraepelin places so much reliance on the mannerisms, the negativisms or obedience, and the speech peculiarities because these are *signs*, motor phenomena, closer to objective medical "facts" than the more private cognitive, perceptual, or emotive events.

He closes typically, with his expectations and the actual results. The catatonic cases generally improve. "But even in the most favorable event a certain degree of dullness and want of freedom will probably remain in the spheres of emotion and action." Then the result:

When the patient had been eight months in the asylum, we were able to discharge him substantially improved. He was not very accessible, but fairly intelligent and free from delusions. Now, two years later, he is actively engaged in his business. The delusions may disappear completely [4, p. 154].

(Kraepelin seldom gave delusions much importance diagnostically or prognostically.)

It is well to contrast the diagnostic features he emphasized in this lecture with the more general statements he made later. In the Eighth Edition of his textbook, and probably as a result of Bleuler's teaching, Kraepelin wrote that dementia praecox was marked most characteristically by two psychopathological features.

On the one hand we observe a *weakening of those emotional activities which permanently form the mainsprings of volition* . . . the result . . . is emotional dullness, failure of mental activities, loss of mastery over volition, of endeavor, and of ability for independent action.

The second group of disorders, which gives dementia praecox its peculiar stamp . . . consists in the *loss of the inner unity* of the activities of intellect, emotion, and volition in themselves and among one another . . . emotions do not correspond to ideas, the patients laugh and weep without any recognizable cause, without any relation to their circumstances and their experiences, smile while they narrate the tale of their attempts at suicide . . . it is just this disagreement between ideas and emotion that gives their behavior the stamp of "illness" [9].

The student of Bleuler will recognize immediately the close similarity of these features to two of the fundamental symptoms enunciated by Bleuler: affect disturbance and disturbances of association. These more *psychological* conceptions, directed to processes behind the symptoms and signs, however, were not typical of Kraepelin's interests or ideas. Even in his textbook where groups of patients were "melted down," as it were, to provide common denominator descriptions, he would never rest his weight on the psychological features alone. He had learned the main diagnostic lesson of syphilitic dementia, that the most diverse psychological phenomena could be associated with a single etiological agent. He therefore kept his eye always on the course, on the patient's trajectory.

His preference for composite portraits, for groupings of signs from many cases (the method of clinical presentation he used in the various editions of his textbook), resulted in broad *clinical pictures,* to which any one individual could contribute but a part. The assumption was that the underlying disease process came through only fractionally with the single example but could be seen in its complete dimensions with the group. Also, the lack of individual case detail in most of his writings again signaled his relative indifference to the psychological or physiological *processes* behind the clinical pictures, which, as Freud demonstrated on the psychological side and Wernicke on the neurological, only the details could be expected to illuminate. Further, subsequent investigators have complained that the method of composite portraiture made difficult any comparison with other bodies of clinical experience.

One feature of his usual descriptions of the dementia praecox cases is not so prominent in our example. The cases were generally as striking for their *retention* of some faculties as for their loss of others. Consciousness, recall, orientation, comprehension were more often than not intact—remarkably so when put beside the profound difficulties of attention and judgment, strange ideas firmly adhered to, hallucinatory interruptions of perception, emotional dullness, and disconnections of the stream of thought. This *contrast* within the mental state was not put down as the fundamental or identifying feature of the condition but it stands as perhaps the most *puzzling* one.

Our case example is, however, perfectly characteristic of his method and ideas in one respect. Little or no attention was paid to the patient's environment or experience. Dementia praecox was accepted as the *nonpareil* model of endogenous psychosis. It had the quality of *fate,* not to be swerved from preordained ends. We must ask whether this impression of the isolation of dementia praecox patients from environmental events was a facet of the overwhelming power of an endogenous disease process or whether it was a manifestation of *withdrawal* from life and *uncommunicativeness* about what has been happening to the persons involved. In short, was the classic poverty of historic detail in the stories of these patients clinical fact or artifact?

The individual case material quoted here also makes clear his *clinical methods.* They were preeminently objective. As I have indicated, he was more interested in signs that all observers can share than in symptoms, which depend on the patient's description of his inner state. The patient was himself treated as an object, observed, talked about, in his very presence and perhaps at the sacrifice of some finer feelings. This is the common practice in medicine; concern is with disease, which the patient "gets" or "has." The disease is not his "fault," remains separate from the personality, and therefore comments about it should not be taken "personally." Such a psychiatry or medicine favors traits or signs of sufficient obviousness to cross the barriers between patient and physician, and, as Sullivan was to emphasize, subject to distortions by that passage. Obviousness tends to be equated with importance, as in politics or advertising.

The method also depends upon *face-to-face interviews* in which the authoritative physician searches for objective signs and repeats his examinations until satisfied that a decisive course has been established and a prognosis can be made [10]. Then a distinct disease process is assured—an active metabolic process to explain the deteriorating course of dementia praecox and a "constitutional" one in the case of manic-depressive psychosis. (It seemed less necessary to have an "active" disease agent at work in the nondeteriorating conditions. In addition, the best evidence was, and still is, that inheritance plays a more important role in manic-depressive psychosis than in dementia praecox.) Treatment was not discussed, except along the lines of social and psychological manipulations. Definitive treatment must await fuller understanding of the hypothetical disease entities.

Genetic and Neurological Findings

Kraepelin's principal causal hypothesis for many cases in the psychotic group, of a metabolic process on a genetic base, remains the shining hope he left it. The hope has been stimulated further by the therapeutic promise that pills and injections have always held out to mankind and in recent years partly realized. The young man entering psychiatry from a medical education studded with chemical discoveries plunges naturally into its pursuit.

Kraepelin himself and the European centers of psychiatry that so felt his influence moved steadily toward a *genetic* explanation of whatever physical processes were hypothesized. Before Kraepelin, a *general* tendency to morbid inheritance had been assumed. With the laying down of acceptable diagnostic boundary lines, *specific* inheritance became a possibility. Here was an acid test of the Kraepelinian "diseases": Would they preserve their integrity from generation to generation? The basic plan of the investigations has been simple, although there are immense difficulties in execution. Groups of families of psychotic patients have been searched for the degree of concordance, or joint occurrence, of the psychosis among near and far relatives; the expectation being for a substantially more frequent occurrence of the psychosis in the patient's identical twin, for example, than in an ordinary sibling or distant cousin. In fact, a sharp drop in incidence between the identical twin relationship and two-egg or ordinary siblingship has been the most impressive single finding, for both dementia praecox and the manic-depressive psychoses. It has compensated partly for the results defying easy analysis along conventional Mendelian lines. The work has excited an enormous volume of criticism from psychologists, sociologists, and statisticians, but the claim of significant genetic influence on the major psychoses remains one of the most substantial in psychiatry.

The other major organic hypothesis of Kraepelin's day, that the identification and localization of brain functions would best illuminate psychiatric disorders, continues the basis for many investigations, without exciting the almost religious devotion of more exclusively chemical interests. To Kraepelin, neurology seemed as helpless to deal with the multifaceted pathology of chronic psychosis as it had been with hysteria. He turned instead to diffuse poisonings or poorly circumscribed infections, just as Freud turned away from "neurologizing" to processes of symbolization, distortion, and the broad concepts of wishes and instincts. The ideas of modern neurology and neurophysiology are, however, as different from those of Kraepelin's contemporary, Wernicke, as Hughlings Jackson's were from those of the "bump" anatomists, the phrenologists Gall and Spurzheim. Further, chemical and neurological hypotheses are not only compatible but mutually dependent; already a localizing brain chemistry or chemical neurology appears that will render the old distinctions practically, as well as theoretically, obsolete.

Critical Signs and Composite Portraiture

We have seen that Kraepelin organized his patient material not only etiologically but by *critical signs* and clinical *"pictures,"* that is, by giving special weight to some phenomena, particularly catatonic ones, and by his "composite portraits." The baffling fact of the changeability of psychiatric signs and symptoms, their simple inconsistency, led him to look for constant, hopefully indelible features, which could be marks of a disease. Critical signs, of such appeal to the detective physician seeking the invader in the mudstain, had been elusive; the hysterical stigmata for one generation of psychiatrists were like mist to the next. But by settling attention on certain groups of patients Kraepelin intensified the search. Its principal results were in the work of Eugen Bleuler: Signs gave way to fundamental symptoms, and these, in turn, to psychological processes. Janet and Freud mark out the same path from Charcot's "disease," hysteria.

The method of composite portraiture or *clinical pictures* appeals more to the artist than to the detective in physician or psychologist. The number of elements to be employed demands a gradual building up, a sensing and sketching, a rounding off as well as filling in suggestive of the artist's task. It also invites charges of prejudice and subjectivity. In recent years these have been rebutted by the use of statistical techniques, such as factor analysis, which allow apparently objective manipulation of enormous numbers of individual items in a search for traits and clusters of traits. The resulting clusters or syndromes have on the whole reproduced Kraepelin's groupings. Is this because he made fundamental distinctions, or because the modern investigator selects items for his computer unknowingly restricted to the very signs and symptoms Kraepelin himself employed? *Random* procedures enter only parts of the new techniques—not, for example, the procedures for selection of the material to be managed statistically. We have as yet no way of sampling the *whole* range of behavior, because the universe of psychiatrically relevant behavior has expanded enormously, and continues to grow. The serious investigator seeking truly representative data wrestles with a wet elephant.

Nevertheless, more than any other individual, Kraepelin gave modern psychiatry its *structure* [11]. The principal investigators since, including Freud, have worked largely within the distinctions he made. (How fitting a monument to this enthusiastic hobbyist of *botany!*) This is a matter of immense importance. By providing psychiatry with a structure, he made possible observations that were referable to at least partially understood and agreed-upon areas. Data increasingly different from the type that he himself had observed could be collected on this or that group of cases, whose meanings and limits were at least provisionally set. If much complaining and reserving judgment on the fundamental nature of the categories persisted and their meaning gradually altered, still a significant moratorium on the old arguments occurred. If this was no peace treaty, it was at least a truce. And if it was as much a truce of exhaustion as of triumph, no one else could mobilize sufficient experience and fresh distinctions to carry the field against him. Kraepelin had said, let us accept these distinctions for a while and, working within them, discover what genetic, psychological, chemical, and sociological correlations we can; there must be some provisional organization if psychiatry is to go forward at all. This was one source of the outpourings of work in new directions that accompanied and followed his lifetime.

PIERRE JANET*

Pierre Janet united the enormous variety of symptoms and signs of hysteria and obsessional neuroses under a few psychological concepts [12]. He did not seek the model for psychiatric illness in medical pathology as Kraepelin had done; psychological phenomena were searched for *psychological* principles and processes. His guiding concepts were suggestibility, dissociation, idea, function, consciousness, action, and mental energy rather than stigmata, disease, course, syndrome, or cortical lesion. The phenomena he investigated, however, were the traditional ones: somnambulisms, fugue states, contractures, obsessions, anesthesias, delusions of persecution, and disturbances of vision, respiration, and alimentation. He did not move deeply into fresh divisions of mental life, as would Freud, nor did he explore the social envelope, with Meyer. Janet was the great encyclopedist of symptoms and signs of neurosis.

The intellectual world was ripe for Janet, whose work quickly found a place in the textbooks of the day and even in a series of lectures at Harvard. He was that richly educated

* Leston L. Havens, "Pierre Janet," *Journal of Nervous and Mental Disease* 143:383, 1966. Copyright © 1966, The Williams & Wilkins Co. Reproduced, as revised, by permission.

hybrid, the physician-psychologist, whose doctorates of medicine and philosophy accredited him to both body and mind. Freud, in contrast, was a briefly trained psychiatrist and an amateur psychologist; his American invitation came from the less prestigious Clark.

Janet brings us the variety of hysterical and obsessional phenomena, a garland of exotic psychopathology, lovingly, aesthetically described. He had the collector's mind, holding examples up for the reader's appreciation, delineating the critical features, returning each to its neat compartment. We are led from simple to complex symptoms, the patient's ideas are solicited and noted down, and Janet turns the material over and over again in the search for common features. His theoretical constructions were readily understood and clarified much that had seemed random and diverse. The intelligibility and attractiveness of his writing—as well as the undisturbing nature of his ideas—were vital qualities in the setting of ignorance and malice toward mental diseases that prevailed, and often still prevails.

Somnambulisms

The first case examples are from his lectures on hysteria. Somnambulisms were described at the outset because they illustrated in manageable compass a large variety of typical hysterical features [13]. The modern reader needs to tone down his usual response to Victorian melodrama.

We come back to the common story of a young girl twenty years old, called Irene, whom despair, caused by her mother's death, has made ill. We must remember that this woman's death has been very moving and dramatic. The poor woman, who had reached the last stage of consumption, lived alone with her daughter in a poor garret. Death came slowly, with suffocation, blood-vomiting, and all its frightful procession of symptoms. The girl struggled hopelessly against the impossible. She watched her mother during sixty nights, working at her sewing machine to earn a few pennies necessary to sustain their lives. After the mother's death she tried to revive the corpse, to call the breath back again; then, as she put the limbs upright, the body fell to the floor, and it took infinite exertion to lift it again into the bed. You may picture to yourself all that frightful scene. Some time after the funeral, curious and impressive symptoms began. It was one of the most splendid cases of somnambulism I ever saw.

The crises last for hours, and they show a splendid dramatic performance, for no actress could rehearse those lugubrious scenes with such perfection. The young girl has the singular habit of acting again all the events that took place at her mother's death, without forgetting the least detail. Sometimes she only speaks, relating all that happened with great volubility, putting questions and answers in turn, or asking questions only, and seeming to listen for the answers; sometimes she only sees the sight, looking with frightened face and staring on the various scenes, and acting according to what she sees. At other times, she combines all hallucinations, words, and acts, and seems to play a very singular drama. When, in her drama, death has taken place, she carries on the same idea, and makes everything ready for her own suicide. She discusses it aloud, seems to speak with her mother, to receive advice from her; she fancies she will try to be run over by a locomotive. That detail is also a recollection of a real event in her life. She fancies she is on the way, and stretches herself out on the floor of the room, waiting for death, with mingled dread and impatience. She poses, and wears on her face expressions really worthy of admiration, which remain fixed during several minutes. The train arrives before her staring eyes, she utters a terrible shriek, and falls back motionless, as if she were dead. She soon gets up and begins acting over again one of the preceding scenes. In fact, one of the characteristics of these somnambulisms is that they repeat themselves indefinitely. Not only the different attacks are always exactly alike, repeating the same movements, expressions, and words, but in the course of the same attack, when it has lasted a certain time, the same scene may be repeated again exactly in the same way five or ten times. At last, the agitation seems to wear out, the dream grows less clear, and, gradually or suddenly, according to the cases, the patient comes back to her normal consciousness, takes up her ordinary business, quite undisturbed by what has happened [14, pp. 27–31].

We recognize the elements that Charcot and psychoanalysis were to make familiar: an emotion, in this case despair, following on dramatic and moving events, then a change in consciousness at the onset of crises or attacks of illness that repeat, often many times, ideas of the traumatic events, finally awakening, amnesia, and apparent indifference to the remarkable happenings of a few moments before. The dramatic coloring of both the precipitating events and the attacks that repeat them is greatly emphasized. We are invited to observe and admire; the hysterical patient is so typically compared to an actress. In fact, the artificial element is too much suggested by Janet's description. He must add that no actress could rehearse these scenes; to observe them is to feel not only a masterful performance but the pressure of an illness, even desperation. Janet, like Charcot, underscores at once the theatrical *and* medical interest of hysteria.

Attention is called to the heightening of function. She remembered and repeated every detail. She appeared not merely to imagine the original scene but to hallucinate it. Another patient, in waking life paralyzed from the waist down, at night nimbly climbed among rooftops. Memory, imagination, motor skills were sharpened and inspired. We are asked to notice also the variety of ways in which the traumatic scenes returned. In one attack she observed, in another, participated. Still another patient described a whole scene in words, or fell sick with paralysis, vomiting, or a lump in the throat. These last, Janet suggested, represent the same memories and ideas as the somnambulisms. Ideas, pale creatures for the rest of us, are carried up into hallucinations, fits, changes in feeling and movement.

This is *suggestibility,* which Bernheim argued was the essence of hysteria. So possessed by some ideas were the hysterical patients that all other associations, observations, and memories appeared shut out, the patients living through the idea of the moment. Nor did the idea need to be reintroduced in its original form. A mere hint, a word, or the fragment of a sensation sufficed; the train of images, acts, feelings, attacks, tics was set in motion automatically, independent of the patient's familiar will. These several features comprised suggestibility: the fact of ideas themselves, their ready triggering off, the automaticity of the resulting sequence, and the vividness of the ideas' expression. (Like Kraepelin, Janet did not regard the particular *content* of the ideas as of much importance.) Plainly, not everyone was suggestible in this sense, although special circumstances—for example, the contagion of a crowd—might greatly lower the average man's immunity.

The other side of suggestibility, of heightened function and recall, was amnesia and forgetfulness. The shutting out of parts of the patient's internal life was as striking a feature of hysteria as the portions being, at other times, dominant and vividly expressed. Janet noted that the amnesia covered both the attacks and the actual events they repeated. (This further strengthened the link between attack and event, already related chronologically and by internal similarities.) What we can call the emotional equivalent of amnesia, *la belle indifference,* also covered both attack and event; the patient returned to her ordinary life as if nothing had happened. Many nonhysterical neurotics produced or exaggerated their symptoms when attention was called to them, the conscious mental life of such patients appearing to participate. But when hysterical patients became conscious of their signs, they were "indifferent," or the signs diminished, sometimes even disappeared. The average man's impulse is to crow; the patient has been "discovered" and drops the symptom. Yet hard-bitten malingerers do not act this way; they have been attending all along and are not surprised by the disclosures. Hysterical phenomena gained their greatest power independently of conscious mental life, perhaps *because of* their isolation from conscious mental life. (This observation has a long reach: A true witch, the Inquisition asserted, did not know she had the devil's patch; psychoanalysis, five centuries later, would have the treatment goal of making unconscious content conscious.) We should record carefully that the shutting out covers affective responses or feeling states as well as thoughts, the stuff of mental content, and memories of both the trauma and the attacks. Janet also observed a connection between anesthesia and amnesia. The loss of sensations was often accompanied by a loss of memories related to the sensations, and modifying the traumatic memories (changing them by hypnosis, merely recalling them, or discharging the affects associated with them) often modified the symptoms.

The conception of a *condition seconde* (subconscious, or the later unconscious) had been mentioned by Charcot; it was made explicit by Janet, and expanded, differentiated, and changed in significance by Freud. Similarly, "forgetfulness" would become the modern "repression" and "denial." The clinical observation of mental states which were sharply separated by amnesia or a change in personality was the extreme and therefore recognizable instance of what is noted every day: "I cannot remember, report, or bring to consciousness all I know, feel, or perceive. I am forgetful!" Consciousness is a little light playing over fragments of a larger mental life. Janet was not ready for this broadened statement of subconsciousness, nor for the Freudian hypothesis that divisions of mental parts were due to conflicts or antagonisms between them. He concentrated on the dramatic clinical instances. Their careful description made forgetfulness an undeniably major feature of hysterical states.

The somnambulist was asleep to his ordinary life. But the forgetfulness or unconsciousness of hysterics was not a complete or steady sleep. A patient with tunnel vision can still play ball. Hold the anesthetic hand behind the patient's back, put a pencil in it; the patient "feels" nothing but associates to "writing," "lead," "pens," and even "pencils." Furthermore, the anesthetic hand can itself write or gracefully adapt to different objects. Still another patient's arm is anesthetic; apply ice to it, and the vessels below contract, whitening the skin, indicating there must be sensory transmission. The patient might report *feeling* nothing but have images of something ice-like. (Alfred Binet was also a great student of these phenomena [15].) The point is, sensation does not get to the hysterical person's *awareness* but it does get to the spinal cord and brain. In Janet's words, there is a restriction of the hysteric's field of consciousness; the waking will excludes certain movements, feelings, ideas, and sensations. This powerful formula takes in the effects of chloroform or ether or distraction. The conscious will being put to sleep, functions return—for instance, the visually tunneled patient can play ball (for most of playing ball is automatic, unwilled movement anyway), or symptoms are occasionally reduced when attention is drawn to them (awareness being turned on a hitherto avoided function or body part, the latter may wake up to join the conscious will).

Janet also noticed that if the hysterical patients were distracted or the examination conducted when they were just awakening, contact *could* be made with the apparently forgotten psychic parts. The anesthetic hand would write messages, answer questions, even as the patient was talking of something else, and the content of the messages suggested attitudes, memories, and feelings quite different from those of the speaking self. These dissociated psychic parts might temporarily capture the whole personality (as in the somnambulisms), exist apart from the personality (seemingly in a hand or ear), and occasionally enter and color it (as when the patient felt sudden, unexplained emotions or had ideas that seemed to come from nowhere). The split-off parts were *powerful,* were *organized,* and could be *contacted.*

Fugues

Fugues last longer than somnambulisms and lack the persistent change of consciousness so obvious in the latter. A lapse of consciousness may usher in the fugue, but it disappears immediately to leave the appearance of wakefulness, of complex and purposeful interaction with people and things. We are asked to accept that one unfamiliar with the old self would not find the new person of the fugue state so remarkable as to call a policeman or a doctor. In Janet's description below, mark the features uniting the fugue with somnambulisms and other hysterical "accidents."

The subject is a boy of seventeen, Rou., son of a neuropathic mother, rather nervous himself, who already had, when he was ten years old, tics and contractures in the neck. . . . At thirteen he often went to a small public house, visited by old sailors. They would urge him to drink, and, when he was somewhat flustered, they would fill his imagination with beautiful tales in which deserts, palm trees, lions, camels, and negroes were pictured in a most wonderful and alluring way. . . . When his drunkenness was over, the stories seemed to be quite forgotten; he never spoke of travels, and, on the contrary, led a very sedentary life, for he had chosen the placid occupation of a grocer's boy, and he only sought to rise in that honourable career.

Now there come on quite unforeseen accidents, almost always on the occasion of some fatigue or a fit of drunkenness. He then felt transformed, forgot to return home, and thought no more of his family . . . he had but one idea left in his head; namely, to get to the sea, enlist in a ship, and sail away towards those enchanting countries of Africa. . . .

I will dwell on only one of his fugues, which is particularly amusing, and was of extraordinary duration, for it lasted three months. . . . A bright idea had occurred to him; not far from Melun, at Moret, there are canals that go more or less straight to the south of France, and in those canals there are ships laden with goods. He succeeded in being accepted as a servant on a ship laden with coal. . . . He was badly fed, often beaten, exhausted with fatigue, but, though you would scarcely believe it, he was radiant with happiness. He thought only of one thing—of the joy of drawing nearer to the sea. Unhappily, in Auvergne, the boat stopped, and he was forced to leave it and continue his journey on foot, which was more difficult. In order not to be resourceless, he hired himself as a helper to an old china mender. They went slowly along, working on the road.

Then, one evening, an unlooked-for event took place again. The day's work had been a success; the two companions had earned seven francs. The old china mender stopped and said to R., "My boy, we deserve a good supper; and we will keep today's feast; it is the fifteenth of August." On hearing this, the boy heedlessly said: "The fifteenth of August? Why it is the feast of the Virgin Mary, and the anniversary of my mother's name-day." He had scarcely uttered these words when he appeared to be quite changed. He looked all around him with astonishment, and turning to his companion, said, "But who are you, and what am I doing here with you?" The poor man was amazed, and was quite unable to make the boy understand the situation; the latter still believed himself in Paris, and had lost all memory of the preceding months. They had to go to the village mayor's, where, with great difficulty, the matter was made more or less clear. The mayor telegraphed to Paris, and the prodigal child was sent back home. Is not that name, which suddenly evoked the memory of his mother and awakened him likewise, a pretty conclusion of a fugue? [14, pp. 51–53].

The critical features are five: (1) some change in consciousness, whether due to drunkenness or fatigue, (2) other neurotic phenomena, in this case tics and contractures, (3) an idea, the sailor life in enchanting Africa, (4) amnesia for the episodes, and (5) trauma, but in a new sense: a series of molding (or, if you prefer, misleading) experiences, the companionship of the old sailors, not a single frightening or depressing event. The meaning of idea, too, is enlarged: a wish for the future, not a memory of the past.

The fugue, entailing as it does to some measure a fresh personality and not merely isolated symptoms or the reenactment of scenes, allowed Janet to contrast the usual personality of the patient with the surprising creations of hysteria. Rou. was a grocer boy and ostensibly content. His dreams of foreign lands were not part of everyday existence, not shared with friends. He led a sedentary life and "only sought to rise" in his career. Such sharp contrasts between one personality and another were even more dramatic in the closely allied state of multiple personality. These recurrent, sometimes lifelong, fugues expressed still more fully organized and separate individualities, less restricted to a single idea or wish than the classic fugues. As one personality the patient might be irascible, vindictive, self-centered; as another, self-sacrificing, amiable, even saintly. The very sharpness of the contrast suggested a relationship between the two. Perhaps one was the opposite of the other, even formed as a reaction to the other, or perhaps together both represented a whole human being, one portion "civilized" and the other "uncivilized." The implications of these contrasts were to be developed under the detailed study of hysterical patients' mental content that psychoanalysis introduced. The fugues and cases of multiple personality first made them recognizable.

The contrast between fugues and "normal" personality or among the various alternating individualities was often between forgetfulness, lethargy, or depression, on the one hand, and heightened function, liveliness, and ready memory, on the other. These last did not always dominate the *normal* person, nor were they always the features to which the patient and relatives were accustomed. Frequently the vigorous and attractive personality emerged only in the fugue states, whether spontaneously or after being hypnotized, as with the famous Marceline, whom Janet's brother and then Janet attended. (Periodic hypnotic treatments improved the dull, plaintive personality she had always had and to which she regularly returned.) These observations shook the whole foundation of normative psychiatry. What the patient brought to the illness (his or her premorbid personality) had been largely accepted as the standard against which determinations of disease were to be made. A change from the normal, at least one that showed up in a hospital, police station, or psychiatrist's office, must be a change for the worse. But plainly many of the fugue and alternating personalities represented changes for the better. Very soon Adolf Meyer was to make the radical extension of this line of thought: Perhaps even some acute schizophrenic illnesses were advances over the patient's previous personality achievement. Henceforth the clear delineation of normal standards would be a *goal* of psychiatric thought, not its settled achievement.

Comparison of the usual and fugue personalities had a different and very significant impact on Janet's conception of the normal and diseased. What struck him as the most obvious and pervasive abnormality of *all* patients was their ennui, laziness, depression, or, at its most profound, their "abulia." This was what most distinguished them from a vigorous normal personality. Some degree of ennui or lowered energy he saw as the common denominator of all psychic abnormalities, a concept later to be made the capstone of his explanatory system.

Janet was too keen and honest an observer to ignore what had originally escaped his own ideas. He discussed patient after patient freed of neurotic symptoms or depression only when she was in love with someone else's husband, taking dangerous risks, stealing, or back with a homosexual lover [16, pp. 917–931]. He well knew the disdain "erudite psychiatrists" have for such observations and he, as erudite as any, could only hope the future would make something of them [16, p. 889]. His own theoretical structure did not encompass these facts, and his concepts of the normal and ethical were disturbed by them, but, as he wrote of one patient changed by a "love-adventure," "How can we ignore the medical value of the perverted love which transformed this young woman for three years?" [16, pp. 917–931].

Recall the "pretty" ending of the fugue described above. The old china mender suggested he and Rou. celebrate "today's feast, the fifteenth of August." The boy then associated to the Virgin Mary, his mother's name day, and, presumably, his mother, and awoke. Here was an inadvertent occurrence of what would be termed the method of free association. The separate personalities were not completely separate; they could be broken into associatively. Delicate strands appeared to connect psychic parts, along which the sensitive clinician could run stronger lines to join the dissociated elements.

Hysterical Anorexy

Janet remarked that somnambulisms had once been all the rage; by 1905 they were old hat, and the latest thing was hysterical paralyses. Today both have lost their interest. It is the visceral disturbances of alimentation, respiration, circulation, the so-called psychophysiological reactions or psychosomatic states that get first call. Janet closed the clinical sections of his *Major Symptoms of Hysteria* by reviewing them. At once the formula drawn from the somnambulisms must be changed.

Hysterical symptoms and signs are mental fragments dissociated from conscious, voluntary control, but most visceral functions are never conscious or under voluntary control. Indeed, these hysterical visceral disorders seem to occur when ordinarily involuntary functions are invaded by consciousness, or, at least, by ideas that may be conscious.

Today's "anorexia nervosa" was at that time often called "hysterical anorexy," to "designate a disease both mental and physiological, very long and very complicated, which consists chiefly in the systematic refusal of food, in certain digestive disturbances, and in a consequent inanition" [14, p. 228]. It almost always occurs in women and "is one of the facts of the special pathology of the girl of eighteen" [14, p. 229].

Mu . . . presented her first gastric disturbances after the death of her brother, who succumbed rapidly to pulmonary phthisis. . . . It is thought quite natural that the girl, whose stomach is diseased, should be careful of what she eats. . . . She resigns herself to everything and shows herself a patient of exemplary docility; moreover, save for vaguer and vaguer pains in her stomach, she seems to enjoy perfect health; her tongue is clean, her stomach and abdomen normal; the only thing she may suffer from is obstinate constipation. . . . The family at length become disquieted at the indefinite prolongation of these treatments and ultra strict diets, which do not seem very well justified. They suspect hypochondriac ideas and obstinacy, and their attitude becomes quite modified. Now they try to allure the patient by all possible delicacies of the table, they scold her severely, they alternately spoil, beseech, threaten her. The excess of the insistence causes an exaggeration of the resistance; the girl seems to understand that the least concession on her part would cause her to pass from the condition of a patient to that of a capricious child, and to this she will never consent. . . .

Now the girl scarcely ever speaks of her pains in the stomach, but she repeats that she will eat when she is hungry and that she is never hungry. . . . In fact she seems to be in very good health and shows much strength and activity. . . . Supported by this conviction, our strange patient struggles with all those around her, by every possible means. She seeks a support in one of her parents against the other, she promises to do wonders if her family is not too exacting, she has recourse to every artifice and to every untruth. It is the period when such patients hide victuals in their pockets, fill their cheeks and throat with them, to go and spit them out in the lavatory, when they learn to vomit immediately what they have just swallowed. . . .

Lastly comes on, sooner or later, but sometimes only after years the . . . period of inanition. Organic disturbances begin to appear, the breath is foul, the stomach and abdomen are retracted, there is an insuperable constipation. . . . The patients who no longer leave their beds remain in a semi-delirious, semi-comatose condition. At this stage they behave in two different ways; some continue to be delirious, and, as Charcot said, have but one idea left; namely, to refuse to eat. Others, fortunately begin to be frightened. . . . You know that the dog cannot be called back to life when it has lost forty per cent of its weight; the hysterical can still be saved at fifty and above. There is a limit, however. . . . It is the melancholy period when those poor girls ask to eat and it is too late. It is true that things generally take another turn, and an intercurrent disease comes on, broncho-pneumonia or almost phthisis, which simplifies the situation [14, pp. 230–233].

(The social events Janet recounts are largely drawn from the writings of Lasègue [17].)

He then reviewed the "essential phenomena" [18], dismissing one after another of the previous explanations and seeking the widest possible generalization.

Lasègue, who with Gull had given the first accurate description in the mid-nineteenth century (when so many new syndromes were being recognized), emphasized the fixed ideas. One patient wanted to die; another feared the sensation of a ball in her esophagus; still another would not eat the flesh of living creatures. Charcot one day discovered tight around the waist of a self-starved young girl a rose-colored ribbon. He extracted the confession that this was the length of waist she must not exceed: "I prefer dying of hunger to becoming big as Mama." Charcot was enthusiastic and searched avidly for ideas about obesity. But, Janet complained, there were so many of these ideas, they appeared to have little in common, and other phenomena were of at least equal importance. Above all, he did not relate the social events, so sensitively described, to any persistent ideas. In Janet's mind it was as a *class* of phenomena that ideas gained their importance, pointing to a *diagnosis* or *pathological process*. One of his patients told him how ridiculous she thought the idea of eating, "how much she wondered to see people gather for the dirty operation" [14, pp. 242–243]. He listed this remark under "dissociations of the social idea of alimentation." No *particular* reasons for the disgust were sought. Here we meet again the classificatory, symptom-centered, pathological orientation of objective-descriptive psychiatry.

Anesthesia had been the most popular choice for a pathognomonic or stigmatic sign in hysteria; indeed, the magnetists made it the underlying process explaining other phenomena. The anorexic patients reported that their food was tasteless. Anesthesias were noted on the tongue, cheeks, esophagus, and on the skin over the stomach. Janet mentioned Pavlov's studies: "The saliva secreted by a dog varies with the object presented to him, with the taste and smell of that object" [14, pp. 237–238]. Since the anorexic patients taste or smell little, "it is very likely that their digestion will be disturbed; perhaps the gastric juice is different, too." (Pavlov later developed a psychiatric theory, not unlike Janet's, of higher and lower levels and weak and strong nervous energies.) On the other hand, the anesthesias were never complete; digestion could be demonstrated despite them; and even animals without stomachs try to feed. The anesthesias are "more elementary and more general disturbances" than the fixed ideas, but he could not rest on them his whole understanding of the condition.

Janet was most impressed by the devotion to exercise and movement many anorexic patients showed. One played all day at shuttlecock; when locked in her room, she was found doing violent gymnastic exercises. Gull, Lasègue, and Charcot had noticed this, and their explanation was the popular one: The patients want to convince others that they are strong and do not need to eat more. Janet's patients denied such an aim or the related goal of keeping thin, and, typically, he accepted their conscious denials [19].

Accompanying the love of exercise he noted "a general excitation to physical and moral activity, a strange feeling of happiness, an euphoria." "The need of food goes with the feeling of weakness and depression; persons depressed by neurasthenia are great eaters. The exaltation of the strength, the feeling of euphoria, as it is known in the ecstatic saints, for instance, does away with the need of eating" [14, pp. 241–242].

This is how I propose to you to represent it to ourselves, without, however, pretending to explain it. The function of alimentation, if we consider it on its psychological side, is one of the most considerable systems of thoughts that exist in the brain of an animal. It comprises fundamental phenomena, such as the feeling of weakness, of depression, and the fear of death. Besides, it comprises numberless secondary phenomena, such as the sensations and motions connected with all the parts of the organism that play a role in alimentation, from the hands, lips, and tongue to the rectum and anus; lastly, it also comprises phenomena of improvement, as the images of pleasant aliments, the habits of eating cleanly, and the mixture of certain social phenomena that usually complicate our alimentation. There is in the hysterical a dissociation of this system, which may totally or partially withdraw from consciousness. In complete anorexy, you will find the loss of all the elements, I have just described, the loss of the sensation of weakness, replaced by a pathological euphoria, the loss of the sensations of the organs, but also, more than is generally believed, the loss of the movements. These patients can no longer cleanly convey their food to their mouths, they can no longer masticate, and above all, they can no longer swallow, nor can they go to stool. . . . Hysterical anorexy is, at bottom, a great amnesia and a great paralysis. Alimentation has become, as it were, a somnambulistic phenomenon which can only be effected in the second or somnambulistic state. . . . This phenomenon is lost to the normal and waking consciousness" [14, pp. 242–243].

Janet is proposing that the anorexic illness represents the dissociation not primarily of an idea or a sensation but of a system or complex of physiological events, fears, movements, sensations, and ideas, what he calls a *function;* hence the term *functional lesion.*

He did not relate the euphoria of the anorexic patients to

the beautiful indifference of the more typically hysterical ones, or to mania, in which overactivity, euphoria, and grandiose ideas combine. Later workers added to this list of manic features a tendency to deny unpleasant facts by substituting their opposites (strength for weakness, wealth for poverty) and the unconscious ideas of being eaten, eating others, sleeping, and dying, which suggest profound similarities between the manic and anorexic patients—and anorexia nervosa was moved away from the neuroses and closer to the psychoses. Undoubtedly, as both Bleuler and Jung remarked, there were many psychotic patients among Janet's neurotics. (Janet excluded from the neuroses only the most obvious dementias, patients whose mental life had been reduced to a "dust-heap" [20, p. 313].) The modern conception of psychosis, moreover, depends upon a still greater range of observations and differentiation of concepts than Janet achieved.

In this flood of new achievements it is easy to lose sight of what Janet accomplished [21]. The meaning of both idea and trauma was extended, the concept of functional dissociation introduced, and the gamut of neurotic symptoms and signs clarified and ordered: He significantly shaped what subsequent generations have called neuroses.

Psychasthenias

We take up now Janet's other principal group of neuroses, what he called the psychasthenias: today's obsessional states, some anxiety neuroses, depressive reactions, and hypochondrias. He again constructed the syndrome from meticulous descriptions of the individual symptoms, broadening the latter to include several of what we term character traits, and then summating in a few general features, as he did for hysteria with suggestibility and forgetfulness. The clinical material is anecdotal as before, but behind the selected vignettes are many years of close observation, careful questioning, and thorough follow-up (often for 15 or 20 years [16, p. 15]) of a large number of cases, so characteristic of objective-descriptive psychiatry at its best.

One feature immediately separates the obsessional patients from the hysterics. The hysteric appears not to know what troubles her, has forgotten the trauma, conflicts, and emotions which preceded the symptoms, and may even be indifferent to the symptoms, whereas the obsessional patient is "embarrassed, constrained, has trouble expressing himself but knows perfectly well what torments him. Instead of those around the patient understanding the subject of his fixed idea, he himself tells us the content of his obsession and can fill in all the details" [20, p. 17].

What is it that torments him? (We write *him* now, for these illnesses affect men as often as, perhaps more often than, they do women, another contrast to hysteria.) It is fancied crimes, sacrilegious thoughts, and sexual perversions which the patient fears are about to be acted upon. The *hysterical* attacks are typically filled with "events of the common life, the death of an infant, the absence of a loved one" [20, p. 17]. Compare the description of the somnambulist Irene with the account that follows:

A man of '40, after much circumlocution, revealed what torments him day and night. Two years ago he lost his father and uncle for whom he had the greatest affection and veneration: he misses them, that is natural. Will he be obsessed by the image of their figure, like an hysteric mourning her father? No. He is obsessed by the thought of the soul of his uncle. But what is frightful is that the soul of his uncle is associated, juxtaposed, or confounded (we know that these patients express themselves very poorly) with a repugnant object: human excrement. . . . He makes a thousand variations on this pretty theme, utters cries of horror, pounding his chest. "Can one imagine anything as bad, to think that the soul of my uncle is sh——" [The polite elision is typically Janet's.] [20, pp. 17–18].

The contemporary mind, educated by psychoanalysis, immediately grasps the less affectionate and venerative feelings toward the father and uncle *not* perfectly known to the patient. We surmise that the obsessions express these unconscious attitudes and that the embarrassment and anxiety are reactions of the polite, conscious side of his nature to the hostile attitudes. We emphasize the contradiction or conflict implied. Note what Janet sees: that the obsessional patient *does* know more of the content of his mental life than the hysteric and reacts to this knowledge with widespread embarrassment and shame. There is no cleanly split-off, forgotten complex of ideas. The symptoms are chronically present, at the very center of consciousness, endlessly thought about, added to, elaborated, justified, rationalized, or concealed (while the hysterical patients may show off their symptoms, apparently oblivious). Consciousness is not clouded but clear. In place of hysterical inattention and distraction, there are constant "efforts of attention." Indeed, when psychasthenic "ticquers" are distracted, their tics *decrease*.

In place of indifference, the obsessional patients feel a pervasive discontent—a moral, psychic, and physical hypochondriasis. Instead of suggestibility and the quick removal of symptoms, no reassurance satisfies; the patients must be forever verifying their honesty, cleanliness, sanity, perceptions, what they did last. The personality and the symptomatic elements are in much closer touch with one another than is characteristic of hysteria. The psychasthenic is losing a certain freedom and voluntary control of his thoughts, but, unlike the hysteric, he struggles to retain it. Perhaps this sheds light on why the obsessional rarely carries out the feared acts, while the somnambulist nightly repeats the traumatic scene.

There is not only a collaboration of the whole personality, Janet writes, but a heightening of thinking, reasoning, comparing, correcting, and remembering. While the hysterical patients are forgetful, many obsessionals recall the most minute details. We expect the somnambulists accurately to revive past experiences during the sleepwalking, but the obsessionals remember wide awake. (Janet does not remark that, while memories are present, emotions, excluding anxiety and depression, generally are not; the patients do not repress their thoughts, but they isolate their feelings: The man of 40 was conscious of thinking of his dead relatives as excrement but not of his hating and despising them.) This is a "lucid madness." Early he suggested "a certain degree of intellectual culture plays a role in its development" [22]. Later he noted obsessions could be found in people without any education [20, p. 54].

The sharpest possible contrast to hysteria occurs when the obsessional patients *cannot* remember. Instead of indifferently letting the split-off fragment go, there is a mania for interrogation, research, rumination, explanation, recall. These mental operations take on almost independent life, without practical end or closure, often an "arduous rethinking of the obvious" [23]. The patients doubt their mental capacity, feel incomplete, may mistrust all those about them, too, redoubling their mental efforts.

Behind these striking differences between hysteria and psychasthenia Janet suggests a deeper-running similarity: Both groups of patients cannot hold their ideas in full consciousness. The hysteric's ideas slip away into amnesia, from which they can be retrieved but to which they readily return. The psychasthenics do not forget, but they lose "a certain degree of the *perfectionnement* of the ideas" [20, p. 63]. These patients have at one moment full possession of their thoughts ("I know perfectly well I did not commit the crime"), but then the certainty diminishes and the ruminative doubting resumes. This is a partial dissociation. Janet struggles to conceptualize the psychasthenic's experience of reduced certainty, clearness, consciousness, and memory. He settles on the unexpected phrase, a loss of the "function of the real."

In attempting to understand this conception it is as important to note what he does *not* emphasize as what he does. The remarkable *content* of the psychasthenic patient's mental life is very little discussed. He states, for example, that homosexuality is a frequent preoccupation but quickly sets aside this "delicate question" [20, p. 20]. He discusses the "sickness of fiancés": "There are young girls tormented by the thought that they do not really love their fiancés, who make desperate efforts to 'really love' and end up, under pressure of this striving for perfection, detesting them" [20, p. 21]. The detestations themselves are left unexplored. Similarly, he doubts that the patients' self-discontents, their anxieties, senses of incompleteness, and agonized efforts to think and remember themselves out of uncertainty, guilt, annoyance are basic to the condition. All these phenomena, he asserts, are *secondary* to failures in action, failures in completing specific functions. The phobic patient, whom Janet includes among the psychasthenics, is not paralyzed because of fear; he is afraid because he is paralyzed. (Compare the James-Lange theory of emotion: We do not smile because we are happy; we are happy because we can smile.) He asserts that the patients typically overcome their fears if the object of fear is brought to them [20, p. 161]; but they cannot act on their own. There is a mysterious power which inhibits action.

The paralysis (which he compares with hysterical paralyses) especially affects *social* acts [20, pp. 81–84]. The patients are unable to participate casually in social relationships; they are detached, above it, tend to dominate or be dominated. There is a general lack of easy contact with present life and reality. The patients feel separate, are preoccupied with the past or future, cannot throw themselves fully into the here and now;

the present has the effect of an intrusion. They cannot love [16, p. 499]. At the condition's worst, the patients lose a sense of their own reality or the world's. (Again Janet includes within psychasthenia many psychoses short of dementia; later he understood delusions of persecution as the result of similar failures of action [24].) He is suggesting that the function disturbed in psychasthenia is among the highest and most complex of human functions, the ability to grasp and work with current reality. This is the "function of the real" [25].

Recall his conclusion from the case of hysterical anorexy. There was a loss of the ability not only to take food into the patient's mouth but to taste, digest, excrete, feel hungry, tired, or sad. Inadequate substitutive acts came forward as partial compensations: The anorexic patients were frantically busy; the psychasthenics' endless thinking fills in for lack of appropriate action and feeling. (Janet conceptualized symptoms as a falling back from higher levels of function; later clinical evidence would suggest that symptoms could also be a falling *forward*—away from simpler, inhibited, functions.) Now we can understand the place he assigned consciousness and its restriction in the genesis of mental illness. The hysterical cases experienced changes of consciousness and were unable to bring back into awareness certain memories and ideas. It was tempting to believe that this restriction of consciousness was the weak link in the psychic chain, allowing fragments to slip away into the *condition seconde* (as Freud's associate Breuer believed). But in fact Janet understood failures of consciousness as only signals of a disintegrated psyche, just as an adequate consciousness was only one indicator of an integrated, fully functioning psyche, free and energetic enough to recall, attend, and act. He mentions that nervous crises are likely to occur at the time of falling asleep or waking up [20, pp. 280–281]. He does not make responsible the change in consciousness accompanying those times, the sleep-time relenting of censorship and the ego, in modern language, which allows unconscious material to break through. He writes instead of the failure of the act of sleeping. It will not be long before psychiatry is concerned with conflicts over the *wish* to sleep.

Neuroses are disorders of *function*, the most complex sequences of acts, Janet conceptualized. They are not illnesses of nerve, muscle, brain parts, or even such psychic parts as emotions, sensations, will, consciousness, or understanding; they are disorders of the highest integrated and integrative functions depending on the coordination of all these and many others. Weakness of the highest integrated activities releases the simpler responses below (compare Sherrington, Head, Jackson, and Pavlov). Hence the difficulty of anatomic localization, for the *lesion* in neurosis is not at the level of spinal cord, midbrain, or even some discrete portion of the cortex, but in the relationship, coordination, and integration of many areas. (Again, in modern language, mental illnesses are disorders of the *ego*, the name psychoanalysis gave the integrating and executing activities of the personality.) Hence, too, the importance of training, education, ideals, symbols, and relationships in the genesis of neurotic disturbances and in their treatment. The psychotherapies are nothing else than the name we give treatment directed toward these integrated functions. The nineteenth century discovered a hierarchically organized nervous system, of higher and lower functions in levels, demanding an increasingly complex coordination as one ascended the cord and brain, or, from the viewpoint of psychology, as one went from relatively simple reflex functions to the most complex human acts. It was at the upper end of this ascension, Janet argued, that psychiatry found its disorders and treatments.

Thus, because psychiatry is concerned with the final, most complex adaptive behaviors and because these behaviors are in continual evolution both in the life of the individual and in the larger movements of society as a whole, it is not surprising, Janet suggests, that psychiatric disorders are most evident whenever fresh adaptations are required, as in puberty. When we do not evolve the new functions, when our development is arrested (or, as psychoanalysis would say, fixated), neuroses occur. The form of these varies as the functions demanded by adaptation vary.

Finally, we catch a glimpse, in Janet's discussions of the social disabilities of psychasthenics and of these patients' relationships to reality, of the developments in psychiatry that have the greatest contemporary momentum. We meet everywhere today efforts to define the ideal or healthy relationships between individuals and all the steps short of that ideal, as well as their consequences for others, especially in the family. This social psychology now forms part of psychiatry as the concepts of object relations that have sprung from psychoanalysis, as interpersonal psychiatry, and as much of existential analysis. Late in his life [26] Janet himself presented a hierarchy of the functions of the real, a schema of steps or stages between removal from and full contact with reality. (Earlier he had presented and illustrated the steps back from impotence to the capacity to love: first erection or ejaculation, then both, next gratification without interest in the partner, then desire, and finally curiosity and gallant behavior [16, pp. 988, 1023].) It was the nature of neuroses, Janet argued, to strike at these highest functions of mature relatedness.

Janet's Contributions

We can sum up Janet's contributions and place them between what preceded and followed with a simple illustration. Before Janet, *tics* had been separated from the signs of nerve, cord, or brain lesions by several investigators. "Tics reproduce in exaggerated form certain complex, physiologically ordered movements applied to an end. They are, in some measure, caricatures of acts, of natural gestures," Janet wrote [20, p. 97]. They are likely to occur at inappropriate or inopportune times, giving an impression of absurdity, and, Charcot noted, they frequently bear a relationship to traumatic events.

Janet brought tics into a group of symptoms and signs, psychasthenia. He noted their similarity to other "impulsions" (what we today usually call "compulsions") and to the doubts, recriminations, desires for precaution, perfection, expiation, compensation, and repetition that accompanied and were often expressed in the tics and in other psychasthenic phenomena. A syndrome (now included under the term *obsessive-compulsive neurosis*) was thus described which has remained, except for the loss of some psychotic patients and symptoms, largely intact since.

Janet also noted both a difference and a similarity between the dissociation of hysteria and that of psychasthenia. The psychasthenic patients were conscious of their tics, and, like the hysterics, had lost voluntary control over them. The psychasthenics were ashamed and tried to conceal the involuntary movements, which increased when the patients attended to them. The hysterics, on the other hand, were both unconscious and without voluntary control. Janet insisted that only a rare case fell between the diagnostic groups [16, pp. 643–644], but it was not uncommon for a hysterical case later to develop psychasthenic symptoms [16, p. 815]. Janet sought sharply defined disease states, but the results of his own long-term observations and of his differentiation of the dissociation idea into types of dissociation (which psychoanalysis would extend) were already beginning to move psychiatry away from the concept of disease *entities* toward that of disease *processes*.

Janet also described the *genesis* of tics in the patient's yearnings and daydreams (much as he did with the 17-year-old Rou., whose fugue was the fulfillment of his wish to be a sailor).

One young lady worked all day by the side of a window look-ing on the street. Her liveliest wish was to quit her monotonous work and go into the street that she constantly observed. [We do not hear from Janet what she saw or wanted to do there.] Cease-lessly she raised her eyes from her work and turned her head to the left in order to watch what happened in the street. Little by little she sensed that her head turned itself constantly to the left; she even pretended to have on a hat which was too heavy on that side [20, p. 109].

Finally, Janet illustrated abundantly that tics were *arrested* acts, begun but stopped short of completion. The bored young lady jerked her head to the left but then had to jerk it away again. The patients were not able to come into a full relation-ship with the objects of their desire. Psychoanalysis would soon elucidate the conflicts and inhibitions standing against the full relationship.

Hysteria, Janet insisted, could not be simply the product of a special susceptibility or suggestibility to ideas, for many of the patients had no ideas of their "accidents." It was obvious to both Janet and Freud that the *conscious* ideas of the patients did not encompass the phenomena of hysteria. Freud then searched, first by hypnosis and later by the method of free asso-ciations, for *unconscious* ideas and was led forward to the idea of unconscious yearnings, attitudes, convictions, and expecta-tions. Janet searched for what *besides* ideas was dissociated, and in what ways. He left behind the old conception of single ideas, resulting from trauma and splitting off from mental life, for that of dissociated functions or systems within which many sensations, acts, fears, and ideas were included.

Hysteria was therefore the disease of *coconsciousness*, sepa-rate, organized centers of attention, receiving impressions and able to be communicated with, in control of the personality (as in the somnambulisms or fugue states) or capturing a leg, arm, or the function of eating. (The distinction was not between conscious and unconscious or between ego and id, for each hysterical function had its own consciousness, organizing principles, and capacities for communication; the hysterical ego, like the personality, was already split. We will find Sullivan using the same conception to understand and treat the schizophrenic ego.) In psychasthenia, the dissociations were less complete. The remainder of the personality reacted to the separated elements, tried to justify them, agonized, felt incomplete. The separated elements themselves were less massive than in hysteria, merely an impulse or a thought, not taking over the whole personality of the patient. Finally, in dementia, the personality "fell in ruins" [20, p. 343], reduced to its smallest elements, to reflexes, scattered impulses, gestures, and pieces of thought. "In many psychoses, in confusions, in toxic deliria, in dementias, the curve descends very low, as far as the elementary intellectual activities or reflex activities," he wrote. The type of disintegration depends on the elements separated, the completeness of the separation, the degree of remaining contact and influence, which determine the position of any illness in Janet's "hierarchical table" [27] of mental maladies. All mental illnesses, he claimed, were manifestations of various degrees and types of integrative failure, failure of what a later generation called "the synthetic function of the ego." Illnesses were distinguished by the types of dissociative process, not by dissociation itself or the individual's wishes, ideas, or unconscious attitudes—the subjects of psychoanalysis. Janet was concerned with the *pathological forms of consciousness:* splits in consciousness, as in hysteria; failures to be fully in touch with reality, as in psychasthenia; radical discontinuities of attention, as in dementia [28]. Objective-descriptive psychiatry was typically concerned with the form as opposed to the content of behavior. It could therefore accept from psychoanalysis the concept of mental or defense mechanisms (indeed much of ego psychology) to the point of making them an integral part of diagnosis, while fantasies and wishes remained outside.

The final expression of the integrated psyche is, Janet argued, successful action. The disintegrated psyche cannot complete its life tasks. Obsessional symptoms occur whenever skills are absent, are being learned, or are blocked from use. In Meyer's language, the patient has ineffective habits. Neuroses involve failures of competence or mastery.

At this point Janet's creative impulse expired. Why does the neurotic psyche dissociate? What determines the type of dissociation? What maintains the dissociation? What are the blocks to successful action, to full involvement? What is the energy Janet described as rising and falling? (Henry Ey was to write that Janet's system lacked "a motor, the instinct" [29]. These were the next great issues of psychiatric research. His own answers largely repeated the questions. "It is a special moral weakness, consisting in the lack of power on the part of the feeble subject to gather, to condense, his psychological phenomena, and assimilate them to his personality," he wrote in 1901 [30, p. 502]. Perhaps, he said, intoxication, fatigue, hereditary predisposition, emotional shocks, or family irritations [30, p. 526; 16, pp. 560–572] could produce it. Throughout, he emphasized the *weakness* of consciousness, will, the integrating forces, not the *strengths* of unconscious elements and conflicting forces, as Freud was to do. The future lay with penetrating the very weaknesses and inhibitions to action that Janet had described.

Janet did not have Charcot's or Freud's relentless curiosity, their eagerness to throw caution, order, and convention to the winds and follow the surprising, scandalous, and unexpected [31]. Much that mental patients did and felt disgusted him; he called them weak, degraded, lazy. (Psychiatric investigation has repeatedly been slowed by such revulsions of frightened disbelief.) Undoubtedly, too, he was rendered cautious because investigator after investigator, even the great Charcot, had made extravagant claims as to therapy or final causes, only to find that the patients' suggestibility had picked up the investigator's hopes and eagerly confirmed them; Freud had the same lesson to learn. Still, it is remarkable that Janet does not move toward a conception of mental illness as conflict, for he notes again and again, in his discussions of psychasthenia particularly, that the patients are horrified by the urges they find in themselves. We must suspect that he himself was horrified.

Charcot's was a bustling kitchen, as we will now see, alive with noise, smells, explosions, and excitements, like the great Salpêtrière itself. Janet's was a neat, well-stocked pantry, with everything in cans. Nevertheless he gave us the account of neuroses most easily brought into relationship with general principles of *neurological* development and function; and if he did not answer (indeed he hardly asked) the questions to which psychoanalysis would address itself, still, the ideas he developed do not contradict the *depth* psychological answers that were forthcoming; they foreshadow, in fact, one whole group of those answers, what is called today ego psychology. Moreover, in an age ignorant and malicious enough literally to bury alive people suffering from psychological stupors, his grace and clarity did useful and enduring service [32].

2

BEGINNINGS OF PSYCHOANALYSIS

CHARCOT*

WILLIAM OSLER said, "Know syphilis and you know all of medicine." Know hysteria or schizophrenia and you come round, more or less the worse for wear, to most of the critical observations and fundamental disagreements in psychopathology. Each has accumulated over the years a great variety of clinical phenomena, its own character types, intricate mechanisms, and a host of ideas. Both defy every effort to settle on a single explanation or on one main fact. There have even been times recently, as there were in the 1890s, when the two seemed more alike than different,

* Leston L. Havens, "Charcot and Hysteria," *Journal of Nervous and Mental Disease* 141:505, 1966. Copyright © 1966, The Williams & Wilkins Co. Reproduced, as revised, by permission.

secret twins in several masks who by gestures or tone of voice reveal a deep identity. Both are diagnoses, and therefore passé, setting much of the present generation to wriggling. In addition, the concept of hysteria resembles the people to whom the term itself refers, but grown a great deal older: an aging actress, still capable of titillating us, called into service at desperate moments, temperamental to the point of provoking endless disputes, historical, tattered, but seeming to embody a wide and significant current of observation and experience. Listen to her and you will learn much of what there is to know about human nature.

The most prominent features of the syndrome, a chronic course typically beginning in puberty, with changing bodily symptoms of many kinds, dramatic episodes with intense emotion, often some alteration of consciousness, and a persistent but elusive connection to desire, passion or love—all were collected and described many centuries ago. The Greeks cleverly connected them by one idea, of a diseased uterus, unsatisfied, angry, and hence wandering through the body, episodically to disturb the individual or an organ [1]. The fits of hysteria appeared to begin with pains in the lower abdomen, the excited uterus required satisfaction, and it then attacked perhaps the throat, the stomach, or a limb. In men the seed creates the love of procreation, Plato wrote, and the organ of generation "seeks, by the raging of the appetites, to gain absolute sway."

. . . The same is the case with the wombs and other organs of women; the animal within them is desirous of procreating children, and when remaining without fruit long beyond its proper time, gets disconnected and angry and wandering in every direction through the body, closes up the passages of breath, and, by obstructing respiration, drives them into the utmost difficulty, causing all varieties of disease, until at length the desire and love of the man and the woman, as it were producing and plucking the fruit from the tree, cause the emission of seed into the womb, as into a field, in which they sow animals unseen by reason of their smallness, and formless [2].

Union, copulation, and insemination, these were Plato's therapies. Would that treatment had always been as benign! Down through the centuries almost every organ charged with the disease, most especially the genitals and uterus, has been extirpated in the effort to remove the offending condition. Further, hysteria was thought to be a feminine condition and therefore recipient of the attitudes so widely accorded the "second sex." If hyperfemininity is loved, and the female hysteric is often femininity magnified and caricatured, it is also derogated, its flightiness and variety no fit subject for the serious counsels of medicine.

Jean-Marie Charcot stands across both great objective schools of psychiatry, objective-descriptive psychiatry and psychoanalysis. There were two currents of exploration in Charcot, each running to high tide independently of the other: one neuropathological, disease-centered, nosographic; the other psychological and social, having to do with ideas, traumatisms, and dissociations, and springing from clinical histories and hypnotic experiments, just as the first current sprang from the clinic and the dissecting room. He fashioned a neurological, syndromic account of hysteria on the basis of his examinations of patients, either epileptic or copying epileptics, that had later to be corrected by his student and colleague Janet, whose descriptions were given in Chapter 1. At the same time, Charcot listened to historical details that, once put together and conceptualized, made possible the start of psychoanalysis.

Like Kraepelin, he taught by lectures. These were crowded, dramatic presentations; students came from all over the world, and with them poets, artists, curiosity seekers. Psychiatry's alliance with literature and art was coming to flower.

The general points were developed from specific examples.

As with Kraepelin, the patient was introduced and then discussed.

R, aged 44 years, clerk in an oil factory, entered the Salpêtrière May 12, 1884, or about a year ago. He is a large strong man, of firm muscles; was formerly a cooper, and endured without fatigue arduous toil [3].

In the lecture from which this is taken, Charcot proposed that hysteria was not restricted to women, and further that it was not restricted to effeminate men. Hysteria bears the marks, he argued, of a real disease and is not the random outpourings of wayward female intuition. This great advocate of the lawfulness and significance of hysteria pleads that if it occurs in a vigorous man, it must be taken seriously! Psychoanalysis had begun its troubled relationship with women.

The patient's father, now 76, suffered for six years with undescribed nervous attacks. A great-uncle and two daughters of this uncle all had epilepsy. Three of the patient's children were ill; one had nervous crises, another had attacks of hysteroepilepsy, and the third was feeble in intelligence. How often the investigator indicates his etiological biases by the clinical material he gives first. For Charcot, as for Kraepelin, the roots of hysteria lay in defective heredity.

Evidence of the defective "constitution" appeared early in the patient's life.

While a child, he was very timid, his sleep was troubled by dreams and nightmares, and besides he was addicted to somnambulism. He would often rise in the night time and go to work, and the next morning he would be much surprised to find his job done. This state continued from 12 to 15 years. He married at 28 years of age. We do not find in his antecedents either syphilis or alcoholism, vices from which coopers are not always exempt. He came to Paris when 32 years old, working at first with his father, who was employed as shop clerk in an oil refinery [3].

Then the "accidents" began. When 32 he lacerated himself with a razor. "A vein was cut, and the blood spurted; under the influence of the hemorrhage and the fright, the patient lost consciousness and fell to the ground." For two months he was pale and could not work.

In 1882, consequently about three years ago, he was lowering a barrel of wine into the cellar, when the cord which held it gave way; the barrel rolled down the stairway and would certainly have crushed him if he had not jumped to one side; he did not, however, save himself sufficiently to avoid a slight wound of the left hand. Despite the fright which he experienced, he was able to get up and help raise the cask. But five minutes afterward, he had an attack of loss of consciousness which lasted twenty minutes. Coming to himself, he was unable to walk, so weak had his limbs become, and he was taken home in a carriage. For two days, it was absolutely impossible for him to work; during the night his sleep was disturbed by frightful visions and interrupted by cries of: Help! I am killed! He went over again in dreams the scene in the cellar. He had nevertheless resumed his work, when ten days after the accident, in the middle of the night, he had his first attack of hystero-epilepsy. Since this time, the attacks returned almost regularly every two months; and often in the interval, during the night, whether at the moment of first sleep or about the time of waking, he would be profoundly disturbed by visions of ferocious animals [3].

There is defective heredity, Charcot argued. To this occurs an accident, some external event, perhaps trifling, but experienced as a "traumatism." The subjective element is of great significance.

It is always necessary, alongside of the traumatism, to take account of the factor which very probably has played a more important part in the genesis of the accidents [here he means the subsequent symptoms] than the wound itself. I refer to the terror experienced by the patient at the moment of the accident, and which found expression shortly afterwards in loss of consciousness followed by temporary paresis of the inferior extremities.

Indeed, the most important element appeared to be the *psychic* one, for it occurred in cases of hysteria without evidence of traumatic events.

The prominence of emotion in hysteria had long been recognized. Indeed a popular synonym of the term was and remains "intensely emotional" or an emotional outburst, especially when "hysterics" is meant. Robert Carter, a contemporary of Charcot, made the diagnosis depend on excluding epileptic characteristics and including "some evident exciting cause, such as sudden fright, disappointment, or anger" [4, p. 1002]. The disorder was hypothesized to be so common among women because they were thought to be more emotional, a curious idea that probably arose from special meanings of the term *emotional* and the fact that men did most of the writing.

Emotion began and was then shut off as the patient lost consciousness; he awoke unable to walk. However, when he again lost consciousness, in sleep, there was evidence of continuing terror, now in his dreams. The same visions and fears infiltrated the period between waking and falling asleep, a condition of *diminished* consciousness. One feature of the dreams was noted: "He went over again in dreams the scene in the cellar."

The patient resumed work. Shortly after, the first attack of "hystero-epilepsy" occurred. Between attacks the nightmares continued.

Disposition, accident, traumatism, emotion, the cutting off of emotion as the patient loses consciousness, weakness, free intervals, nightmares, and then the attacks—these are the critical elements. In the intervals between attacks there is evidence of the terror continuing in such states of reduced consciousness as sleep. The patients also had a characteristic attitude toward their symptoms, *la belle indifference,* and the indifference was often interrupted by *labile* affect, as Sydenham had noted two centuries before [4, p. 222]. This patient was not amnesic for the accident or for the attacks. He remembered his terrifying dreams and described the conditions of the accident as well, but not every patient remembered.

He entered a hospital, was transferred to the Salpêtrière, the venerable Paris asylum where Charcot worked, and was then examined and described. The foci of this objective description are three: hysterical *stigmata*, that is, the allegedly permanent phenomena; hysterogenous *zones*; and the *attacks*. Subjective phenomena are largely ignored.

The patient is pale, anemic, has but little appetite, especially for meat, to which he prefers acid foods; in short, the general condition is far from satisfactory. The *hysterical stigmata* in this patient are very well marked. They consist in *a double anesthesia in patches* of great extent, for pain (pinching, pricking) and for cold. Sensorial anesthesia in general does not exist, except to a very mild degree; taste and smell are normal; hearing is nevertheless quite perceptibly blunted, especially in the left ear; the patient hears no better when the sonorous object is applied to the cranium. As far as vision is concerned, the symptoms are much plainer, and alone suffice, in a measure, to enable us to affirm the hysterical nature of the affection. He presents, in fact, on both sides *a notable contraction of the visual field*, more marked, however, on the right [3].

Anesthesia, the failure to report sensation, was, he argued, the most dependable stigma of hysteria. It had also been for the Inquisition: The judges searched for a "devil's claw," that patch of skin where the patient did not feel the iron. The judges were instructed to expect that the patch would move and, for the most reliable diagnosis of witches, that the victim herself would not know she had the patch. Thus a mobile anesthesia, unknown to the patient, had been diagnostic of hysteria for centuries.

This was a *neurologist's* examination. The physician had only to elicit the signs; he stood back to observe. Empathy, understanding, rapport, if they were goals at any time, must not affect the examination.

We are, however, told that the patient *reacted*. In fact there were points or zones which touched off attacks. These last, with the stigmata, established the diagnosis. The attack was orderly, in stages: aura, unconsciousness, disorganized movements (but with some persistent features), and the passionate and recovery periods.

Lastly, to finish what I say of the permanent stigmata, there exist in R *two hysterogenous* points, the one cutaneous, seated below the last right false ribs, the other deeper, in the popliteal space of the right side, at a point where the patient has a cyst, which is the seat of extreme pain of spontaneous origin. There does not exist in this patient any testicular point. Pressure exercised over the spasmogenous points, whether accidentally or voluntarily, produces all of the phenomena of the neck, with the sensation of a ball, hissings in the ears, and beating in the temples, these two last phenomena constituting, as you know, the cephalic aura. Those points whose excitation may provoke the attack with singular facility are, on the other hand, but feebly spasm-checkers (spasmofrenateurs), that is to say, their excitation, even when intense and prolonged, arrests but imperfectly the attack in the process of evolution [3].

The modern reader will not miss the sexual implications of the points' location. The diagnosis of hysteria was often made only when a testicular point had been found. Then the patient entered the attack, its movements sometimes suggestive of coitus. The sexual implications were not lost on Charcot either, but for the most part they remained part of his *informal* teaching, the corridor remarks his students recalled, not part of the lectures. Such matters made up the *psychiatrie de concierge*.

Then the attacks.

The patient loses consciousness and the *paroxysm* proper begins. It is divided into *four periods* which are quite clear and distinct.

In the first, the patient executes certain epileptiform convulsive movements. Then comes the period of great gesticulations of salutation, which are of extreme violence, interrupted from time to time by an arching of the body which is absolutely characteristic, the trunk being bent bow fashion, sometimes in front (emprosthotonos), sometimes backward (opisthotonos), the feet and head alone touching the bed, the body constituting the arch. During this time the patient utters wild cries. Then comes the third period, called period of passional attitudes, during which he utters words and cries in relation with the sad delirium and terrifying visions which pursue him. . . . Finally he regains consciousness, recognizes the persons around him and calls them by name, but the delirium and hallucinations still continue for some time. . . . Then he comes to himself, and the attack is over, although it is generally sure to be repeated a few minutes later, and so on, till after three or four successive paroxysms, the patient at last completely regains the normal state. Never during the course of these crises has he bitten his tongue or wet his bed [3].

Although this last remark directed the observer's suspicions away from true epilepsy, Charcot did not distinguish clearly between hysteria and epilepsy, another condition in which focal lesions are often difficult to demonstrate at the autopsy table. Bernheim and Janet were to say later that many of Charcot's cases had learned their hysteria within the clinic itself [5].

The young hysterics, living in the Salpêtrière held the epileptics when they fell and nursed them during their post-seizure confusion. The hysterics were, as Charcot's assistant Pierre Marie said, subject to powerful impressions. "In 1899, about six years after Charcot's death," wrote one of his successors, "I saw as a young intern the old patients of Charcot who were still hospitalized. Many of the women, who were excellent comediennes, when they were offered a slight pecuniary remuneration, imitated perfectly the major hysteric crises of former times" [6]. Janet was to argue that suggestibility was a more reliable sign of hysteria than anesthesia or attacks and that this very suggestibility allowed the patients to be molded by the clinic's expectations.

Undoubtedly the epileptic patients gave an order and regularity to the symptoms of Charcot's cases beyond what the hysterical material alone would have provided, whether due to imitation or intermixture. A similar suspicion must attach itself to Kraepelin's "dementia praecox," the case examples of which for a long time included instances of syphilitic dementia. Clinical concepts do not mature in isolation. Independent ideas emerge, as do adults, only after long periods of imitation, influence, and confusion.

Experimental Hysteria

Charcot's stigmata, his stages of the attack, and much else of his objective descriptions soon lost their credibility. Today we can recognize in the patients much that *Janet* observed; Charcot's accounts seem either products of deception or anachronisms. But his explanations! Watch as that great, free mind attacks hitherto insoluble problems.

In the hysterical cases, he wrote, "there is without doubt a lesion of the nervous center, but where is it situated and what is its nature?" "Certainly it is not of the nature of a circumscribed organic lesion of a destructive kind as would have been the case in the diverse hypotheses we have passed in review. We have here unquestionably one of those lesions which escapes our present means of anatomical investigation, and which, for want of a better term, we designate dynamic or functional lesions" [7].

Now, how do these elusive lesions occur? He approached the problem both experimentally and clinically. The English physician Reynolds had already described paralyses *dependent on ideas*. Charcot, as well as others, had suggested a link between the ideas and emotions incident on traumatisms, on the one hand, and the occurrence of some hysterical symptoms, on the other. But, between the two groups of facts, "many links remained obscure." "Evidently this is a subject which would gain in clearness and precision if it could be submitted to experimental investigation" [7].

We know that in subjects in a state of hypnotic sleep it is possible—and this is a notorious fact now—to originate by the method of suggestion, or of intimation, an idea, or a coherent group of associated ideas, which possess the individual, and remain isolated, and manifest themselves by corresponding motor phenomena. If this be so, we know that if the idea suggested be one of paralysis, a real paralysis virtually ensues, and we see in such case that it will frequently manifest itself as accentuated as that arising from a destructive lesion of cerebral substance.

The hysterical girl, Greuz, who is now before you, presents on the left side the usual complete hemianesthesia; on the right side there is no appreciable perversion of sensibility. We shall be able, then, on this side, easily to observe any perversion of sensibility which may occur during the evolution of the perversions of motor power which we are about to provoke. I may inform you in passing that this girl has been subjected only four or five times to the influence of hypnotism, so that in her case there is wanting the influence of training, produced in subjects frequently hypnotised. Further, I can assure you that the phenomena which you notice today are exactly the same as in our first experiment.

Greuz is put into a somnambulic state by means of slight pressure exercised on the eyeballs for a few seconds. The peculiar rigidity of the members which you observe produced by light touches over their surface, or even by movements performed at a distance (somnambulic contracture), is of a somatic nature which, as you know, enables us to appreciate when the sleep is well established. Then, in order to determine the production of the phenomena which we have purposed studying, I proceed by affirming in a loud voice, "Your right hand is paralyzed," saying to the patient in a tone of conviction, "You cannot move any part of it, it hangs by your side." The patient demurs to some extent. "But no," she replies, "you are mistaken. My hand is not in the least paralyzed, you see I move it." And really she does move it, though very feebly. Then I insist, and always with an accent of authority. I repeat a certain number of times my first affirmation. You notice that after a few minutes' discussion the paralysis is definitely established [7].

The experimental "brachial monoplegia" was then described and compared with very similar paralyses occurring spontaneously in two hysterical men. The limb was flaccid, all active movement abolished, and sensibility had disappeared in the whole arm, each a characteristic feature of the hysterical states. The *idea*, your right hand is paralyzed, had in the hysterical subject been accompanied by an actual paralysis and anesthesia of the limb.

We cannot attend closely enough to this moment in the history of psychiatry. A clinical syndrome was being reproduced artificially, that is, by an experimental procedure, under the control of the physician. Undoubtedly this had happened by chance many times before and even been recognized for what it was, but Charcot unmistakably linked the clinical and experimental phenomena and repeatedly demonstrated them. This was a discovery comparable to the reproduction of human and animal disease in the laboratories of Pasteur and Koch. In the psychiatric instance the etiological agent was not a cholera vibrio or tubercle bacillus but an idea, a suggestion, and the path between the experimenter and the subject was not the test tube and the alimentary canal but the mental d emotional relationship between patient and physician.

Through Charcot's lifetime and since, several arguments have raged around the discovery. Is hypnosis only a special instance or manifestation of hysteria, and are only "hystericals" hypnotizable? Any clear answer has been prevented by the vagueness of both the hysteria and hypnosis concepts. If hypnosis depends on establishing a relationship similar to that which hysterics establish (for example, the ready transference of feeling for parents to others around them), then indeed the two share a common process or mechanism, just as many of the signs and symptoms of the one can be reproduced in the other. However, many subjects appear to be hypnotizable who never show the *disease* hysteria, that is, the full-blown chronic state, with all its bodily manifestations, sexual difficulties, special fantasies, affects, and chronic course. But perhaps these hypnotizable subjects are latent or potential hysterics, the circumstances of whose lives have never favored the development of the whole condition. So the argument goes. (Note that it continues partly because of the very common psychiatric practice of using a term, in this case *hysteria,* in two senses at once, to refer to both a symptomatic entity and a psychological process.) The argument takes on redoubled vigor when a second issue is introduced. Perhaps hypnotism is only a special instance, not of the hysterical, but of the normal, a state of *heightened suggestibility.* Now the problem is to separate the hypnotic from the everyday. This effort has gone forward with great momentum recently. Many hypnotic phenomena are reproducible in almost anyone, can be imitated without hypnotic preparation, and may not merit the term *hypnosis;* true hypnotic events may be distinguishable only subjectively [8]. We have, then, three overlapping but probably not identical circles, the normal, the hypnotic, and the hysterical. This is the contemporary position: There are common elements among these otherwise separate states.

The demonstration was not, however, completed by comparison with spontaneously occurring hysteria. Both might be the result of *simulation* or *malingering.* It was necessary to repeat the experiment or one like it using a simulator for comparison. There was no question that simulation occurred in hysteria; indeed it was an especially common event there. The issue was, did anything else occur? This Charcot set out to answer experimentally.

He induced catalepsy, in this case the maintenance of a

limb in one position, in a hysterical subject and compared it with the outstretched arm of a vigorous normal man instructed to simulate. To make the comparison more exact, a pressure drum was attached to the outstretched limb of each subject and a pneumograph applied to the chest, to provide tracings of the respiratory movements. The simulator maintained for a brief time the same tracings as the cataleptic, but soon the simulator's outstretched hand trembled, wavered, and began to record large oscillations, while the cataleptic's graph was flat. Similarly, the cataleptic's respiration was even, while the normal man's quickly became irregular, corresponding to the indications of muscular fatigue noted in the limb tracing.

In short you see that the *cataleptic patient* is unacquainted with fatigue; the muscles yield, but without effort, without voluntary intervention of any sort. On the other hand, the *man who simulates* succumbs under the double test, and finds himself betrayed on both sides at the same time: first, by the tracing given by the limb, which reveals the muscular fatigue; and second, by the respiratory curve, which betrays the effort made to hide its effects [9].

Charcot compared the effects of hypnosis in a hysterical subject with the effects of simulation; to this author's knowledge the comparison has not been repeated. In experiments comparing hypnotized normals with simulators, the latter can be brought to perform in ways at least very difficult to distinguish from hypnotized subjects, but only if their motivations, the suggestions, and instructions given them are alike. Moreover, if the suggestions and instructions are similar enough, and the resulting behavior is identical, who but the simulators themselves are to say that they have not been hypnotized? [8]. Note that the objective grounds for distinguishing simulated from hypnotic behavior are being shifted to the instructions, suggestions, and motivations given or aroused in the subjects and to the relationship between experimenter and subject. It is characteristic of recent psychiatric work to undertake what is essentially a sociological analysis.

Charcot's attempt to separate hysteria and malingering could not settle that difficult problem. On the one hand, the exploration of hysteria, psychologically and socially, was just beginning. On the other, the exploration of malingering and other delinquent states was to be postponed longest of all. Even contemporary studies on simulation use normal subjects pretending to simulate, not "real" impostors or criminals!

The Innovative Process

Trauma, emotion, fixed ideas, free interval, recurrence of the fixed ideas in nightmares, hypnoid moments, then the symptoms—how was this sequence to be understood? Charcot took his lead from the experimental hysterias already produced.

In clinical hysteria the pathological ideas seemed often to spring from trauma. A lorry had almost struck a hysterically paralyzed girl, and she dreamt of having been run over; and between trauma and symptoms occurred emotions, incubation period, hypnoid moments, so that if the pathological processes in hysteria and hypnosis were the same, the first must be slower and more complicated. Here is another birth moment of much modern psychiatry:

> This problem, bristling with difficulties of every kind, we must now proceed to face. I do not promise you, be it understood, a solution of all points, but in endeavouring to reach our aim we shall perhaps encounter glances at truths whose practical consequences ought not to be disdained. To arrive at the point to which I wish to lead you, I shall have to take a course apparently devious, and must return once more to a subject which has already occupied our attention. I mean those remarkable paralyses which have been designated *psychical paralyses, paralyses depending on idea, paralyses by imagination.* Now, observe, I do not say *imaginary paralyses,* for indeed these motor paralyses of psychical origin are as objectively real as those depending on an organic lesion . . . [7].

The paralyzed girl and the paralyzed cooper had both lost the use of their legs. Each paralysis occurred after a fright. The expression of their fear had been cut short in the girl's case by the need to help her mother; the cooper had gone quickly to lift the fallen barrel. Then the two had seemed well. But later, nightmares occurred in which the fixed ideas of paralysis and danger appeared, and symptoms. Most important, the ideas and related emotions were both recurrent and unknown to the patients when awake, who seemed, if anything, blasé.

Among certain subjects it is possible by means of suggestion or intimidation to create a group of coherent associated ideas that become *fixed* in their minds as a sort of parasite, which remains *isolated* from everything else, but which can be projected externally in the form of related motor phenomena. . . . The suggested idea or group of ideas is guarded in its isolation from the control of that great collectivity of personal impressions that have been accumulated and organized for a long time and that constitute the conscience or, more properly, the ego [6].

Trauma seems to set this process of fixation and isolation into motion. Ideas and feelings touched off by the trauma quickly disappear from association with the "great collectivity" of conscious personal impressions, disappear into a different state, what Charcot called the *condition seconde,* from which they emerge in states of weakened consciousness, sleep, and the hypnoid moments.

We have here a phenomenon of unconscious or subconscious cerebration, mentation or ideation. The patient, in a case of this sort, is aware of the result, but he does not preserve any recollection, or he only preserves it in a vague manner, of the different phases of the phenomenon. Questions addressed to him upon this point are attended with no result. He knows nothing or almost nothing. Briefly one can compare the process in question to a sort of reflex action, in which the centre of the diastaltic arc is represented by regions of the grey cortex, where the psychical phenomena relative to voluntary movements of the limbs are situated. By reason of the easy dissociation of the mental unity of the *ego* in cases of this kind, these centres can be set in operation without any other region of the psychic organ being interfered with or forming part of the process [10].

The whole process of disappearance, fixation, transformation into dreams or bodily symptoms, or the dozen other transformations Freud was to detail, takes time, so that an interval of elaboration or incubation is required.

Charcot called his hypothetical process dissociation—and wondered whether it did not result from a weakness of mental life. Perhaps some minds form fresh impressions too readily, cannot hold them in the perspective of their other ideas and feelings, and lose the fresh impressions to another, less logical and connected level of mental life. Consciousness, attention, awareness in these patients seem scattered, weak, dreamy; as Janet wrote, the patients cannot keep their attention long on reality. It was a disease of the ego, modern thought would say; the great organizing agent of mental life nods and stumbles. Charcot and Janet did not know why; they spoke of hereditary tendencies and low levels of energy. The pathological sequence and process would have to be pursued farther back in time before much else could be said. However, a magnificent step had been taken. It was possible now to connect the most diverse phenomena, up to then utterly obscure. As Freud wrote, the medieval demon (and the wandering womb, too) had been replaced by a psychological formula.

•

The pictorial artist, the great classifier and visualizer Charcot was not the preeminently *verbal* man Freud was, from whom great sentences and paragraphs, articles and books sprang with discipline and spirit, like fresh armies forever eager to respond to the smallest impulse or largest purpose of their master so earnest and yet so light. Still more important, the type of objective examination and attitudes Charcot and Kraepelin brought to diagnosis precluded securing many fantasies and memories. Reach often enough for the hysterogenous zone, search with the needle for the anesthetic patch, and there is either no time to listen or the patient will not talk. Thus the next steps waited on fresh methods [11].

BREUER AND FREUD

In taking the step from objective-descriptive psychiatry to psychoanalysis, we can use a distinction Wölfflin makes in his account of the development of artistic perception. There is a movement, he argued, from "linear" to "painterly" perception, away from the edge or line of objects and toward what is within the edge. In the classic period, "the eye is led along the boundaries and induced to feel along the edges," while with the baroque (Rembrandt is the most extraordinary example), "seeing in masses takes place where the attention withdraws from the edges, where the outline has become more or less indifferent to the eye as the path of vision, and the primary element of the impression is things seen as patches" [12].

We cannot press the analogy to visual art very far, but it will move us in the right direction. Through much of nineteenth-century psychiatry, a distinct *outline* of conditions was sought; emphasis was on whatever distinguished a group of patients, the external features separating one group from another, like an edge. These prominent phenomena, particularly signs (objective events such as catatonic movements that all can observe at once), lend a distinctiveness, a sense of precise outline to the descriptions. They are the farthest thing from later preoccupations with internal states, ideas, subjective reports, and understanding the whole person; these fill up the outlines provided by what we call objective-descriptive psychiatry.

I will discuss in Chapter 6 the extraordinary temporal development of psychiatry, the gradual extension of interest to whole lifetimes, considered in more and more detail, and to illnesses searched out through the generations. Kraepelin and his associates extended the generational studies; in addition, they followed up illnesses through whole lifetimes. Now Charcot's little sequence, trauma, emotion, idea, interval of elaboration, hypnoid moment, and emergence of the symptoms, is taken up into the great Freudian historical sequences that are pushed back to the start of life. Moreover, what was one pathological process, dissociation, differentiates into a host of special mechanisms—conversion, projection, introjection, and the others—that explained the various sequences observed. Charcot begins and Freud develops, at first with the help of Joseph Breuer, the new dynamic, historical, intrapsychic psychiatry.

The Case of Anna O.

Breuer's treatment of Anna O., from which the next discoveries emerged, took place between 1880 and 1882. It is unlikely that the treatment would have resulted in the advance, as similar therapeutic efforts in the past had not, if Breuer had been ignorant of the clinical sequences being discovered in hysteria, and if he had not been a friend of Freud. The outcome would have been even less likely had Freud not been a student of Charcot or finally if, as a struggling young practitioner of neurology, Freud had not been referred many neurotics and found unsatisfactory their treatment with the available methods of electrotherapy, hydrotherapy, massage, and rest-and-feeding cures.

The first facts about the patient seem conventional enough, but their number and variety should alert us to one of the principal features of the new investigations, their *duration* and *in-*

timacy. Breuer's patient was not merely examined. Symptoms were not only described or sequences of symptoms related. Breuer evokes the half-waking world of the patient, collects the mental contents of that world, learns to elicit further contents, and then pursues specific lines of association. The inner reaches of mental life were being broken open.

Anna O., a 21-year-old girl of "powerful intellect" and "great poetic and imaginative gifts" lived a monotonous existence relieved only by systematic daydreaming, her "private theatre." (There is no good evidence that Anna had great poetic gifts, but it is characteristic of hysterical patients to excite enthusiasm in their doctors.) She had never been in love except with her father, of whom she was "passionately fond," and she fell ill soon after he contracted a chest abscess that caused his death less than a year later. Giving her whole energies to nursing him, she gradually succumbed to weakness and distaste for food, both partly the result of a severe cough of "nervous" origin. Breuer was then called in and undertook her treatment.

He diagnosed a state of "altering consciousness." In the primary condition she recognized her surroundings, was melancholy and anxious but otherwise was her familiar self. In the *condition seconde* she hallucinated black snakes and was "naughty," abusive, and amnesic for events in the first condition. The "absences" had begun early in the illness and grown longer and more pronounced. Then her father died, and "a violent outburst of excitement was succeeded by profound stupor."

She improved briefly, but:*

* This and the following quotations cited to Note 13 are excerpted from Chapter 2, Case Histories: Case 1, Fraulein Anna O. (Breuer) in *Studies on Hysteria* by Josef Breuer and Sigmund Freud, translated from the German and edited by James Strachey in collaboration with Anna Freud assisted by Alix Strachey and Alan Tyson. Published in the United States by Basic Books, Inc., by arrangement with The Hogarth Press, Ltd.

Some ten days after her father's death a consultant was brought in, whom, like all strangers, she completely ignored while I demonstrated all her peculiarities to him. "That's like an examination," she said, laughing, when I got her to read a French text aloud in English. The other physician intervened in the conversation and tried to attract her attention, but in vain. It was a genuine "negative hallucination" of the kind which has since so often been produced experimentally. [Hypnotically.] In the end he succeeded in breaking through it by blowing smoke in her face. She suddenly saw a stranger before her, rushed to the door to take away the key and fell unconscious to the ground. There followed a short fit of anger and then a severe attack of anxiety which I had great difficulty in calming down. Unluckily I had to leave Vienna that evening, and when I came back several days later I found the patient much worse. She had gone entirely without food the whole time, was full of anxiety and her hallucinatory absences were filled with terrifying figures, death's heads and skeletons. Since she acted these things through as though she was experiencing them and in part put them into words, the people around her became aware to a great extent of the content of these hallucinations [13, p. 27].*

Like Janet's somnambulist, she was "acting through" events, events which required Breuer's talking cure to uncover. Breuer had so far remained largely outside the patient's mental life. Like the consultant who blew smoke in her face, he had *examined* her. Soon he began to move inward.

I have already said that throughout the illness up to this point the patient fell into a somnolent state every afternoon and that after sunset this period passed into a deeper sleep—"clouds." (It seems plausible to attribute this regular sequence of events merely to her experience while she was nursing her father, which she had had to do for several months. During the nights she had watched by the patient's bedside or had been awake anxiously listening til

* All quotations from Freud in this book, not otherwise credited, are taken from *The Standard Edition of the Complete Psychological Works of Sigmund Freud*, rev. and ed. by J. Strachey. London: Hogarth and Institute of Psycho-Analysis, 1962. Reproduced by permission of Sigmund Freud Copyrights Ltd., The Institute of Psycho-Analysis, and The Hogarth Press, Ltd.

the morning; in the afternoons she had lain down for a short rest, as is the usual habit of nurses. This pattern of waking at night and sleeping in the afternoons seems to have been carried over into her own illness and to have persisted long after the sleep had been replaced by a hypnotic state.) After the deep sleep had lasted about an hour she grew restless, tossed to and fro and kept repeating "tormenting, tormenting," with her eyes shut all the time. It was also noticed how, during her *absences* in daytime she was obviously creating some situation or episode to which she gave a clue with a few muttered words. It happened then—to begin with accidentally but later intentionally—that someone near her repeated one of these phrases of hers while she was complaining about the "tormenting." She at once joined in and began to paint some situation or tell some story, hesitatingly at first and in her paraphasic jargon; but the longer she went on the more fluent she became, till at last she was speaking quite correct German. The stories were always sad and some of them very charming, in the style of Hans Andersen's Picture-book without Pictures, and, indeed, they were probably constructed on that model. As a rule their starting point or central situation was of a girl anxiously sitting by a sickbed. But she also built up her stories on quite other topics. —A few moments after she had finished her narrative she would wake up, obviously calmed down, or, as she called it, "gehaglich" (a neologism suggesting the German word meaning comfortable). During the night she would again become restless, and in the morning, after a couple of hours sleep, she was visibly involved in some other set of ideas. —If for any reason she was unable to tell me the story during her evening hypnosis she failed to calm down afterwards, and on the following day she had to tell me *two* stories in order for this to happen [13, pp. 28–29].

Note clearly upon what behavior of Breuer, what psychiatric method, these observations depend. He must visit her regularly and at different times of day. He must listen to her "few muttered words." He must first "accidentally but later intentionally" repeat these words and then allow her to tell the stories. He must note, too, that stories accumulate if untold and affect her mood. He does not intervene actively yet; he does not, for example, hypnotize her, nor does he see his way among the stories. He was largely the passive investigator, being taught by the patient, and teachable because he was available, devoted, and willing to listen.

Sometimes, however, she was not willing to talk. At one point, like the consultant, he attempted "forcibly breaking into her mental life." The content of her absences then changed into terrifying hallucinations. Also when he left her bedside for several days she became distrustful and resisting, and his intrusions required more forcible efforts. Then he urged, pleaded, gave drugs, and she had to satisfy herself of his identity "by carefully feeling my hands."

She began to relive, in the absences, the successive events of the previous winter, day by day.

I should only have been able to *suspect* that this was happening, had it not been that every evening during the hypnosis she talked through whatever it was that had excited her on the same day in 1881, and had it not been that a private diary kept by her mother in 1881 confirmed beyond a doubt the occurrence of the underlying events. This reliving of the previous year continued til the illness came to its final close in June, 1882 [13, p. 33].

The *separation* between her two conditions, the relatively normal one and that of reliving the past winter, was not complete. Charcot had already reported intrusions into sleep from nightmares repeating traumatic memories, and Janet demonstrated that contact could be established with the *condition seconde* at certain times. Breuer noted, in addition, that moods and an occasional misperception carried into normal life from the secondary condition. Anna would be angry with him for no apparent reason; then they would recall she had been angry with him a year before. What at first had seemed an inappropriate affect was found appropriate, but to the mental content of a different period.

He had now to relieve her, not only of the current "imaginative products but also of the events and vexations of 1881." He must have felt himself falling farther and farther behind when he came upon a still earlier set of memories from the period in which she nursed her father, July to December, 1880. But while the work grew, its rewards multiplied, for the discharge of these memories appeared to affect her symptoms.

It was in the summer during a period of extreme heat, and the patient was suffering very badly from thirst; for, without being able to account for it in any way, she suddenly found it impossible to drink. She would take up the glass of water she longed for, but as soon as it touched her lips she would push it away like someone suffering from hydrophobia. As she did this, she was obviously in an *absence* for a couple of seconds. She lived only on fruit, such as melons, etc., so as to lessen her tormenting thirst. This had lasted for some six weeks, when one day during hypnosis she grumbled about her English lady-companion whom she did not care for, and went on to describe, with every sign of disgust, how she had once gone into that lady's room and how her little dog— horrid creature!—had drunk out of a glass there. The patient had said nothing, as she had wanted to be polite. After giving further energetic expression to the anger she had held back, she asked for something to drink, drank a large quantity of water without any difficulty and woke from her hypnosis with the glass at her lips; and thereupon the disturbance vanished, never to return [13, pp. 34-35].

Anna had said nothing at the time of the "trauma"; idea and feeling had been shut off because she wanted to be polite.

Here is the "cathartic method," widely used at the time, from which psychoanalytic technique would develop. "Each individual symptom in this complicated case," Breuer wrote, "was taken separately in hand; all the occasions on which it had appeared were described in reverse order, starting before the time when the patient became bedridden and going back to the event which led to its first appearance." To do this and also to talk out the two other sets of experiences, her current imaginative products and the events from the previous year, he began hypnotizing her in the morning, asking her to concentrate on the symptoms treated at the time and to report all the occasions on which they had occurred. These he would jot down. During the spontaneous hypnotic period of the subsequent evening she would go over the memories in more detail, assisted by his notes.

On this laborious route he reached the starting point of her absences. He had already noted that many of the symptoms arose when she was nursing the father, especially during "frights." He had also noted that "dread" of a memory inhibited its recall and that only forcible measures could overcome the inhibition. On the last day, helped by rearrangement of the room to resemble her father's sickroom, she reproduced the scene that follows.

Her father was in a high fever, the mother away; a surgeon was awaited from Vienna. The girl, sitting by the bedside, fell into a "waking dream" and "saw a black snake coming towards the sick man from the wall to bite him."

She tried to keep the snake off, but it was as though she was paralysed. Her right arm, over the back of the chair, had gone to sleep and had become anaesthetic and paretic; and when she looked at it the fingers turned into little snakes with death's heads (the nails). (It seems probable that she had tried to use her paralysed right arm to drive off the snake and that its anaesthesia and paralysis had consequently become associated with the hallucination of the snake.) When the snake vanished, in her terror she tried to pray. But language failed her: she could find no tongue in which to speak, til at last she thought of some children's verses in English and then found herself able to think and pray in that language. The whistle of the train that was bringing the doctor whom she expected broke the spell.

Next day, in the course of a game, she threw a quoit into some bushes; and when she went to pick it out, a bent branch revived her hallucination of the snake, and simultaneously her right arm became rigidly extended. Thenceforward the same thing invariably occurred whenever the hallucination was recalled by some object with a more or less snake-like appearance [13, pp. 38–39].

Immediately after the scene's recall she was able to speak German. Her other symptoms vanished. Soon after many returned, but she was to enjoy later a vigorous and productive life [14].

This little scene must engage our close attention because Breuer made observations that enlarged significantly *the sequence of relevant events in hysteria*. The scene was not traumatic in the traditional sense. There was fear, suspense, danger, but the seemingly crucial event was not outside the patient but within: She dreamt that a black snake would bite her father. In addition, she attempted to ward off the snake but could not; her arm was paralyzed. Further, this paralysis had a physical basis, the arm having gone to sleep hanging over the chair. When a bent branch or stick later recalled the dream snake, she partly lost consciousness and the arm again stiffened.

He also observed that some of her symptoms did *not* appear during absences, that is, during states of changed consciousness, but during an *affect* in waking life. This had been Charcot's observation, too, and others', but the *nature* of the affect was now a little clarified.

A dispute, in the course of which she suppressed a rejoinder, caused a spasm in the glottis, and this was repeated on every similar occasion.

She began coughing for the first time when once, as she was sitting at her father's bedside, she heard the sound of dance music coming from a neighboring house, felt a sudden wish to be there, and was overcome with self-reproaches. Thereafter, throughout the whole length of her illness she reacted to any markedly rhythmical music with a tussis neurosa [13, p. 40].

The words *wish, suppressed, self-reproaches* occur. The observation of *conflicting* values, attitudes, or wishes has been made and would soon be linked to the idea of separated or *dissociated* mental events.

Symptoms may develop without absences, apparently under the impact of feelings alone. The symptoms, pursued associatively, during a hypnotic state, lead to forgotten memories. The latter are organized temporarily, must be followed up systematically, if they are to be followed up at all, and sometimes result in the discharge of affect. The recovered memories are of "little scenes"; within the little scenes, however, the psychological events of closest association to the symptoms are dreams or feelings, perhaps wishes. (Breuer makes this last observation without in any way emphasizing it; nor does he point to the fact that the scenes are *family* scenes.) The physical symptoms often begin with actual physical disabilities or sensations; the mental event is not asked *to create* a physical one. Absences and symptoms recur if the patient is reminded of the dreams or feelings originally associated with them. Objects in the contemporary environment may closely enough resemble the dream objects, as the bent branch resembled the dream snake, to trigger off whatever is associated with the latter. Memories and the affects linked to them are *accumulated* if not discharged—after a missed cathartic treatment, Anna had *two* stories to relate. Hypnosis or threats and urgings are necessary to overcome an occasional reluctance to remember, or at least to communicate the memory: Now hypnosis is being used, not as Charcot used it to reproduce symptoms, but to enlarge mental associations and permit their being shared. The effective psychotherapist or investigator cannot stand apart from the patient but must take up the patient's mental content and struggle against powerful forces to enlarge it. Finally, symptoms diminish or even disappear after the memories and feelings are recovered and communicated. Many decades earlier Mesmer had produced his cures when he could develop an emotional crisis or storm; his elaborate and romantic settings were designed for that purpose. The new cathartic method wedded an interest in emotion with an even greater interest in the *specific mental content* (ideas) discharged.

The Link Between Charcot and Freud

Breuer's *method*, however, remained very close to Charcot's. It was symptom-centered, hypnotic, and objective. The patient was examined under hypnosis, associations to the symptom were collected, and the relationship that grew up between the doctor and patient was largely ignored. Indeed, Breuer broke off the treatment not only because it was apparently successful but because he learned that Anna had grown to love him; when they parted she underwent a dramatic pseudopregnancy. These facts are omitted from his account, in part because he wanted to believe they were *artifacts* of a method that was meant to keep the physician outside the patient's illness. Plainly, though, it was drawing him more and more into it.

In his explanations of what he had observed, Breuer also remained close to the ideas Charcot and Janet made familiar: Hysterical symptoms result from the sequence predisposition, trauma, idea, emotion, in a state of altered consciousness, for which the model is hypnosis; and, as Janet illustrated, there might be not one trauma but many, and not one unconscious idea but many. Breuer shared Janet's conviction that the change in consciousness reveals the patients' *weakness,* but in Breuer's theory it was a proneness to "hypnoid moments" that allowed psychic elements to slip out of integration, going their dissociated ways. His explanation of the occurrence of psychic paralysis after a condition of fright and physical paralysis was also the one popular at that time: Things that occur together stay together, stamped into the nervous system as habits or learned responses. However, Breuer's *observations* raised issues that would throw aside in some respects and refine in others these early efforts at explanation of psychopathology.

Anna would not tell every doctor what she told Breuer. The production of associations varied with confidence in the doctor. Even with Breuer she experienced at times a "dread of recall," and sometimes, when he tried to break in, she began hallucinating and became terrified. It was as if her memories were *sensitive* and protected by some active force.

A *dream* appeared in the pathogenic sequence leading to the symptoms. Further, the examples of symptom formation from the incidents of the threatening rejoinder and the dance music involved wishes, suppressions, self-reproaches, shame, and anxiety, in contrast to the usual *external* trauma. Perhaps what was important about many trauma was not their superficial or apparent impact but their capacity to evoke fear, shame, self-reproaches, anxieties, and conflicts. If so, situations not apparently traumatic might be. The whole concept of traumatic hysteria was extended. Perhaps, too, the patients' dreams and other fantasies suggested what the apparently traumatic events meant to the patients and why they were so anxious or ashamed.

The perception of real external objects like the bent branch set off absences and paralysis. Patients were sensitive, perhaps conditioned to various external stimuli, so that past reactions were being repeatedly revived under the impact of the present. Therefore, the *condition seconde* or unconscious was not impervious to external impressions but let in some and shut out others—indeed, was hypersensitive to some. Similarly, the bank of memories and affects could be broken into by the *physician's* efforts, at first awkward and inadvertent, later more gentle and intended, but in either case apparently *painful* to the patient and seemingly resisted on that account. The patient's cooperation was a function not only of the attitudes and personality of the doctor but of what sore points he touched. Also, the points he touched were often *tender,* not only sore to touch but loving. Anna fell in love with Breuer and imagined herself pregnant, perhaps by him. Freud was to wonder whether indeed she loved the physician. Perhaps Breuer's presence had lit up an old love that had been, like the painful memories, unconscious.

Breuer noted that *both* buried affect and idea needed discharge if the patient was to change: both catharsis and insight. This was not Breuer's or Freud's discovery; at least Janet preceded them, and it was implicit in Charcot's realization that both emotion and idea entered the *condition seconde*.

The doctor was entering minefields of the past. No wonder Janet wrote, as the old mesmerists had written, that doctors forming close and prolonged relationships must expect trouble and stick with the patients until the work is done.

•

One pays tribute to Joseph Breuer with an easy pleasure. He came and went swiftly in the development of psychiatry, demanding no reorganization of our ideas or feelings, no great commitment of mind and heart; he does not demean or patronize or upset us much. He simply gave sound value and went his way. The value was observations; he moved psychiatry forward by the freshness of his observing eye. Earlier in his career he had made a significant contribution to the new physiology of the nervous system. Now his solitary case report stands as a critical bridge in the development of the new psychiatry. Modest, clear-seeing, recording with integrity phenomena he could not conceptualize, this good physician demonstrated what a brilliant and patient man, a Jenner or a Sydenham or a Breuer, can contribute from the shifting but fertile ground of clinical experience. He was the clear fine calm before the storm.

3

FREUD AND PSYCHOANALYSIS

T HE TALKATIVE, friendly, exciting hysterical patients not only offered a scientifically *accessible* mental
life, not too terrifying, contemptible, or incomprehensible; they also liked to talk to the doctors and the doctors liked
to listen to them. Since a great many were lively women, and
most doctors were males, the element of sexual interest undoubtedly held doctor and patient together through frightening times. Knowledge of hysteria therefore advanced quickly
beyond knowledge of other conditions—indeed, served as a
model for understanding many mental illnesses, just as the
understanding of physical disease followed and was modeled
on ideas about infectious disease. But while the knowledge of
hysteria advanced, it raised vexing questions. The hysterical

patients are suggestible; they are persuasive and manipulative, as well. They had led Charcot into a scientific blunder of major proportions. Anna O. frightened Breuer right out of psychiatry. Freud's data were the same patients' mental content of fantasies and memories, perhaps the most elusive and exotic data in all psychiatry. Would he be able to find firm ground among these subjectivities?

The high drama of Freud's case reports is not, however, a matter primarily of this issue, or even of the clinical stories, so like novellas that he apologized to the scientific community. We are struck immediately by Freud's method of work. This boundingly ambitious man urged, cajoled, massaged, tricked, hypnotized his patients; yet he could listen like a tomb. Here was another Charcot: brilliantly aggressive, bold to the point of folly, at the same time subtle, perceptive, quick to recognize any break from the familiar. He would dare to tell his patients the most outrageous things and yet listen as long and patiently as anyone had before.

He possessed to the highest degree what Napoleon called the supreme desiderata of generalship: complete patience and utter decisiveness. We can question whether he had the same emotional flexibility but we need to understand at the start this striking power: both to act and not to act.

The clinical material that follows reveals Freud adding to the pathogenic sequences now familiar from Charcot and Breuer; he will push them farther back in time and farther into forbidden mental territory. Simple pathogenic sequences will grow complex and interrelated. At the same time, the once aggressive procedure of investigation and therapy will become passive and neutral. This change in method was totally unexpected and needs to be outlined in advance.

Mesmer had observed that physical contact with the patients stimulated their emotional crises; similarly, both Freud and Janet made use of the patients' relative freedom and comfort of associating and emoting when relaxing during physical massage. Later Freud pressed the patients' heads to elicit thoughts and feelings, as if he were appealing to a concrete level of mental life able to respond to the attempted squeezing out of psychological products. Then hand-head contact was abandoned, and the patients were urged to associate to symptoms or fragments of a dream. Finally, with the classic technique, the symptom was no longer pursued; patients were asked to say only "what came to mind." The doctor was superficially less present. He could not be seen or felt, he did not question, but in another sense he was more present; a relatively undefined *presence* lay behind, which was perhaps larger for not being any particular face or set of hands. And just as there was no particular question to answer or symptom to hold in mind, so there was a general insistence on speaking freely (this soon proves more "demanding" than almost any *specific* inquiry). In short, while everything seemed calm, peaceful, and "free," the clinical situation had become crowded with implicit demands and restrictions elbowing themselves forward from within the patient. What had happened was that the doctor's passivity shifted the focus of activity, and restrictions on activity, to the patient. This was a radical change.

CONFLICT AND DISSOCIATION

The first clinical examples will seem small-gauged, even trivial, hardly more than refinements on Charcot, Janet, Breuer, and many others we could credit. Then this largely quantitative change will collect enough details, push far enough back in time, above all demand consideration of so many forces, tendencies, interests of the patients that the quantitative change seems qualitative. Our concern will have gone from single symptoms after one or a few hypnoid moments to so many subconscious ideas, linked in so many complicated ways, and to so many events, that we must give up altogether talking about ideas, even about complexes, and use, as psychoanalysis came to, such terms as *infantile neurosis* to depict this many-sided, interrelated, feeling-idea-drive-and-event-filled what-should-we-call-it; perhaps neurotic *formation,* for one is moved toward geological or archeological analogies. Yet these geological or archeological analogies fail us too, for the formation has a fluid or elastic, active quality that suggests more the complex chemical processes, flowing into and out of one another, that have been demonstrated in living tissues. The point is that we are being asked to think about psychological illness in a new way. Where objective-descriptive psychiatry followed symptoms temporally and related them to other symptoms, psychoanalysis revealed that symptoms are like tips of icebergs; the very prominence of the tips demands much larger foundations. These foundations, in turn, cannot be separated easily from the foundations of better-functioning aspects of the personality. Pathological processes do not lie apart from normal processes—to be quickly and sharply separated from them—but overlap with them, make use of them, just as pathological processes in biochemistry make use of routine metabolic pathways, turning them in destructive directions. The human capacities for fantasy and solitude can be taken up into a bizarre autistic life, special interests of childhood into perversions, the love of parents, twisted a little, into marriages like wars. But we reach this knowledge only slowly, through an accumulation of clinical details.

In one of Freud's first case histories he reported that a group of memories was associated with the patient's fear of eating. As a child "she had been forced under the threat of punishment to eat the cold meal that disgusted her, and in later years she had been prevented out of consideration for her brothers from expressing the affects to which she was exposed during their meals together" [1, p. 89]. We have again the report of a past experience allegedly productive of feelings that were not expressed; the example differs from Breuer's dance-music scene principally in the former's having been a *repeated* experience. Like Breuer, Freud made "a thorough clearance of this whole array of agencies of disgust" and noted that the eating inhibition disappeared. In Freud's example, the affect needing discharge, disgust, was more clearly identified than in Breuer's. Further, it was not a wish in the usual sense but an emotion brought on during a little scene, just as Anna's fear occurred during the dream. The material suggested that another affect, disgust, may contribute to symptom formation. It made a little clearer, too, that not only wishes and memories may need to be brought into awareness but also the reactions to them, what came to be called the *defenses* against them.

Such contents of the pathogenic sequences suggested a process at work, conflict, which might lead to that other, already familiar, process, dissociation. A young female patient hallucinated the smell of burnt pudding. She had also a nasal catarrh and anesthesia and was fatigued and depressed. She reported that the burnt pudding sensation began while she was looking after her employer's children and had just received a letter from her own mother, which the children snatched from her. Just then some pudding was actually burnt. The smell persisted [1, pp. 114–115].

Freud proceeded on the assumption that some *conflict of feelings* "elevated the moment of the letter's arrival into a trauma." He assumed that there was a sum of excitation, blocked from direct discharge, which could be triggered off into the formation of a symptom. How else could such a trivial moment become traumatic? He then guessed and suggested to her that she was in love with the employer and that she was afraid of being revealed. She immediately agreed and spoke of her shame that others should laugh at her hopes. Plainly this wish and its conflicted feelings were not deeply suppressed or forgotten—were in fact promptly confessed! But she said she had wanted to drive the wish "out of my head and not think of it again; and I believe latterly I have succeeded" [1, p. 117].

Freud then searched for the origin of these conflicting inclinations. (He began this search casually, like a man entering a little park, but it was a clinical forest he entered, in which to work for the remainder of his life.) Sometime before her symptoms started, she had talked confidentially with the employer. "He unbent more and was more cordial than usual and told her how much he depended on her for looking after his orphaned children; and as he said this he looked at her meaningly" [1, p. 118]. Or so she had believed. With this little encouragement her love flowered.

But why the intense prohibitions? Why could she not enjoy the fantasy in secret? Or in public: who knows what, with other circumstances and personalities, might have developed between them? Two other "little scenes" returned. In both, the employer had been angry, once directly with her. The hope of love was crushed. "He can never have had any warm feelings for me, or they would have taught him to treat me with more consideration" [1, pp. 120–121]. But while her hope was crushed, it was not extinguished. Both parties to the conflict, one pushing her to love the employer and one away, had been heightened and rendered more incompatible. And Freud speculated that the little scenes were *traumatic* (which now meant productive of symptoms) not only because they increased the conflicts by strengthening one side or the other but because in the traumatic moment she briefly became *aware* of these conflicting inclinations and could not tolerate the awareness. We will shortly take up the few details illuminating this last step.

The traumatic moment contained not *one* emotion but at least two; not one idea but at least two ideas; and the several ideas and emotions were related in a way that suggested conflict. Moreover, there was the familiar lapse of consciousness, but it was limited to loss of consciousness *of the conflict*, which in turn, Freud argued, was preceded by awareness of the conflict. Finally, the conflicting elements had previously been born and nurtured through "little scenes." The conflicting elements did not spring full-grown from the final trauma. Charcot's pathogenic sequence was now sprouting like a giant tree.

Another patient's symptoms began when she saw her uncle in bed with a cousin [1, p. 130]. (Actually it was not her uncle but her father, but such revelations of family life were still unacceptable.) Repeating this to Freud did not relieve the symptoms. He assumed there must be earlier memories. She then recalled the uncle's trying to get in bed with *her*, and some fragments suggesting that the cousin and uncle had been intimate before. The finding was, again, of earlier, perhaps related events. These events had not themselves, however, produced symptoms. He suggested to the patient that during the final trauma she had thought, "Now he is doing with her what he wanted to do with me that night and those other times" [1, p. 131]. (Note he did not suggest she *wished* it.) He assumed that this thought induced disgust, was excluded from her mind, and generated the symptoms.

But why should the final event have produced symptoms when earlier scenes had not? Perhaps the final scene was clearer, its similarities to the original experiences of the uncle's attempted seduction greater (like the similarity of the bent twig to the snake). Certainly the patient was older, more knowledgeable, and herself now sexually more mature than she had been. An event is productive of symptoms, he suggested, because it brings together incompatible elements of sufficient energy to generate the symptoms, like the mechanism of a nuclear explosion. And her wishes may now have grown stronger and more difficult to contain.

Similarly, another patient's sister died, and a series of re-membered episodes, attitudes, and actions were united in sug-gesting that the patient loved her brother-in-law [1, p. 156]. At the moment of the sister's death she became aware, "Now he is free to marry me." The idea was instantly dismissed, and later symptoms began.

Two large areas of clinical observation are coming gradually into view. One has to do with wishes and the other with pro-hibitions. Freud's examples again and again contain sexual elements, more specifically sexual elements in connection with family members, still more specifically relationships be-tween daughters and fathers. (Was this a function of the type of cases he saw, of *his* relationships with the patients, or of their intrinsic nature?) Secondly, the prohibiting function was a little clarified. Disgust was not apparent until the meaning of the various little scenes had become more or less conscious to the patient. Disgust was, in short, a function of her aware-ness. This datum is difficult to mark out sharply; it would nevertheless serve importantly in Freud's conceptual recon-struction of these events. The disgust function, he would argue, was part of the *conscious* personality which reacts and prohibits, what he termed the ego and the superego. His ob-servations suggested that the ego was not stirred to action until awareness had been aroused.

What began to grip his mind was at once familiar and very fresh: not the traumatic events themselves, not the lapses of consciousness, not even the particular feelings involved, but the patients' fantasies (and dreams) and the patients' reactions to them. Fantasies and dreams seemed to reflect wishes, at least those fantasies that persisted, and around the wishes stood a company of chaperones, fear, shame, guilt, disgust, which allowed some wishes only limited and properly attired access to conscious mental and social life. A *dialectical* process was being described: wish confronting counterforce; symptoms, the synthesis; a process operative across a host of impulses, conditioning situations, precipitating events, degrees of consciousness, and directness of conflict. The mind seemed like a turbulent assembly, for introducing issues, effecting compromises, and finding workable lines of action sufficiently harmonious to prevent breakdowns. Students of the brain were already aware of its multifocal activity, the great avenues of input, communication, and action, the convergence of many fibers often on one fiber, and the final, common spinal pathway which must express the neuronal consensus. It could be no surprise that breakdowns, conflicts, and blockages should occur.

The psychotherapeutic aim must be to bring into awareness as many psychic elements as possible, clarify their relationships, and hold them in consciousness against the psyche's effort to dismiss and forget. Contrast this with the old *catharsis*. Now it was not just emotions that were being sought but a holding-in-awareness, and not just a single feeling and idea but many and conflicting ones, and ones that led back into the past. Plainly investigators had not been unassisted in these efforts. It was Anna who led Breuer from related memory to related memory. And one of Freud's patients quite plainly told him to be quiet and listen, for the key facts would emerge. The patient's mental operations included a relating or synthesizing tendency (just as the investigator's did) that justified the latter's waiting and listening. But spontaneous mental operations were also discursive, disruptive, defensive; hence the symptoms and hence the need to intervene; the unassisted organism was not able to hold the related ideas and affects together. Charcot and Janet had been right to mark dissociation down as the first principle of symptom formation.

Several ideas and feelings must be held in awareness, against the pressure of their conflicts, and the successive events originally leading to the ideas and feelings traced out like tributary streams until the sources of conflict and the symptomatic results of conflict had been exposed and run dry. The cathartic method brought the traumatic *moment* back and into the treatment. The new associative method brought the *successive moments* of symptom formation back and into the treatment and tried to hold their contents in awareness. Surprisingly, treatment must repeat the trauma. Like the trauma it must bring conflicting forces into consciousness, but, unlike trauma, *hold* them in consciousness until some solution other than dissociation and symptom formation could be found. Like trauma, treatment causes pain—this bringing together of forces in conflict hurts and must be resisted. Further, just as there was generally not one trauma but successive trauma, so treatment is not all done within a moment but must be worked over the same ground again and again. What began as a single, simple process of catharsis and insight becomes prolonged, repetitious, many-sided, much-resisted; and rather than healing insights and abreactions we approach an intellectual and emotional *reliving*, a kind of historical reconstruction in which the patient is a little reconstructed, too.

Charcot, Janet, and Breuer had pointed fingers at the hypnoid moment that often followed trauma and fright and preceded the emergence of hysterical symptoms. The lapse of consciousness was like falling asleep or falling under hypnosis. The hysterical attack, its hypnotic equivalent, and the dream were entered similarly. Now Breuer's own observations, and those of Janet and Freud, suggested that the hypnoid moment was only a dramatic instance of a much more ubiquitous *unawareness*, or, as Janet said, a restriction of consciousness that fell across broad stretches of the patient's past and present. Consciousness was not a strong, steady beam but a flickering light. "Hypnoid moment" suggested occasional lapses, but the more intimately the patients were known, the more they seemed to have forgotten or could not attend to or must see darkly or not at all.

And the clinical evidence made increasingly clear that this weakness of consciousness did not so much usher in dissociation as spring from them. The evidence suggested not only some change of consciousness at the moment of symptom formation but the even earlier occurrence of discordant ideas and feelings, a quarrel within. The splitting had already begun. The resulting fragments were not passive products of an inherently weak structure but active elements in a personality reduced and disorganized by conflict. This was the first great fruit of Freud's work. Even the discovery of memories and ideas hitherto concealed but seemingly related to the hysterical symptoms did not have comparable importance. For they did not necessitate a *dynamic* psychiatry. Psychiatry had begun the study of mental content to fill in the space between the ideas and events on the one hand and the symptomatic results on the other. It was associationistic, for the clinical material suggested that experience had established *persistent* relationships; the little scenes brought together psychic elements which thereafter tended to set one another off. But associationism by itself need not be dynamic. Its minimum demands are for a plastic organism, one that experience can shape, even a tabula rasa on which *only* the hand of experience writes. A dynamic psychology or psychiatry demands that psychic events enter into relationship with one another, for which associationism laid down some of the rules, and that they enter a dynamic relationship, conflicting, competing, cooperating, discharging, holding back, all of which presumes centers of energy separate but in contact with one another. Paradoxically, psychoanalysis passed beyond associationism and became a psychology of drives, motivations, energy, instincts, and their relationships by pursuing the method of "free association."

The study of symptoms led back through contiguous, similar, or simultaneous ideas (the associationist principles) to *wishes,* which in retrospect appeared to select and order the ideas. Ideas had affects or charges attached to them that pressed for discharge, and the more or less specific aims and objects of these charges were as readily thought to be *inherent* as built up through association. In addition, the ideas themselves were as easily seen as expressions of bodily states as the other way round: It was as easy to say the patient felt heartbroken because her heart skipped a beat as it was to say her heart skipped a beat because she felt heartbroken; that argument would lead nowhere. In fact it was more convenient to think of a common energy able to charge ideas *or* bodily organs than of the two linked by associationist principles. Memories emerged spontaneously, sometimes explosively, as if powered by forces pressing for expression. Where nothing emerged spontaneously, one discovered shame, disgust, or some prohibiting force, which, having been expressed in its turn, allowed the blocked energies to emerge. Internal forces seized now this idea, now that, and reorganized mental life along this principle or that, processes which themselves suggest the play of Freud's own mind in all its vigor and dynamism. The patterns and repetitions could be traced far back into the life of the organism. The associationist connections by contiguity and similarity became the paths along which the psychic forces traveled, with switch points, as Freud said, allowing the train of excitement to veer on unexpected lines and charge with energy different fragments of perception and thought. In essence, the mind could split, for there are active, unharmonious parts, and life experience may bring disharmonies to birth or at least heighten and expose them.

THE DORA CASE: REVERSAL OF AFFECTS AND DISPLACEMENT

However great these steps, they were not the end. Contemporary students will miss any mention of transference, the very laboratory of psychoanalysis. Touching on "historical reconstruction," as I have done, only hints at the revolution this concept brings to therapeutic practice. And the concepts of sexual development and of the development of the defenses! Freud poured out ideas in a volume still difficult to absorb.

At first glance Freud's Dora story presents nothing new:*

It is merely a case of "petite hystérie" with the commonest of all somatic and mental symptoms: dyspnoea, *tussis nervosa*, aphonia, and possibly migraines, together with depression, hysterical unsociability, and a *taedium vitae* which was probably not entirely genuine [2, pp. 23–24].

Most of the case material only corroborates what Freud's earlier cases suggested: that into the familiar pathogenic sequences of Charcot and Janet must be put conflicting affects and sexual desires. Even the volume of family detail that Freud presents can be matched from earlier reports.

Her father told me that he and his family while they were at B—— had formed an intimate friendship with a married couple who had been settled there for several years. Frau K. had nursed him during his long illness, and had in that way, he said, earned a title to his undying gratitude. Herr K. had always been most kind to Dora. He had gone walks [sic] with her when he was there, and had made her small presents; but no one had thought any harm of that. Dora had taken the greatest care of the K.s' two little children, and been almost a mother to them. When Dora and her father had come to see me two years before in the summer, they had been just on their way to stop with Herr and Frau K., who were spending the summer on one of our lakes in the Alps. Dora was to have spent several weeks at the K.s', while her father had

* This and the following quotations cited to Note 2 are excerpted from Fragment of an Analysis of a Case of Hysteria in *Collected Papers of Sigmund Freud*, edited by Ernest Jones, M.D., volume III, translation by Alix and James Strachey. Published by Basic Books, Inc., by arrangement with The Hogarth Press Ltd. and The Institute of Psycho-Analysis, London.

intended to return home after a few days. During that time Herr
K. had been staying there as well. As her father was preparing for
his departure the girl had suddenly declared with the greatest determination that she was going with him, and she had in fact put
her decision into effect. It was not until some days later that she
had thrown any light upon her strange behavior. She had then
told her mother—intending that what she said should be passed
on to her father—that Herr K. had had the audacity to make her a
proposal while they were on a walk after a trip upon the lake.
Herr K. had been called to account by her father and uncle on the
next occasion of their meeting, but he had denied in the most em-
,phatic terms having on his side made any advances which could
have been open to such a construction. He had then proceeded to
throw suspicion upon the girl, saying that he had heard from
Frau K. that she took no interest in anything but sexual matters,
and that she used to read Mantegazza's *Physiology of Love* and
books of that sort in their house on the lake. It was most likely, he
had added, that she had been over-excited by such reading and
had merely "fancied" the whole scene she had described [2, pp.
25–26].

This is a lively beginning but still quite familiar. Almost at
once, however, material is introduced along two less well-worn
paths. Dora's father put the blame for her symptoms on the
psychic trauma of Herr K.'s alleged proposal. In elaborating
the relationship between the two families he revealed his close
affection for Frau K., the poor opinion he held of his own
wife and Herr K., and Dora's former "worship" of Frau K.
After the incident Dora wanted to separate the two families,
and her father did not.

We are presented a tangled and intense set of family connections. In unraveling them Freud talked not only with the
patient but with her father, repeatedly during the treatment.
Most important, he did not treat the patient as sick and the
parents as well, so often the practice, but applied a cool eye to
both. This was a clinical *investigation*, aggressive, detached,
skeptical.

Second, the experience with Herr K. could not explain the specific form her symptoms had taken, for some had appeared years before, even as early as her eighth year. "If, therefore, the trauma theory is not to be abandoned, we must go back to her childhood and look about there for any influences or impressions which might have had an effect analogous to that of a trauma" [2, p. 27]. Not only are the patient's family and family connections thrown open to clinical investigation, but so is the patient's whole past, and with it her whole personal experience. Freud is saying, I will not keep the study of mental illness within narrow confines of family propriety, or present or recent history, or those parts of personal experience deemed suitable for polite conversation; I will follow where the trail leads.

Once before Herr K. had kissed Dora, when she was 14. She had felt intense disgust and run away. Describing these events to Freud she experienced the pressure of Herr K.'s body against her chest. Freud suggested two psychological processes by which the disgust and sense of pressure came into being. Dora should have felt, he writes, sexual pleasure and excitement from the kiss, rather than disgust. This *reversal of affect* is "entirely and completely hysterical. I should without question consider a person hysterical in whom an occasion for sexual excitement elicited feelings that were preponderantly or exclusively unpleasurable; and I should do so whether or no the person were capable of producing somatic symptoms" [2, p. 28].

This is typical Freudian hyperbole. He will show on many occasions that almost any phenomenon can be pressed into the service of many psychic purposes, that little if anything is pathognomonic, to use the medical expression, "entirely and completely" of something else. Indeed the two psychological processes he is introducing at this moment in his narrative, the reversal of affects and the soon-to-be-described displacement, both disclose fresh combinations of psychic elements offering a bewildering array of possibilities. Thus, far from supporting pathognomonic phenomena the Freudian concepts *dissolve* many apparently fixed connections, as between a symptom and particular diagnosis. The old explanatory sterility of most pre-Freudian psychiatrists gives way rapidly now to a blazing glory of concepts among which it is difficult to choose.

Not only did Dora *reverse* the pleasurable feelings Freud expected her to respond with after Herr K.'s embrace (for Freud had met Herr K., too, and he was young and "prepossessing"), but, Freud argued, she *displaced* the sensations she had. Pleasure had been turned into disgust. Disgust is a sensation of the mouth, and although the kiss could explain that, perhaps something else was at work. Dora declared she could still feel the pressure of Herr K.'s embrace on the upper part of her body. She also reported an unwillingness to walk past any man engaged in eager or affectionate conversation with a woman. Freud hypothesized that the three—disgust, the sensation of pressure on the upper part of her body, and the avoidance of men engaged in affectionate conversation—all sprang from one source: feeling Herr K.'s erect penis against her body. *She* denied it. He went farther and argued that any disgust she might have felt as a result of genital contact sprang, in turn, from the closeness or association of urinating with the penis and defecating, and that disgust with urine and feces was in part a learned response (the conditioning of civilization) and in part our narcissistic reaction to giving up something once part of ourselves.

Our minds bridle at this rush of the master's thought. We protest, "But she denied it," which he overruns with "If her fear of the male genital were so great as to need displacement, she *must* deny it" and by reference to other cases in which he claimed the direct connection was uncovered. Experimentalists and commonsense, practical people are reduced to fresh disgust of their own, but the fact is, Freud had discovered something, however casual—even cavalier—his demonstration of it.

Fear and fascination toward the penis occur often in the mental life of both men and women. The negative component can be so strong that attention turns sharply away and displaces any impression left over from contact with the penis. These impressions may persist, even preoccupy mental life. Both horror and fascination, both repulsion and attraction, seem to lie, as it were, "close together," in the sense that there can be rapid reversals or transitions between the two. More commonly, when one is uppermost, perhaps monopolizing awareness, a more prolonged inquiry discloses the opposite twin close by. Unfortunately, in the development of these ideas, man's often silly pride in his penis and his consequent inability to understand how any woman in reasonably good health could be disgusted with it, no matter how wantonly or inefficiently the man uses it—this silly pride and blindness led many psychiatrists to expect all women to respond with instant adoration to all male efforts. Thus were the investigators and therapists, including Freud himself, victims of the very complex Freud had discovered. But that is regularly the case, evidence of the importance of the discovery, and reason for no surprise. However, especially at the present time when the extent of discrimination against women is coming into view, it is important to mark both the complex's significance and the easy way it is used to put women down.

For the purpose of this chapter, it is also important to underline two other things: both that Freud did not *prove* what he claimed about the origin of Dora's symptoms and that he *did* make it possible to consider his claims in any later cases which appeared. It may be that this *opening up of inquiry* is the major general contribution made to psychiatry by Freud. Certainly he observed and conceptualized with extraordinary freshness; from an experimental point of view, however, he

proved very little. As he said of himself, he was a conquistador, invading new lands and bringing back tales from exotic
places. Soberer types could shrug the tales off or go see for
themselves.

I did not find it easy, however, to direct the patient's attention
to her relations with Herr K. She declared that she had done with
him. The uppermost layer of all her associations during the sessions, and everything of which she was easily conscious and of
which she remembered having been conscious the day before, was
always connected with her father. It was quite true that she could
not forgive her father for continuing his relations with Herr K.
and more particularly with Frau K. But she viewed those relations
in a very different light from that in which her father wished them
to appear. In her mind there was no doubt that what bound her
father to this young and beautiful woman was a common love-
affair. Nothing that could help to confirm this view had escaped
her perception, which in this connection was pitilessly sharp; *here
there were no gaps to be found in her memory.* Their acquaintance with the K.s had begun before her father's serious illness; but
it had not become intimate until the young woman had officially
taken on the position of nurse during that illness, while Dora's
mother had kept away from the sick-room. During the first summer holidays after his recovery things had happened which must
have opened everyone's eyes to the true character of this "friendship." The two families had taken a suite of rooms in common at
the hotel. One day Frau K. had announced that she could not keep
the bedroom which she had up till then shared with one of her
children. A few days later Dora's father had given up his bedroom, and they had both moved into new rooms—the end rooms,
which were only separated by the passage, while the rooms they
had given up had not offered any such security against interrup-
tion. Later on, whenever she had reproached her father about
Frau K., he had been in the habit of saying that he could not
understand her hostility and that, on the contrary, his children had
every reason for being grateful to Frau K. Her mother, whom she
had asked for an explanation of this mysterious remark, had told
her that her father had been so unhappy at that time that he had
made up his mind to go into the wood and kill himself, and that

Frau K., suspecting as much, had gone after him and had persuaded him by her entreaties to preserve his life for the sake of his family. Of course, Dora went on, she herself did not believe this story; no doubt the two of them had been seen together in the wood, and her father had thereupon invented this fairy tale of his suicide so as to account for their rendezvous [2, p. 32].

It is not surprising that this cool-headed, sharp-eyed girl should have come to some damning judgments of her father. "He was insincere, he had a strain of falseness in his character, he only thought of his own enjoyment, and he had a gift of seeing things in the light which suited him best" [2, p. 34]. Still worse, Dora felt "handed over" to Herr K. "as the price of his tolerating the relations between her father and his wife." Herr K., we discover, sent Dora flowers every day for a whole year, gave her valuable presents and all his spare time; yet the parents could deny any "love-making"!

Nothing is more characteristic of Freud than his dissatisfaction with any first-given explanation. Most would have been content to stop here, Dora's distress amply explained. She had every reason to be outraged, not only with Herr K. but with her parents as well; and since she could not complain openly, the whole set of ideas and feelings must be driven into the *condition seconde* and then out again as symptoms. We would have had a nice case of traumatic hysteria, along traditional, if somewhat racy, lines.

But watch Freud's next step:

[Dora] was right in thinking that her father did not wish to look too closely into Herr K.'s behaviour to his daughter, for fear of being disturbed in his own love-affair with Frau K. But Dora herself had done precisely the same thing. She had made herself an accomplice in the affair, and had dismissed from her mind every sign which tended to show its true character. It was not until after her adventure by the lake that her eyes were opened and that she began to apply such a severe standard to her father. During all the previous years she had given every possible assistance to her father's relations with Frau K. She would never go to see her if she thought her father was there; but knowing that in that case the children would have been sent out, she would turn her steps in a direction where she would be sure to meet them, and would go for a walk with them. There had been someone in the house who had been anxious at an early stage to open her eyes to the nature of her father's relations with Frau K., and to induce her to take sides against her. This was her last governess, an unmarried woman, no longer young, who was well-read and of advanced views. The teacher and her pupil were for a while upon excellent terms, until suddenly Dora became hostile to her and insisted on her dismissal. So long as the governess had any influence she used it for stirring up feeling against Frau K. She explained to Dora's mother that it was incompatible with her dignity to tolerate such an intimacy between her husband and another woman; and she drew Dora's attention to all the obvious features of their relations. But her efforts were vain. Dora remained devoted to Frau K. and would hear of nothing that might make her think ill of her relations with her father. On the other hand she very easily fathomed the motives by which her governess was actuated. She might be blind in one direction, but she was sharp-sighted enough in the other. She saw that the governess was in love with her father. When he was there, she seemed to be quite another person: at such times she could be amusing and obliging. While the family were living in the manufacturing town and Frau K. was not on the horizon, her hostility was directed against Dora's mother, who was then her more immediate rival. Up to this point Dora bore her no ill-will. She did not become angry until she observed that she herself was a subject of complete indifference to the governess, whose pretended affection for her was really meant for her father. While her father was away from the manufacturing town the governess had no time to spare for her, would not go for walks with her, and took no interest in her studies. No sooner had her father returned from B—— than she was once more ready with every sort of service and assistance. Thereupon Dora dropped her [2, pp. 36–37].

Far from preventing or interrupting her father's relationship with Frau K. or her own tie to Herr K., she had done everything to preserve or even nourish them. The apparently traumatic situation was one Dora herself desired! Frau K.'s children, for example, were largely neglected by their mother; Dora substituted for Frau K. on many occasions; and this threw Dora still closer to Herr K., for *he* was a devoted parent.

Freud concluded that Dora was in love with Herr K. Very quickly he learned from her that others had observed signs of this love for several years. Again, however, Dora herself denied the feeling. If she had been in love, and she might have been, she said, it was all over since the scene by the lake.

But Freud had now grasped the value of turning her denials and complaints toward others back against herself. She complained that her father's ill health was only a pretext for rendezvous with Frau K.; Frau K. used illness to the same end. And so did Dora! Dora had had gastric pains, fits of coughing, and aphonia, and in most of these symptoms' appearance and disappearance there was a clear relationship to Herr K. She could not talk when he was gone; she could only write; and so on through a number of symptoms and episodes. But what, Freud asked, lay behind the *present* illness, for which he was treating her? What purpose did it serve? He then told Dora its aim must be to detach *her father* from Frau K.

I felt quite convinced that she would recover at once if only her father were to tell her that he had sacrificed Frau K. for the sake of her health. But, I added, I hoped he would not let himself be persuaded to do this, for then she would have learned what a powerful weapon she had in her hands, and she would certainly not fail on every future occasion to make use once more of her liability to ill-health. Yet if her father refused to give way to her, I was quite sure she would not let herself be deprived of her illness so easily [2, p. 42].

So it was not only Herr K. Dora wanted, but her father as well! And once again, the symptoms were not floating, as it were, on the surface of the patient's mind, ready to be washed away by the first wave of insight, but anchored deep into the structure of the patient's relationships and yearnings. If Dora's symptoms arose out of love of her father, and if love of her father could not be consummated, what could cure Dora?

Dora now found herself intensely preoccupied with thoughts of her father's affair with Frau K. Speaking again and again to Freud of the affair did not relieve this *obsessive* trend of thought, nor did discussing it with her brother, who took a more commonsense view. "If father has found a woman he can love," the brother said, "we should be glad, for mother understands him so little." Dora agreed in principle but was no less obsessed. (We can suspect what may have made the brother so understanding!)

Freud then supposed, as he would of hysterical *conversion* symptoms, that behind this obsession must lie unconscious forces. He supposed further that the unconscious ideas were likely to be either *extensions* of the conscious ideas or their *opposites*. By extension he meant an unconscious idea which, if present, would make her preoccupation "understandable." In fact, he wrote, Dora was acting more like a jealous wife than a daughter, acting more like a displaced lover than anything else. Indeed there was evidence of an unusually close bond between father and daughter, or at least of circumstances that could have fostered it: In his illness the father would sometimes allow only the daughter to nurse him; she had been very early his confidante. Freud concluded that Frau K. had displaced not the mother so much as Dora.

In a deeper sense, however, Frau K. had displaced the mother, Freud believed, in *Dora's* affections. Here, he suspected, was a still more unconscious idea.

When Dora talked about Frau K., she used to praise her "adorable white body" in accents more appropriate to a lover than to a defeated rival. Another time she told me, more in sorrow than in anger, that she was convinced the presents her father had brought her had been chosen by Frau K., for she recognized her taste. Another time, again, she pointed out that, evidently through the agency of Frau K., she had been given a present of some jewellery which was exactly like some that she had seen in Frau K.'s possession and had wished for aloud at the time. Indeed, I can say in general that I never heard her speak a harsh or angry word against the lady, although from the point of view of her supervalent thought she should have regarded her as the prime author of her misfortunes [2, pp. 61–62].

In a footnote on the case written much later Freud gave as the reason for Dora's failure to complete treatment his failure to analyze the homosexual element. Never, he wrote, had he conducted a psychoanalysis without coming upon a "very considerable current of homosexuality" [3].

Who then was the critical figure in Dora's neurosis? Father, Herr K., or Frau K., who may indeed only have been standing in for the unsatisfactory mother? Freud seemed to vacillate. The timing of the start of her obsession, plus considerable material collected in association to a dream, pointed to the importance of Herr K. But in proposing to her, Herr K. had used the same words that, she had learned shortly before, he used in proposing to a servant, and he had denied his feelings for her. Then she had fallen sick, becoming preoccupied with her father and his relationship with Frau K. Similarly she may have been thrown back on her feelings for Frau K. after Herr K. had disappointed her; clinical evidence of homosexual feelings often follows heterosexual failure. In any case she broke off treatment after she had confessed her humiliation by Herr K.

The father said she would come back, but he had never been straightforward either. Freud suspected the father had supported the treatment only so long as he hoped Freud would "talk" Dora out of her belief that there was something more than a friendship between him and Frau K. (He was not the first parent to find a "sick" child too frank or deep-seeing for the parent's comfort!) Freud suspected also that he might have kept the girl in treatment if he had acted differently, "if I had exaggerated the importance to me of her staying on, and had shown a warm personal interest in her"—in short, played a part to provide the affection she longed for. But, he wrote, "I have always avoided acting a part, and have contented myself with practising the humbler arts of psychology. In spite of every theoretical interest and of every endeavour to be of assistance as a physician, I keep the fact in mind that there must be some limits set to the extent to which psychological influence may be used, and I respect as one of these limits the patient's own will and understanding" [2, p. 109].

Nor was he sure Herr K. could have done much better. There was every reason to believe her slap was not final, that greater perseverance on Herr K.'s part might have reversed her feelings. But Freud suggested that the result of such perseverance was uncertain; it was typical of Freud to present two quite opposite possibilities. Even if Herr K. had rewon her, "she might just as well have been merely provoked into satisfying her craving for revenge upon him all the more thoroughly." "Incapacity for meeting a *real* erotic demand is one of the most essential features of a neurosis." On the other hand, sometimes "the onslaught of a violent emotional excitement" can overcome "the barrier erected by repression." "It is possible for a neurosis to be overcome by reality." "But we have no general means of calculating through what person or what event such a cure can be effected" [2, p. 110].

WISH AND FANTASY

A wealth of possibilities! These Freud showers on us with a boundless hand. And as the number of Dora's possible loves comes to light, conflicting with one another, masking one another, even standing in for one another, we see the focus of

Freud's concerns shifting. At the start of the case report he interviewed relatives and lovers, asked questions, constructed a sequential history of symptoms—in short, sought a factual account of Dora's illness in the tradition of the medical descriptive psychiatry he had learned. But soon the associative method took first place, with its quite different goals and operations. After the initial chapter describing the clinical picture there were two more on Dora's dreams, which comprise the bulk of the report. Freud's interest had moved from symptoms and relationships to wish and fantasy. The new method was superbly adapted for surfacing fantasies, poorly adapted for checking facts.

With this in mind, we can understand his vacillation. The strength of the different wishes surfaced can be at best roughly calculated. Some are plainly substitutes for others. In the realm of fantasy, Dora speaks of Herr K., but she may mean her father or indeed someone else. The unconscious world is not exclusive, logical, orderly. It permits displacements from one to another, condensations of one person with another, the simultaneous presence of opposites, and the overriding of space and time.

This is not to say that wish and fantasy are not real. They are very real, in fact powerful engines not only of mental life but of what happens in the world. Further, Freud believed fantasies represent biological wishes, which he called sometimes sex, sometimes instincts, and if his new psychiatric method did not allow him to measure their strength, it did allow him to uncover their variety and history to an unparalleled extent [4]. The calculation of that strength, he said, would have to wait on endocrine or metabolic methods still unfound. Similarly the new method did no more than hint at the true objects of the wishes or instincts, for it gave no more than names for the objects of the wishes and these names might be condensations or displacements of several objects.

The determination of the true objects waited on a social psychiatry then as yet undeveloped. Wishes and fantasies he had captured; their strength and objects would need other methods.

Inevitably Freud's method misled him about actuality [5]. He had believed his patients' accounts of their infantile seductions and other sexual experiences. Then he grew suspicious and took up the position his method allowed him: that the seductions were fantasies, perhaps memories, perhaps wishes, perhaps both. It has sometimes been suggested that his new statement meant the seductions had *not* occurred and were *only* fantasies. In fact he did not know because his clinical method permitted no clear decision. The study of fantasy eventually led to the closer study of actuality, but that required other methods.

INFANTILE ELEMENTS

The reports of fantasy also led Freud to infancy and to infantile sexuality [6]. He was at pains to show that this material represented not only ideas and wishes, however important these alone might be, but to some unknown extent infantile behavior as well. To this end he called on the large objective-descriptive literature of sexuality and sexual aberration as well as some direct observations of children. In fact, these direct observations were not necessary to his argument, although they supported it. The patients' fantasies were there to be collected by any skeptical person willing to apply the analytic method, and though everyone, including Freudians, would quarrel as to which fantasies, wishes, and childhood periods were most important, their relationships to psychiatric symptoms were far too detailed and striking to be coincidence. As Pasteur had said, the only way one could deny the existence of microbes was to refuse to look into the microscope.

It was true that the difficulties of reporting the data of psychoanalysis were immense. The sheer volume of the material collected over many sessions lasting often many years defied easy organization. Moreover, objectivity demands accurate, complete details, reliable methods of recording, the fullest presentations. But the demands of intimacy were as pressing. The patient's identity must be concealed; the case report must not become an exposure, while, from the standpoint of objectivity, it had to be completely that. Even collecting and recording the material brings objectivity into conflict with understanding. Freud remarked that he did not make notes during the actual sessions with Dora "for fear of shaking the patient's confidence," and for a reason still more significant: He did not want to disturb "his own view of the material under observation" [2, p. 9]. A therapist glued to pen and pad would not receive what Freud received, nor could he grasp and direct the flow of material. The most productive play of intuition demanded a full and free intimacy of minds, a sinking into the material which premature formulations, eager note-taking, too much objective standing back would prevent. Dora's case history was recorded, and from memory, only after the treatment ended. Freud chose to explore and only secondarily to confirm or be secure. The conquistador traveled light because the heavy equipment of experimental confirmation would hold the expedition too close to home.

Indeed the very effort to stand apart from the material for any reason must significantly affect it. The reports of fantasy had not only led to infancy; they had led back to the doctor himself. The young women occasionally paused in their accounts of uncles and employers; Freud wondered whether the pauses did not signal their bringing the same hot misconceptions and curiosities about fathers and employers now to Freud himself and stopping embarrassed at the thought. The physician-investigator who had aimed to bring the pathological products as fully as possible into the treatment situation found they did not remain their foreign, insulated bodies.

From the standpoint of objective science here was a difficulty as great as the difficulties of accurate reporting, or the calculation of the strength of wishes, or the secure location of their true objects. It placed an enormous constriction on the behavior of the therapist. He must not run from these fresh manifestations of the patients' neuroses, as Breuer had done. He must not play into them either, as Freud suggested might have held Dora to the treatment. The therapist must welcome the transferences, for here was a still further surfacing of the neurosis and one perhaps close enough at hand to be dealt with. At the same time the analyst must remain neutral in order not to distort or frighten away the emerging neurosis. It was for these reasons that passivity and neutrality became part of analytic method. They were, so to speak, double magnets drawing the unconscious material into the clinical situation.

What powerful magnets they were! Even in the Dora case, in which they were used so sporadically and briefly, they surfaced an extraordinary network of infantile wishes and memories. Used consistently and for longer periods they would expose powerful and conflicting infantile elements beneath every psychological illness. The resulting developmental conceptions would seem at home in the study of art, religion, history, social organization. Even so-called normal adulthood, when subjected to the same method, seemed only a less narrow victory over the conflicts and fixations of childhood than did more crippled developments. Darwin had placed man in an evolutionary line in which progress was less often fresh starts than gradual modification, so that the most complex creatures had more in common with the simplest than they did with anything outside their developmental line. Freud achieved much the same insight into individual psychological development; elements of the immature clung to the most mature; moreover, evolution could become regression, as when men and women fell back in illness upon their earlier capacities.

The power of the magnets to attract was not, however, any measure of their power to correct. Even when extensively surfaced and analyzed, the infantile neurotic elements, Freud wrote, were abandoned "with the utmost reluctance." Sometimes, too, the very process of surfacing the neurotic elements appeared to make them more virulent, so that the patients "acted out" their illness even more devastatingly than before in their everyday lives. The old mesmerists had warned about this contingency, as did Freud. The ambitiousness of the psychoanalytic exploration and treatment made possible great success but also great failure.

There were ample reasons, then, that this technique of treatment by understanding fantasies and the defenses against fantasies should have been subject to modification from its start. It was attacked as too intellectual, too neutral, too passive, too concerned with fantasy at the expense of reality, too concerned with sexual elements at the expense of values and social relationships. In part as a result of these criticisms, there developed two other great school methods, to which we now turn [7].

4

EXISTENTIAL PSYCHIATRY

K RAEPELIN HAD NO CONFIDENCE that his diagnostic distinctions were the final ones. Like Freud he went on revising his system up to the time of his death, trying to find his way between the need for structure, on the one hand, and the great elusiveness of almost all our knowledge of human nature, on the other. He welcomed Bleuler's nice epitomization of the dementia praecox symptoms; in fact he took Bleuler's major distinctions right into his own textbook. When the Wassermann test appeared, as I have indicated, he watched the number of patients diagnosed as de-

This chapter is reprinted from Leston L. Havens, "The Development of Existential Psychiatry," *Journal of Nervous and Mental Disease* 154:309, 1972. Copyright © 1972, The Williams & Wilkins Co. Reproduced, as revised, by permission.

mentia praecox in the Heidelberg Clinic fall. The straggling, chronic, changeable dementia praecox, it turned out, had picked up in its net some syphilitic dements, so that when there was a clear-cut test for the latter, the dementia praecox rolls shrank. It was not that the dementia praecox concept had proved empty, but that there were soft spots at its edges—some not far from its center—that had to be faced and reworked.

JASPERS

Karl Jaspers knew Kraepelin's work at first hand in Heidelberg, and psychiatric phenomenology, which was to a considerable extent Jaspers' creation, sprang from the limitations of Kraepelin's work. These limitations stuck out most noticeably with the paranoid patients. Kraepelin had put many in the dementia praecox category, but few deteriorated to the degree that catatonics and hebephrenics did; paranoid patients still, even on the back wards of the great state mental hospitals, keep the energy and often the clarity of their minds to the bitter end. Also, many of the paranoid cases, despite elaborate delusions, lived and worked in ordinary life, their illnesses undetected even by those closest to them. Thus if persecutory delusions meant dementia praecox, the category must include people otherwise unremarkable. Then there were paranoid patients whose illnesses seemed exaggerations of their original personalities, precipitates of their life situations, illnesses that seemed to grow bit by bit from their pasts: pathological personality developments. These stood in such contrast to certain other cases on which sickness *fell*, like a blow on the head, that the question inevitably arose: Were these the same illness? Did dementia praecox include both the personality paranoia and this abrupt illness that seemed to come out of nowhere? [1].

Jaspers undertook to distinguish the two, and the clearest

difference that he found pointed the way from descriptive, objective psychiatry to psychiatric phenomenology. The two groups of patients encountered on the wards, examined and examined again, did not seem so different from the standpoint of the objective, outside observer, but their experience, *seen from within,* their subjective experience, did seem different.

In 1910 Jaspers [2] reported four cases of jealousy psychosis—two cases of abrupt origin and two suggesting pathological personality developments. As we review the details of one case, that of Herr Klug, watch how Jaspers continues the Heidelberg study of *symptoms and signs over time,* but now the pathological phenomena are being reported from within. Kraepelin and Bleuler had searched physical movements and the stream of speech for the external forms indicative of specific diseases. Jaspers now brings psychiatry a new field of data, the *forms of inner experience,* at the same moment psychoanalysis is exploring the *content* of inner life.

Julius Klug, a watchmaker, came first to the attention of the *law.* He told the district attorney that his wife was unfaithful to him with a number of men. He felt *wronged,* not ill, and therefore doctors were momentarily absent from the scene. Klug asked for a divorce and was instead referred for psychiatric help.

Typically, there followed threats, protests against the imputation of illness, further requests for legal help, a continuing preoccupation with his wife's alleged adultery, and voluminous correspondence with the authorities. (These patients have professors' minds: They write much, explain everything, and miss the plain points that "simple" people grasp.) The threats gradually became shriller. Klug talked of killing, and three years after the first complaint he was sent to an asylum.

Jaspers next gives the material from Klug's wife. She said he had always been stubborn and quickly excited, but hardworking and reliable; she said that she had made it a policy to give him his way. For more than a decade he had been constructing an immensely complicated astronomical clock, on which he pinned great hopes. Then, for the past three years, *"ist es an ihn gekommen"* [2, p. 576]: It had come to him; he had been seized. In bed alone with her, at the start of the illness, he felt literally squeezed and pressed by adulterous lovers. The German passive construction suggests a new, alien process.

One night, the patient himself described how, after an unsatisfactory party, he heard a noise, as of a door opening, felt a wet cloth over his face, then caught something like whispering or a kiss. There were feelings of bodily movement and pressure. This was "not a dream; the impression was too clear." Yet, he *might* have been "half-asleep" [2, p. 579]. The last points are vital. The "elementary experiences" being described must occur in a clear consciousness, or they can be dismissed as hypnoid and hysterical.

The wife said he claimed that even passing male visitors had had intercourse with her, that their children were a whore's children; he had beaten her, begged her to confess the adultery, but then run away from the men he accused. For his part, he said that she had told him a suggestive dream, there had been rumors, some coincidence of names among the men she knew, and various ambiguities of phrasing. He had tested her by a nighttime visit when he was assumed to be away; she opened the door in her nightgown.

Then Herr Klug is described as he appeared on the asylum ward. Polite, obedient, understanding, he was an exemplary patient, orderly in his habits and willing to answer questions. Little could be suspected from casual observation. Perhaps he was a trifle superior. He dropped hints now and then of feeling that he might fall apart or go crazy, and the poems he wrote repeated the theme of being rescued from situations of great danger: "God does not leave his people" [2, p. 580].

There was a naïve eagerness, too, in his descriptions of the astronomical clock. However, he insisted that he had not been jealous before, and there was nothing remarkable in his family history or the accounts of school, work, or marriage until recently. All these areas are reviewed almost curtly. Jaspers is making the case for an intact personality upon which a pathological process fell.

It was not until the patient and his wife were interviewed together that the psychosis revealed itself. Klug quickly became excited, abused her, and threatened violence. Then his limbs hurt and he had to go to bed.

Jaspers takes us directly to the patient's written accounts, which were later supplemented by an autobiography. These emphasized the unexpectedness and severity of the evening's hallucinatory experiences; the latter were worse than "the worst of murders." In the morning he believed himself poisoned at breakfast, heard a "roaring of waters" [2, p. 583], and had more physical discomfort. The plastic quality of the discomfort is underlined, as were the sensations of pressure in bed. The "elementary experiences" are, above all, alien to everyday life; there must be some miraculous power and intelligence behind their occurrence.

The diagnosis was *paranoia*, and the patient's further course bore it out. The suspicions continued but never extended. No treatment was recommended, only constant observation. He was soon released and returned to watchmaking and his family. Apparently he had learned not to mention his convictions, which burst out only a few times. Once he accused the burgomeister of preventing him from finishing the clock. However, it was finished, even written up in the newspapers. Then he encountered fresh difficulties in selling it, which he blamed on the charge of insanity. The court intervened, praised his extraordinary skill, and awarded him money. There were public discussions of whether the clock should be bought for a museum. The German welfare state of 70 years ago practiced a social psychiatry fit to shame some more recent efforts!

Jaspers finds in Klug's autobiography the combination of grandeur, naïveté, and piteousness so characteristic of the syndrome. (He does not make clear whether these are results of the alien process or the soil on which it grew.) Throughout he emphasizes that the patient's work capacity never suffered, nor did he show any mental weakness. There were no further "plastic" experiences. The ferocity gradually disappeared from his complaints about the wife; she had become old and a "churchgoer," leaving far behind the alleged life of sin [3].

It is the plastic, elementary, vivid, bodily experiences that represent the alien pathological process, Jaspers is arguing. These comprise the indelible nucleus that is elaborated into delusions. Elementary experiences are not continuous with personality development. They break unintelligibly upon it. Personality must be warped and twisted to absorb the manifestations of process.

One lets the patient give a detailed story of himself and his experiences; one enquires when some point is obscure and in this way proceeds through his life, and particularly through the years which are suspect, for the beginning of an illness. As one participates in this experience with an inward understanding, one notices at first that connections are obscure and finally *quite incomprehensible*. One makes a note of these, compares them together, and eventually may find that they can be understood or on the other hand they accumulate and cluster together at some particular time. In that case one has found the most vivid and striking characteristic of the mental illness proper which cannot be demonstrated in any single symptom but which, as one lives into the patients' experiences, impresses itself forcibly on one as a tangible gap in one's understanding [4, p. 829].*

* Karl Jaspers, *General Psychopathology*, trans. from the German by J. Hoenig and M. Hamilton. Chicago: University of Chicago Press, 1963. Copyright in the original work 1923 and 1946 by Springer-Verlag, Berlin, Gottingen, Heidelberg. Copyright © in the English translation 1963 by Manchester University Press, Manchester, England.

There is no understanding Klug's hallucinations, Jaspers insists—no exterior cause, change in circumstances, or even minor occurrences. Later in life no new "connection-points" (to the alien process), no new elementary experiences occurred. The elaboration of ideas and twisting of personality all led back to the original hallucinations. Surely if paranoia were a *personality* disorder, its development would not remain bound to events of barely 12 hours' duration. Finally, in his last, contrasting case illustrations, Jaspers described personalities much more obviously and earlier disordered. Their illnesses *did* appear to flow without break from their attitudes, wishes, and experiences and did have the isolated plastic hallucinations of the first two. To the psychoanalytic complaint that Jaspers appears largely ignorant of his patients' sexual lives or fantasies, ignores the unsatisfactory party that preceded Klug's hallucinations, makes little of the symbolic significance of the astronomical clock, and fails to develop a relationship between the rigidities of character and psychotic developments, he replies that any relationship of similarity, temporal contiguity, or psychic forces that could be established among these elements would still not explain the vivid bodily experiences, would not explain the *form* which the illness took. To invoke the "unconscious" or a breakthrough from the unconscious is simply to invoke words. Worse, to try to explain such phenomena in psychological terms is to overlook the nature of the inner experience, to ignore that one can establish an intellectual explanation but no "inward understanding."

Some experiences cannot be "felt into." The patients themselves experience them as alien. When we get close to the patient, we do not thereby get close to these experiences.

. . . A young man suffering from schizophrenia lived with a woman hysteric who shared many of his hallucinations and anxieties. The patient said of her, "If one gets caught up, one is nervous; once one has the actual experience, one is not at all nervous;

in my case the whole thing is much quieter and clearer" [4, p. 132].

"The 'shouting miracle' is an extraordinary occurrence; the respiratory muscles are put into motion, so that I am forced to shout out, unless I make an enormous effort at suppression, which is not always possible in view of the suddenness of the impulse, or rather I have to concentrate relentlessly on it. . . . At times the shouting is so repetitive that my state gets unbearable . . . since words are shouted, my will is of course not altogether uninvolved" [4, p. 124].

Jaspers is arguing, do not impose an intellectual formula on the material. Respect the differences in experience reported. No one doubts that there are pathological *physical* processes which can break in on mental life. Are not these psychotic experiences more like physical processes than the vast bulk of personal experiences reported? If these arguments carry no force, try achieving an "inward understanding" of the experiences, try "living into the patients' experiences." I tried in the case of Klug, Jaspers says, and I could not.

Jaspers' contribution does not turn on his success or failure with Herr Klug. Perhaps a more empathic observer could have reached an "inward understanding" of Herr Klug's psychosis; some therapists appear to have done so with very similar illnesses. The great point is the test applied. There is no deciding between unconscious process and alien or physical process on the basis of external observation, whether of the brain or the mind. A fresh method is needed, and that, Jaspers suggests, should be one of "inward understanding," "living into the patients' experiences." The *physical* cases should not allow it; the psychological ones should. This is the first step toward the existential method.

Paranoid cases provided the royal road to the exploration of psychosis for both the Heidelberg school and psychoanalysis. These articulate, self-conscious patients, with their great penchant for explaining, served both schools; in fact Jaspers and

Freud each used Schreber's memoirs. Paranoia was like an extraordinary insect fixed in the clear glass of a seemingly intact person. Again it is the *accessible* material, as with hysteria, that shapes the development of scientific ideas. The paranoid patients *did* feel they were subject to an alien influence. Had Jaspers been "taken in" by the psychotic material or were the patients right—subject in fact to an alien process that the psychosis was only an attempt to explain?

The difference between Jasperian and Freudian explanations comes to less and less the more closely we study them. Jaspers would not say that the alien process was physical; he did not know what it was. Of the two, Freud was the one prone to *physical* explanations. He would have been the one more likely to locate the unconscious in the midbrain, for example, and to call psychosis a disturbance of the midbrain. He was forever leaping back and forth between the mind and the body. Jaspers tended to remain on one side or the other.

However, what should interest us about Jaspers is not his ignorance of the cause of psychosis. That he shares with a large and humble company who have learned to be at home with psychiatry's early victories as we work toward larger ones. What Jaspers did was to make clear a fresh difference between psychosis and normal or neurotic life. He did so by studying carefully patients' reports of their experience, as Kraepelin had studied their physical movements, stream of speech, and handwriting, and Freud their mental content. And just as the objective schools of descriptive psychiatry and psychoanalysis fathered detailed methods, so the study of inner experience fathered its own technique.

At first everything depended on finding cooperative, articulate patients in touch with their inner lives. The investigator did little more than ask the patients how they felt and then hope for an intelligible answer. The answers seemed generally to concern symptoms, that is, some discrete pain, anxiety, or peculiarity of experience that caught the patient's attention. (We have already seen how the objective schools also began with these bits of experience.)

A large number of these "subjective experiences" were collected and categorized under a variety of headings. One result was a greater appreciation of how varied human experience is. Phenomena that looked largely identical from the outside were found to have all kinds of inner differences. For example, hallucinations, illusions, fantasies, true perceptions seemed to describe an adequate spectrum until patients developed in more detail what they "saw" or "heard."

In describing sense-experience in false perception, we distinguished illusions from hallucinations and similarly we draw a clear distinction between sense-phenomena and the phenomena of imagery (*i.e.,* between hallucination and pseudo-hallucination). This does not prevent us from finding actual "transitions" in that pseudo-hallucination can *change over* into hallucination and there may be a florid sensory pathology in which all the phenomena *combine.* We cannot reach any analysis, however, unless we attempt sharp distinctions of this sort which provide us with some kind of standard [4, p. 70].

We are given a series of phenomena, with some features in common and others not, a much richer variety of experiences than objective methods revealed. One result was the collapse of neat sortings by the psychological faculty involved; plainly there lie between thinking and perceiving, for example, intermediate or transitional phenomena which defy simplistic categories. The richness of inner life encourages still wider and deeper investigations. What will we find if we extend our interest beyond symptoms, ask questions meant to plumb the whole range of inner experience, place ourselves where we can share the patient's experience, minute by minute? These are the next steps in the development of phenomenology and then existential psychiatry.

MINKOWSKI

I pass on to another case history, which occurred in 1923. At this time a happy circumstance or, more precisely, the vicissitudes of life obliged me to spend two months with a patient as his private physician. I was with him continually, night and day. It is not difficult to imagine the annoyances that such a symbiosis can cause, but on the other hand it creates special conditions for the observer. By allowing him to constantly compare the patient's psyche with his own, it gives him the opportunity to note certain details which usually escape attention.

Briefly, here is the clinical picture. It concerns a man 66 years old who exhibited a depressive psychosis accompanied by delusions of persecution and extensive interpretations. . . .

The patient expresses delusions of ruin and guilt. Being a foreigner, he reproaches himself for not having taken out French citizenship. He sees this as a terrible crime. He claims also that he has not paid his taxes and that he no longer has a penny. An atrocious punishment is in store for him as a result. Someone will cut off the arms and legs of the members of his family and will then leave them exposed completely naked in a barren field. The same thing will happen to him. They will hammer a nail in his head and pour all kinds of filth into his stomach. Mutilated in the most appalling way, he will be led in a large procession to a fair and will be condemned to live, covered with vermin, in a cage with wild beasts or with rats in the sewers until he dies. The whole world knows of his crimes and knows the punishment which awaits him. Also, everyone with the exception of his family will be involved in one way or another. People look at him in a certain way in the street; servants are paid to watch and slander him. All the articles in the newspapers are aimed at him; books are printed expressly against him and his family. The Medical Corps is at the head of this vast movement directed against him [5, pp. 180–181].

Although my patient's case is relatively commonplace from the clinical point to view, the circumstances in which I observed him were not. I have already said that I lived with him for two months. Thus I had the possibility of observing him from day to day, not in a mental hospital or sanitarium but in an ordinary environment. His manner of reacting to normal external stimuli, his ability to adapt to the demands of daily life, the variability of his symptoms and their particular nuances are set out more clearly under such conditions. This circumstance is accompanied by another. We cannot maintain a medical point of view 24 hours a day. We react to the patient as do other people around him. Compassion, gentleness, persuasion, impatience, and anger appear in turn. Thus, in the above circumstances, I not only observed the patient but had the possibility of projecting his psychic life on mine at every moment. It was like two melodies being played simultaneously; although these two melodies are as dissonant as can be, a certain balance becomes established between the notes of the one and the other and lets us penetrate a little further into our patient's psyche. The findings thus noted were psychological on the one hand and phenomenological on the other [5, p. 182].

Here is one of the moments of passage for psychiatry, from the objective, descriptive reporting of Jaspers' informants to the existential encounters that Minkowski begins to experience. The report starts out traditionally; the paranoid and depressive delusional content was familiar enough from a thousand previous examples. However, the necessary materials for preserving the outward, objective position have already been thrown away. The patient is at home, not in a hospital; the doctor does not visit, he stays; there is no desk or instruments or examinational procedures to maintain distance between doctor and patient. Minkowski is able to preserve his professional attitude for a little while, assisted by the "far-out" nature of the patient's communications; in the last paragraph he switches from *I* to *we,* and back to *I* again, taking refuge for a moment in the impersonal plural, but then. . . .

When my children came to visit me one day, I was supposed to have purposely had them bring a change purse with some coins in it. These coins now would be put in his belly. It was shameful to have involved one's children in such an inhuman scheme. Finally he called me a murderer and bestowed on me the name "Deibler." At that point everything fell apart. All that remained were two people who did not understand each other at all and who, as a result, were hostile toward each other. I became angry; he translated his anger in his way by adopting a completely antisocial attitude. He accused me of the most evil deeds and then purposely went into the garden and gathered all the strings and matches that he could find [5, p. 183].

Minkowski does not tell us how he, the doctor, expressed his anger over this silly quarrel, so like a domestic quarrel in its triviality, in its made-up quality, and in one partner's going off to "pick up" compulsively afterward. There is still this professional reticence about the feelings and actions of the doctor. He does tell us that in a calmer confrontation than this angry one he wanted to tell "my partner," "Come on, let's make peace." Again he does not indicate that he *did* say it. However, following this desire of the doctor, the patient underwent a sharp change.

He would react by a fit of simple depression. He would complain of his misfortunes, appeal to our compassion; on the other hand, the interpretations scarcely played a part. It was as if he drew from the arsenal of his pathological attitudes something with which he could establish a certain contact with his fellow men [5, p. 183].

That is not quite right. His delusional, interpreting attitude had also established "a certain contact," such unmistakable contact that Minkowski had gotten angry. However, by contact Minkowski means something *positive,* a greater feeling of liking, sympathizing with the patient, in contrast to the hostility that he had aroused earlier. For a little while Minkowski had been able to stay closer to the patient, break up his endless harangues. For a moment they seemed even to like each other, although it was a liking that did not last long. "As he repeated his melancholic complaints, his moanings, they ceased to move us" [5, p. 185].

Ironically this favorable change had been accomplished by

the collapse of the objective, professional attitude. That brought the two onto fresh ground. Minkowski was not able to see that the breakdown of the traditional attitude and the establishment of a new attitude, which might become professional in its turn, was necessary for the favorable change. Nor did he remark that perhaps the essential point was his having been for a while moved. The insight he had was essentially phenomenological. He knew that living with the patient, encountering him day after day, gave a richer picture of his inner life, that such changes in the position of the observer made it possible to feel more of what the patient felt, almost "experience" the patient's world. The two melodies that Minkowski wrote of might become for a moment one. The phenomenological interest was investigative. The gradually emerging existential interest was therapeutic; it aimed at the changes which Minkowski in his exasperation forced upon his clinical relationship, against his own will. We remember that a similarly great change occurred in psychoanalytic technique when therapists found themselves locked in transference situations that their repeated, steady being with the patient had brought to birth. A clinical "accident," you might say, developed a concept, which in turn shaped changes in technique.

Minkowski wrote that he not only observed the patient, in the traditional objective way; he also compared "his psychic life with mine." There is not a great deal of evidence for this assertion. We do not learn much of Minkowski's psychic life from this report. Nor do the phenomenologists and existentialists often make good, or at least overt, this claim of comparing. Again, we must suspect that the old privacy of the doctor was being put first, despite the existential claim. However, there was a stated *willingness* to compare, which, in principle at least, marks a radical departure. The doctor was to bring his psychic life beside the patient's—not his *knowledge* of disease beside the patient's symptoms, as in objective psychiatry, nor his listening ear, his readiness to grasp hidden connections, as in psychoanalysis, but his own psychic life. This was a degree of equalizing, of egalitarianism, that invites comparison with the great political aspirations of today.

The purpose was not political, however, not equality as a principle of justice or social right. Its end was investigative and medical. Minkowski hoped to understand more by comparing the two psychic lives. It was uncertain how this greater understanding would come about. He wrote metaphorically that there were two melodies being played simultaneously. That by itself does not suggest understanding, or even harmony. But then "a certain balance becomes established between the notes of the one and the other and lets us penetrate a little further into our patient's psyche." He was claiming that the "balance" permitted a movement inward. What is this balance and how does it permit the movement?

At times, after the confrontations and during the brief depressions the patient seemed more normal.

The alternating of symptoms, the diverse forms under which they were presented, establish a current between normal life and the pathological psyche; like a succession of rising and falling waves, sometimes there is an intermission, an attitude of contact prevails, and we cannot help hoping again; at other times the waves mount, everything breaks up, we are submerged once again [5, p. 183].

However, even during the patient's delusions Minkowski caught glimpses of "more normal" attitudes, a "hint of life," and "reality." There was a great deal of intellectual activity involved with the delusions, much to figure out, calculate, which interested Minkowski: The patient realistically perceived that swallowing everything must be very expensive, so he decided to absorb "only parts of the objects in his body; then, with what was left, they would install him in a sideshow at a fair so that he could be the object of public derision." Minkowski could appreciate this concern for economy and the patient's nice ability to reach and accept a compromise.

Yet Minkowski was not concerned with what he could "understand," that is, sympathize or identify with. His own psychic life was being used only for comparison with the patient's, so that whatever matched could be thrown aside. (In watching the development of psychiatry we come to expect this *assumption of the observer's normality* in the early stages of every psychiatric school.) That leaves for study what does not match, whatever seems to lie outside the doctor's familiar mental life. Here is a dramatic example:

From the first days of our common life, my attention was attracted by the following fact. When I arrived, he stated that his final execution would certainly take place the next night. Anxious, he could not sleep and kept me awake. I was consoled by telling myself that the next day he would see that his fears had been without basis. But the same scene was repeated the next day and the next, and after three or four days I had given up all hope; his attitude had not changed at all. What had happened was that I, a normal being, had very quickly drawn a conclusion concerning the future from observed facts. He, on the other hand, had let the same facts go by him without being able to profit from them concerning the same future. I knew now that he would continue to claim that he would be executed the next night—which he did, without any thought of the present or the past. Our thought is essentially empirical. Facts are interesting only insofar as we can base our future behavior on them. This propulsion toward the future was completely lacking in the patient. He had no tendency to generalize and arrive at an empirical law. When I said to him, "Look, you can believe me when I assure you that nothing threatens you; up until now my predictions have always been correct," he would answer, "I admit that up until now you have always been correct, but it doesn't follow that you will be right tomorrow." This reasoning, against which one feels defenseless, represents a serious disorder in the general attitude toward the future. Here time is split up into isolated elements. In normal life they conform to a completely normal integration [5, pp. 185–186].

We must put aside our habit of thinking the doctor and patient meet only now and then and read this passage remembering that not only the patient but also Minkowski was being kept awake all night. Minkowski then discussed the patient's disordered sense of time, to raise the complicated issue as to whether his lack of sense of the future sprang from his delusional belief that execution was imminent or the delusion sprang from the lack of a future; he wanted to decide which was more fundamental. This proved to be an insoluble dilemma, but there was nothing insoluble or a dilemma about Minkowski's *experiencing* the patient's time sense. He did that in the most intimate and painful way possible. He might well have cried out that neither the loss of a future nor the delusion is the basic fact. The basic fact is the loss of sleep, and all the hopelessness and confusion that spring so regularly from that.

How are we to know what is primary, fundamental? Listen to Minkowski wrestling himself toward his own answer.

> . . . Isn't the disorder pertaining to the future a perfectly natural consequence of the delusional idea of imminent torture? This is the crux of the problem. Could we not assume, on the contrary, that the disorder in our attitude concerning the future is of a more general order and that the delusion of which we spoke is only one of its manifestations? [5, p. 186]

> Probably someone will say that basically this is the outlook of a person who has been condemned to death and that our patient reacted this way because of his delusion that he and his family were condemned to death. I doubt it. I have never seen a person who has been condemned to death. I willingly admit that the description we have just given corresponds to the idea that we have of the experience of someone who has been condemned to death. But don't we draw this idea from ourselves? Don't we have it because, at moments, we are all condemned to death—at precisely those moments when our personal *élan* weakens and the door to the future is shut in our face? Can't we assume that the patient's attitude is determined by a more lasting weakening of that same

impulse? The complex idea of time and of life disintegrates, and the patient regresses to a lower level that is potentially in all of us. Thus the delusion is not completely a product of the imagination. It becomes grafted onto a phenomenon which is a part of our life and comes into play when the life-synthesis begins to weaken. The particular form of the delusion, the idea of execution, is in fact only the attempt of that part of the mind which remains intact to establish a logical connection between the various sections of a crumbling edifice [5, p. 187].

The delusion is a secondary or reparative effort in the face of a fundamental breakdown of synthesis, or dissociation, Minkowski argues. The dissociation is the fundamental phenomenon, and its direct expression is the breakdown of the sense of time. We are familiar with both these concepts, of primary dissociation and secondary symptoms, from Bleuler, Janet, and Breuer. We will confront them again in the more modern concept of a weak ego. Do not dismiss either the earlier or the modern version because Freud was able to show that conflict in the case of Minkowski's patient was probably a conflict between destructive impulses toward his family and both his love of them and his conscience. This conflict or crack in the integrity of the personality may be the weakening or disintegrating agent—and therefore more primary than the dissociation. Do not dismiss the earlier concept, for in fact Freud's idea, too, will prove insufficient. It will not explain why the patient's personality was not able to contain the conflicting elements; psychoanalysis itself had to take refuge in the concept of a weak ego, which is hardly more than a return to Bleuler's and Janet's idea by a fresh route. No, it is only when we reach the ground of either social experience or biology that we pierce the dilemma. But that is a later step.

Almost every psychiatric discovery is given *etiological* significance at the time of its discovery. Everyone hopes that he has reached the bottom of things. In describing the changed time sense in schizophrenia, Minkowski had not reached the bottom of things, but he had enlarged the range of observables —and by a method at once new and surprising. He had really experienced the new datum; he really knew what the patient *meant*. Perhaps his discovery was not as impressive as the discovery of *the* cause might have been, but we learn to live with our disappointment in that. The discovery was modest, but it was real and very human. The dissociations that Kraepelin and Bleuler had observed from the outside were now being experienced from the inside—a great confirmation of the importance of this concept. We are not surprised to find the breaks reaching through to the inner experience: If it had been possible to imagine such data before Jaspers and Minkowski, the depth of the fractures might have been predicted. But that would have been speculation. Minkowski had come upon something empirical, convincing.

The development of the method by which he reached the patient's inner experience was not predicted either, any more than the development of psychoanalytic method from hypnosis to head-pressing to free association to analysis of the resistances was predicted. Jaspers had taken the first step in making explicit the *area* of investigation: inner experience. Minkowski now took a second step by staying close enough long enough to the patient to secure more than the fragmentary reports that Jaspers had received. Once trapped with the patient, he found another step perhaps inevitable. It does not seem possible that anyone could have maintained the traditional objective, aloof attitude of Kraepelin under such circumstances; the doctor had either to get out or give in to the feelings so insistently aroused by the patient, who was again and again irritating and then pitiable. This acceptance of the doctor's feelings and open conveyance of them to the patient was a third step toward the full existential method—and the one at sharpest variance with the ideals of traditional practice. We can therefore understand the guarded language with which Minkowski describes it. He hardly acknowledges what he is doing. Certainly, doctors had often found themselves annoyed with patients. A good part of the humor among doctors about medicine expresses that fact. However, to elevate the doctor's emotional response to a principle of investigation and treatment was to fly in the face of a fully accepted tradition.

Psychoanalysis would also acknowledge the doctor's feelings about the patient, the so-called countertransference reactions. But psychoanalysis typically saw those feelings as distortions of the clinical situation, carry-overs from the past, rather than natural outgrowths of the present. Nothing was more typical of the existential attitude than its *acceptance* of the spontaneous, emotional responses to the patient, the incorporation of such reactions into the heart of the method. Where the objective schools saw the emotional reactions and relationships between doctor and patient as disruptive, existentialism was to claim that such reactions and relationships were the very conditions of reliable investigation, and to claim still later that they were also the conditions of treatment.

It is easy to see how such points of difference quickly gave rise to serious, still continuing quarrels. It may not be so easy to see how these insistences of existential psychiatry grew, not only from its own discoveries but also from the discoveries of *objective* psychiatry, both descriptive and psychoanalytic, for both these schools were uncovering the biological and emotional roots of the symptoms. They were insisting that mental, cerebral, rational processes were only part of mental or psychic life, and certainly not the most powerful part. Mental diseases were not purely mental. Freud compared the rational ego to the rider of a great horse, the id, guiding but not always controlling its pace and direction. Thus we should have expected psychiatric efforts to deal more and more directly with emotional responses, or at least to develop increasing skepticism as to how significant any human interaction could be without them. In that respect existential psychiatry was a direct outgrowth of psychoanalytic and biological psychiatry.

Existential psychiatry was also a direct outgrowth of its own method. The attempt to get and stay where the patient was, not to allow any withdrawal into professional objectivitiy or neutrality, not even to allow any "getting out at all" in either a physical or a psychological sense—this holding close to the patient inevitably produced emotional explosions. The craziness of the patients was tolerable only "professionally." That was why the patients were locked away in the first place, and partly why the professional rituals were developed too. The family and society could not stand madness. The ways the doctors stood it were developed as much to protect the doctors as for any therapeutic or investigative reason. We know that the great distance between patient and others initially institutionalized, legislated, and rationalized was very slowly broken down, and that existential psychiatry, this living with the patient for long periods and then feeling what he felt, represents the almost final collapse of those institutional, legal, and rational barriers. However, the *emotional* difficulties of being with the patient remained. It was perhaps these difficulties that had energized the building of barriers in the first place. As a result, Minkowski was as bold and probably unwitting as any of the great explorers, although the dangers experienced did not come from an outraged community, as did Freud's, but from the existential method and its application, like the dangers the Curies and anyone who works with lethal or traumatic materials suffered.

The result of staying with the patient was an emotional explosion, in fact a series of emotional explosions. This is a better metaphor than Minkowski's "two melodies," which suggests something mild, even lyrical. If there were two melodies, they were melodies from Wagner, however much Minkowski preserved his professional veneering of the sleepless, repetitious, irascible, quarrelsome, pitiable, altogether miserable human situation he was involved in. But the new metaphor proves as misleading as the old, because the "explosion" does not break the two people apart; in fact the result is "contact," "a certain balance becomes established between the notes of the one and the other and lets us penetrate a little further into our patient's psyche" [5, p. 182]. Again, what is this balance and how does it permit penetration?

Our first answer was incomplete: The balance had something to do with the discovery of features in common between the doctor and patient, and it had something to do with the patient's desire for compassion and the doctor's capacity to give it. However, there remained a seemingly irreducible stubbornness or stupidity on the patient's part that required all kinds of conceptions about time, personality synthesis, disintegration, and so forth, to come to grips with at all. Like the actual period of contact, understanding was short-lived, giving way to the familiar irascibility in the personal sphere and frantic intellectual activity in the scientific. The penetration was to common elements and then to what was alien—basically ununderstandable, as Jaspers wrote.

This first answer said nothing about the *balance* achieved, except to indicate that it was short-lived. But, having in the meantime underlined the place of emotions in the existential method, I think we can understand what Minkowski meant. Before the explosion, the patient overran the doctor, accusing, abusing, scattering incomprehensibilities everywhere, as busy in that direction as he was in picking up so many things. Then Minkowski's patience gave out. He must have wanted to say "Shut up," and perhaps he did, although we do not know whether he even managed to say "Let's make peace." Like students in clinical supervision, he probably said a great deal more than he reported, dressing the whole cautiously lest we decide he was "subjective" or lacked "understanding." In any case, the patient did shut up and the doctor took his brief command of their relationship. This was the "balance" achieved. The doctor made himself felt, slowed the patient down, insisted on more acceptable behavior from the patient, so that what Minkowski reaches is the patient's capacity to be more than the crazy, bedeviling person he had been.

There are several fruits of this "encounter." We see immediately that the crazy people are not so inaccessible, so removed from personal influence as some biological and psychoanalytic opinions would suggest. (Later the interpersonalists would extend still further this attack on the inaccessibility of crazy people.) We also see the doctor being most effective when he is least professional, which observation must unsettle our comfort in traditional practice, until this unprofessional behavior can be carried up into fresh modes of practice. Most important of all, we see that the "balance" in human relationships—our not taking refuge in professional authority, on the one hand, or the patient's not commanding the doctor by his accusations or pitiableness, on the other—permits closeness, shared feelings, a contact that attracts everyone by seeming peculiarly *human,* desirable, and perhaps even the goal of human life. Or is it an intoxicating vision only for people removed from others either by their oddities or by their professions and little accustomed to everyday closeness? In any case, this ideal of human contact or closeness not only becomes a central part of modern young people's ideals but teaches the psychiatric profession too, so that there is a great concern with improving human relationships, a comprehension of the limitations of many people's capacity for closeness, a dawning realization of how restricted most people are where we would expect them to be strongest. Affection, warmth, and closeness do not seem difficult to achieve, nor do they seem the bugaboo sexuality once was. Gradually both the traditional symptoms of objective psychiatry and the concern with sexuality of psychoanalysis lose their central place to this existential concern both with *contact* and with the closely related personal integrity or *togetherness*.

We have seen how the subject matter of existential psychiatry developed from individual phenomena discussed by willing informants with objective physicians into whole inner states now experienced in explosive contact between people not always recognizably physician and patient. The objective, aloof, and analytic was giving way to a respect for subjectivity, a concern with closeness, and a growing suspicion of everything partial, reductionistic, in contrast to grasping experience whole. At first phenomenology was analytic and reductionistic too. There was a search for the particular experience which explained all others—for example, Herr Klug's pathoplastic hallucinations—just as Kraepelin searched for the critical *external* features. Then a broader view was taken of inner experience; such categories of experience as space, color, time were seen as *primarily* affected (as the facultative movement named diseases mood, behavioral, or thinking disorders). However, this search for a categorical defect also proved narrow, and larger and larger elements of experience were taken up into the explanations. At this point we see the two movements inward, psychoanalysis and existential psychiatry, rapidly diverging, psychoanalysis turning toward fewer and fewer psychic elements more and more sharply defined. The Oedipus complex, castration fear, and penis envy take on growing psychopathological responsibilities, while existential psychiatrists reach for larger and larger conceptions, until they seem as abstract and general as psychoanalysts seem narrow and reductionistic.

The strengths of the schools increase, too. Psychoanalysis gains in precision and explanatory power over broader and broader reaches of historical experience. It finds parallels in primitive society, religion, and humor for what it understands of neurosis. It radically reshapes man's view of himself. Existential psychiatry, all the while growing more abstract, uses its evolving method to get at *feelings* and marshals a great power over feelings which its being-where-the-patient-is brings to light. So, paradoxically, the one, psychoanalysis, at the moment of its seeming almost trivial, finds its data everywhere and gains command of the modern mind. Existential psychiatry, at the moment of its seeming almost abstract and woolly minded, enters the *felt* world of the patient and gains there power to evoke and change feelings. We observe again and again this paradox, this play of opposites, both in developmental processes and in psychosis, and are forced to ask its meaning; it is as if life threw outriggers always to either side to balance movement during change.

BINSWANGER

What follows is a case of Binswanger's, the foremost spokesman for existential psychiatry. See how he goes right to *love* and to what the patient suffers and attempts *now*.

Our patient is a thirty-nine-year-old intelligent woman. She was happily married; but not fully satisfied in her marriage, Protestant, religious, mother of three children, daughter of an extremely egotistical, hard, and tyrannical father and an "angelic," self-effacing, touchingly kind mother who allowed herself to be treated by her husband like a slave and only lived for him.

From the time she was a child Ilse suffered greatly under these conditions, feeling powerless to change them. For three years she had shown symptoms of overstrain and "nervousness." Following a performance of *Hamlet*, the idea came to her mind to persuade her father through some decisive act to treat her mother more considerately. During her boarding school period, the precocious girl had developed a somewhat ecstatic love for her father, and she believed she had great influence upon him. Ilse's resolution to carry out her plan was reinforced through that scene in which Hamlet plans to murder the king at his prayer but shrinks back from doing it. If at that particular time Hamlet had not missed his chance, he could have been saved, Ilse felt. She confessed to her husband that she planned something unusual and was only waiting for the right moment. Four months after the Hamlet performance, when asked for help against her father by her mother, she told her husband that she wanted to "demonstrate to her father what love can do." If he forbade her to do it, he would make her unhappy for the rest of her life; she had to "get rid of that."

One day, when her father had once again reproached her, she told him she knew of a way of saving him, and in front of her father she put her right hand up to her forearm into the the the burning stove, then held out her hands toward him with these words: "Look, this is to show you how much I love you!" [6, pp. 214–215].*

She seemed "oblivious to pain," energetic, and elated despite terrible burns. Her father responded, ameliorated his behavior toward the mother for a few weeks, but fell back again. Then Ilse's fourth child died and she "firmly believed that the loss was the atonement for her love for the *doctor* who had treated the child" [6, p. 215]. "Eight months after the act she was busier and moodier than before" [6, p. 215]. She went away for health cures, grew increasingly grandiose, and with it was convinced that everyone was sneering at her. Then she came to Binswanger's sanatorium.

When asked about the burning, she explained: "I wanted to demonstrate to my father that love is something that overcomes itself, not by words but by deeds. This should have had an effect on him like a lightning bolt, like a revelation, and should have made him stop living as an egotist. When the idea first came to me, it was for my mother's sake, but then I thought if I were to do it for his own sake it would be the right thing. I pitied him, and

---

* Quotations on this page and the next several pages cited to Note 6 are excerpted from Chapter VIII, "Insanity as Life-Historical Phenomenon and as Mental Disease: The Case of Ilse" by Ludwig Binswanger in *Existence: A New Dimension in Psychiatry and Psychology*, edited by Rollo May, Ernest Angel and Henri F. Ellenberger. © 1958 by Basic Books, Inc., publishers, New York.

since then had felt even more love and understanding for him. I guess I must love all men so much because I loved my father so much" [6, p. 216].

The theme of the patient's life, Binswanger argues, is father. Her "almost idolizing veneration of the father" is matched by "energetic rebellion against his tyranny."

. . . The dissonance in this theme signifies an open, never-healing life sore; it could only be resolved by a change in the mind and behavior of the father, by a divorce of the parents, or by eliminating the father. All these roads were blocked by insurmountable external and internal obstacles. Thus, living turns into suffering from the dissonance of its main theme, into grievous floating in the pains of hopelessness. What from the angle of the world appears as hopelessness is, in terms of the "ego," irresolution, indetermination, and shrinking away from decisions. This is the situation Hamlet is in. In his fate Ilse sees her own as in a mirror. The decision which she cannot make for herself she can, at least, make for Hamlet. She believes he should have killed the praying king without consideration of the situation and thus would have saved himself. Only such resolution to act would have saved him "from insanity!" Now the stone starts rolling. In her own situation, the possibility of eliminating the tyrant is excluded. The idea of parricide cannot develop, and, if it did, her love for the father would interfere with the act. Both parents are dead set against divorce. What is left to her is an attempt to persuade the father to change in attitude and behavior toward the mother. The theme that now offers itself is named *sacrifice*. For a sacrifice will offer Ilse the opportunity to prove her love to her father as well as to make the desired "impression." The "sacrifice of love" is designed to overcome the father's brutal tyranny. Through the sacrifice of love Ilse takes the brutality upon herself. It is she who submits to suffering from some brutal pain so that mother does not have to suffer any more. The father himself is "spared" throughout [6, p. 217].

Perhaps the existential language is unfamiliar, but the ideas are not. In psychoanalytic terms she is resolving a *conflict* between love and hate of the father, a conflict that includes the mother. Her solution, the "sacrifice," is the presenting symptom and expresses both sides of the conflict, indeed several sides of what are many conflicts. She indicates to father the pain that his behavior causes her, also how much she will sacrifice for him, and to mother that Ilse is still more servile than the mother, more loving than her mother, but at the same time more effective; *she* can make father a good husband. The sacrificial act serves as the final common pathway of many currents, for a moment joining and expressing them all, as if the central nervous system were a symphony orchestra that must let out its complicated, often dissonant music through one occasional voice.

Whether we emphasize *her* fantasies, *her* attachment to the mother and father *or,* on the other hand, the difficulties of the family situation, we will speak of conflict, on the one hand, or *adaptation,* on the other, favorite terms respectively of the psychoanalytic and interpersonal schools. The one emphasizes problems that patients bring to families; the other, problems families bring to patients. Neither alone can resolve the empirical problem as to where the problems begin or how much weight to give either side. Each presents only the data that *its* method collects, whether fantasies or family facts. Existential psychiatry, for its part, accepts *both* the individual and family contributions to Ilse's tragic situation and then sings its own song, about the patient's *felt* relationship to herself and the world.

Ilse's sacrifice, her solution or adaptation to the conflict, fails. "The life-sore opens again, deeper and more painful than ever" [6, p. 217]. So a fresh solution is called for. The original solution, her sacrifices, had been self-chosen, a decision of the self to reconcile the discordant forces. Now "the self succumbs under the heavy task of pursuing further the leitmotif of its history" [6, p. 217]. The new solution is forced on her and is "self-effacing."

. . . You *must* love all men so much because you love your father so much (*viz.*, delusions of love). This may be complemented by: You *must* attract the attention and interest of *all* people to yourself, because you have attracted the attention and the interest of your father to yourself; you *must* know what impression you are making upon *all* people because you wanted to make an impression upon your father; you must react to everything the others do because you wanted to know how your father reacted to *you*; in short, you must be "in the center of attention" of *all* people (*viz.*, delusions of reference). The lack of insight into the *must* of this loving and attracting-of-attention we call insanity. The cure for such insanity consists in the shaking off of the *must* and in the restoration of the rule of the self [6, p. 217].

The restoration was effected! "Ilse stayed perfectly healthy up to her death at the age of 73. She was able to direct the theme 'salvation' and 'purification' into healthy channels, that is, to confirm it through social work. Advised and counseled by experts over a period of time, she successfully practised as a psychological counselor and at times was also the leader of a psychological workshop group" [6, p. 218]. So Anna O., too, carried forward her life.

However, for a while Ilse's self was effaced in the second, psychotic solution. She gave up her local, particular loved and hated one for the whole world of men. It was a psychotic solution, Binswanger says, because it was not chosen by an integrated self but was forced on her by a dissociated part of mental life, indifferent to the claims of reality. Such are the signs of the "unconscious," psychoanalysis would add, this element of "must" or compulsion, the demand to be met from within, rather than an integrated life-force meeting the world. Further, the unconscious translates father into all men, perhaps expressing a childhood time when father *was* the only man; and so she loves all men, but also is tyrannized over by all men, as she was by the father.

. . . Just as the father's harshness and coldness, inaccessibility to love and sacrifice, turned into a tortuous riddle for Ilse, so the entire environment now becomes an enigmatic power; at one time it is a loving You, one to which she would like to surrender not just her hand but herself altogether; at another time it is a harsh, loveless, inaccessible world which scoffs at her love, derides and humiliates her, wounds her honor. Her entire existence is now limited to the motions and unrest of being attracted and being rejected. But with the pluralization of the You, with the theme extended all over her existence without limit, and with the loss of the original thematic goal, the father, no solution of the problem is possible any more. The theme spends itself on an inappropriate object, it rotates in eternal repetition around itself. The only remaining question is . . . whether the existence will find a way out of this form of self-discussion, return to itself, and so clear the road for new possibilities for a solution or whether it will be blunted in the process by endlessly repeating and stereotyping the discussion as such through acts, behavior, or phrases [6, p. 224].

Note how *polarized* Ilse's world had become. The elements were loving attention and sneering attention, fight and surrender, all men or none. The treatment was to bring this dissociated, compulsive, polarizing power out into the open, challenge its "must," and restore "the rule of the self."

We do not hear much from Binswanger as to *how* he helped Ilse "shake off the must"; it is characteristic of existential writings that technical matters get short shrift beside abstruse, philosophical discussions, despite the great technical problems the existential method generates. However, Minkowski has already prepared us to expect certain elements: a direct, feeling relationship to the patient and an active seeking of the dissociated, unconscious father theme. Binswanger now advances a little farther. It is not enough intellectually to grasp which psychic parts have been dissociated, not even enough to bring them to the patient's attention, he implies. All this is too readily cast aside by fresh "explanation," now on the patient's part, or evaded outright. Nor is it enough to confront the psychotic behavior, as Minkowski did. The "moment of contact" is only a moment; the psychotic material soon flows back over the relationship. A *lasting* contact must be made, what is called *empathy*. However, this empathy of Binswanger's proves quite different from the traditional rapport, therapeutic alliance, and contracts so much talked about and advocated between the doctor and the "normal" parts of the patient. The effectiveness of Binswanger's empathy depends upon rapport with what is *"sick"*! There can be no standing aside from any part of the patient. Only with this deepened empathy can the therapist bring back into the self the lost parts.

First the empathic experience is approached phenomenologically.

. . . We would have to examine to what degree [empathy] is a phenomenon of *warmth*, a phenomenon of the possibility or impossibility of fusing the *chaleur intime* (as in our instance); or a vocal or *sound* phenomenon, as when the poet Hoelderlin writes to his mother that there could not be a sound alive in her soul with which his soul would not chime in; or a phenomenon of *sharing*, as expressed by Diotima in Hoelderlin's *Hyperion*—"He who understands you must share your greatness and your desperation"; or a phenomenon of *participation*, as in the saying, "I partake in your grief" or, lastly, a phenomenon of *"identification,"* as when we say, "I would have done the same in your place" (in contrast to, "I don't understand how you could act that way"). All these modes of expression refer to certain phenomenal, intentional, and preintentional modes of being-together (*Miteinandersein*) and co-being (*Mitsein*) which would have first to be analyzed before the total phenomenon of empathy could be made comprehensive and clarifiable. For this reason alone, the differentiation of psychic life with which we can empathize from psychic life with which we cannot empathize (schizophrenics) loses a great deal of its scientific value, apart from the fact that the limits of empathic possibilities are purely subjective and vary according to the empathic ability and "imagination" of the investigator [6, p. 226].

Then he asks from what base we call the dissociated elements *sick*.

. . . Let us look at our case and specifically at Ilse's sacrifice, and let us see how a layman would react to such an act. He would probably ask himself: Would I have done this, or could I have done this in Ilse's place? And his answer would be: No, no normal person would do a thing like this in our day and time. And in view of the pluralization of the "Thou," he would have felt even more emphatically: "Now this woman has gone completely crazy!" So we see that the judgment on the sickness or health is subject to the norm of the social attitude. If an act, behavior, or verbalization deviates from that norm, it is judged even by the layman as morbid, as a symptom of an illness. However, there may be people who see in the sacrifice the expression of a genuinely religious or ethical self-effacement, of a genuinely ethical readiness for sacrifice and love for one's fellow man; such persons would strongly reject the idea that the sacrifice be considered a symptom of disease. We realize that the norm of behavior is by no means fixed once for all, but that it varies according to an individual's education and culture or to a cultural area. What appears abnormal—or a deviation from the norm—to one person may look to another quite normal, or even like the supreme expression of a norm; the judgment "sick" or "sound" is accordingly formed within a cultural frame of reference. Naturally, the same is true for insanity. What we of the twentieth century consider a symptom of disease was seen by the Greeks as a blow from Apollo or as the work of the Furies, and by the people of the Christian Middle Ages as possession by the Devil. What at the peak of Pietism could pass for an expression of supreme piety would today be considered a phenomenon of morbid self-reflection and morbid guilt feelings, and so forth. But all this cannot alter the fact that a person is judged "sick" wherever his social behavior deviates from the respective norm of social behavior and thus appears conspicuous or strange [6, p. 227].

Carrying this analysis into the relationship between two people, Binswanger asserts that someone is strange or sick because something has come between the doctor and the patient which is experienced as a barrier to communication; the doctor has formed an *idea* of the patient: she is so-and-so; the patient is at least momentarily objectified.

Now Ilse is no longer "someone else" like any other, let alone a Thou, but another strange person and a You which is excluded from the possibility of a purely loving encounter. The barrier to *communicatio* (social intercourse) and *communio* (love), the obstacle, turns into an object (of conspicuousness, avoidance, pity, judgment, etc.). Thereby I separate or remove myself from my fellow men, and the closeness of sympathy and intercourse changes into the distance of objective regard, observation, and judgment [6, p. 228].

If we ask, Why does this objectification interfere with communication? we are immediately confronted with the *secret* nature of the doctor's thought. He cannot tell the patient that she is schizophrenic without the gravest damage to her self-respect and more withdrawal from him. Yet if he keeps his secret, she must suspect something, as he is all the time *judging* her, even if he is only determining "to what extent" she is schizophrenic. Furthermore, this judgment, "she is schizophrenic," imposes a predetermined structure on the world experience that the doctor may attempt to share. He cannot really build up his understanding of it bit by bit as he gets to know his patient, because he has read Minkowski or Binswanger and already "understands" the world experience of the schizophrenic.

No more is there a single essence to the existential method than there is one factor, rule, or attitude of mind that says everything about free association, the psychological examination, or even participant observation, which is the least complex of all the great psychiatric methods. Each is a medley of acts and attitudes requiring description from many angles. However, this *freedom from prejudice or fixed expectation*, this attempt to come naked into the clinical encounter, what Binswanger called "putting the world between brackets," approaches as closely as anything the essence of the existential method, its "fundamental rule." It is certainly the essence of the *phenomenological* method, the "psychological-phenomenological reduction" of the philosopher Husserl: "In the presence of a phenomenon (whether it be an external object or a state of mind) the phenomenologist uses an absolutely unbiased approach; he observes phenomena as they manifest themselves and only as they manifest themselves" [6, p. 76].

ROLE OF EMOTION IN TREATMENT

We have seen that the result of phenomenological reduction, and of our staying not only with the ideas but with the experiences of the patient, is that our *feelings* are engaged. Subject to the same world as the patient (insofar as we can develop empathy), we react much as he does. Or we refuse to accept the patient and, like Minkowski, tell him that something must change, for in practice I can never enter anyone's experience without his adjusting that experience at least a little to fit mine; the empathic movement is never all in one direction. It is, however, *mainly* in one direction, because by a professional encounter, as opposed to friendship or falling in love, we mean this reaching out for the patient. The doctor must make the initial, strenuous efforts precisely because the patient cannot, or else he would not need to see the doctor.

Appreciate how completely existential psychiatry is thus protected from the charge so often made against it: that the existential doctor feels and expresses *whatever* he wants; he is a clinical wild man imposing his views on the patient. Quite the contrary. He is to feel *what the patient feels*. This is the discipline of the existential method. Only when the doctor is deep enough into the patient's feelings, only when he is securely emphatic, does he gain freedom for his own personal responses, just as meaningful transference interpretations in psychoanalysis can spring only out of a slowly, strongly developed transference. The doctor knows that he has gained this freedom because the patient changes his feelings when the doctor presents his. This is the existential meaning of a *relationship:* Insofar as a relationship exists, both parties to it change. Thus, rather than permitting a free or wild exchange of feelings, existential psychiatry insists on a careful, slow, even methodical development of our understanding the patient, the extent of which is judged by the extent of our empathy, of our being able to feel what the patient feels. At the same time, the doctor cannot bring a disembodied spirit to this meeting. If he understands, he will feel what the patient feels and will therefore be affectively present. When he cannot feel what the patient feels, but remains with the patient, there is by definition a clash of feelings which either destroys the relationship or moves it forward on the basis of a fresh understanding. In these encounters both parties must change or they will fly apart.

Such are the elements of the existential method: a focusing on the inner experience of the patient; the shedding of all expectations, all efforts to reach behind appearances, in order to reach that inner experience as fully as possible; the development of feelings as one penetrates the other's world; then the periodic collapse of empathy as one cannot "understand," with resulting clashes that may or may not usher in a fresh understanding; all the while a *feeling* experience during which objective understanding is postponed—in short, so great an emphasis on subjectivity and feeling that we must pause again to make the necessity of this clear.

How is the patient to know (or how is anyone to know) that I am in his world if I stand there *silently, unmoved?* Even my giving a carefully articulated, reasonable account of that world may mean only that I have caught the *idea* of the patient's world without in any way implying I am experiencing it. Or, to use psychological language, I may *isolate* my feelings about the patient's experience and express only my intellectual awareness, and such a limited involvement must carry that much less conviction of "being-together" to the patient. Further, emotional clashes are necessary because, except in the rarest and perhaps nonexistent cases of perfect compatibility, we cannot come to understand one another without exposing those places where we are each dumb to the other's world. (Happy couples must fight.) Finally, only in the occurrence of the emotional clash is there provided the firepower to change each side, and change *must* happen if there is to be new "understanding." This is a genuinely new understanding in that it springs from both parties' having been changed by the encounter; the understanding is possible because they have changed.

I hope the discipline and difficulty of this complex technology are clear. I hope, too, that grasping the existential technique carries with it a beginning understanding of what the technique is meant to achieve. Of course, at the start all that was aimed at was data, reports on the inner experience. Later, as we have glimpsed briefly, there were hopes, largely forlorn, that the method would contribute to the understanding of causes. It does not seem to have done so because the psychotic lesion found, as in Minkowski's case, was the dissociative one familiar to every school. However, what can be more justifiably claimed was an opening up of *"therapeutic"* power resulting from the engagement of feelings. If the doctors could remain within the patient's worlds, "contact" them, challenge and clash with them, and with all the dissociated elements, too, there was at least the possibility that the dissociated elements might be changed, at least led back into the newly integrated personality. The doctor's being where the illness was seemed to make the illness more vulnerable. And being there might make it possible to leave something behind in the patient that the patient could use in times of trouble. Such is the therapeutic rationale of the existential method.

Binswanger occupies a much larger place in psychiatric development than he is usually given. Indeed, it would be difficult to name many greater students of psychiatry. He had profound knowledge of nineteenth-century ideas and, what is perhaps unique, assimilated this knowledge into the discoveries of the twentieth century. He was a moving force in existential psychiatry while to a surprising extent he understood psychoanalysis. He did not have the systematic gifts Kraepelin and Freud and Janet had; nor did he have the gift of discovery Charcot had, or Jaspers' encyclopedic mind. Jaspers seemed to know what was missing because he knew everything else. What Binswanger did was to carry the existential and phenomenological ideas more deeply into clinical material than anyone else except perhaps Minkowski. The clash of these ideas and the clinical material gives us *fragments* of a great psychiatric advance. It cannot be credited to Binswanger as a settled, full achievement, as is the work of Darwin and Freud. We must piece the fragments together, like broken pottery, but this is something we also had to do for Charcot. In regard to clinical techniques especially, the existential literature is very bare when contrasted with the objective and psychoanalytic literature, so that any reconstruction of what the existential doctors actually did must be an imaginative one. However, let us take the fragments once more in hand.

Psychotherapists will recognize Ilse's psychotic experience not only because it has a familiar grandiose-persecutory content but also because of its similarity to a common *transference* phenomenon. Let us pretend that a patient's hostile feelings toward her father are becoming more manifest in therapy; she finds herself searching what is apparent of the doctor's life for some point of criticism. Perhaps the father did not have the present generation's identification with minority groups, and perhaps the psychotherapist is openly prosperous. The patient then complains of her father's bias and, in alternating breaths, of the therapist's excessive concern with his status at the expense of everyone else's. The patient is identified with poor minorities, feels herself put upon, and grows angry with those practicing the discriminations. She has generalized her individual, childhood plight onto the larger, social scene (putting aside whether the generalization fits), just as Ilse psychotically generalized her ambivalent relationship with the father.

We categorize Ilse's generalization as psychotic and the other patient's as neurotic, but in both cases we want to make some change in the generalized material, above all in the conflicting feelings that have not been able to reach a resolution outside psychosis, or in the case of the neurotic patient outside the distortion of a contemporary relationship.

Note that both the existential and the analytic understandings include a heavy debt to the concept "adaptation." Ilse's first solution, her arm burning, had failed. The next solution, her psychosis, does not seem an adaptation aimed at changing the father, except by inference, yet it does seem an attempt to adapt to the conflicting currents within her. However, because the psychotic adaptation is by definition only tenuously related to reality, there falls on it the charge of "sick." But the tenuousness of the relationship to reality is not a product of the generalization. Ilse's "healthy" solution, her social and group work, shares that. When she is well, she not only transfers her attention from father to humanity, as in the psychosis, but also *does* something for humanity. Her healthy solution is thus successfully adaptive to both her inner needs and outer reality.

In order to arrive at that final point, however, she had to complete a real transfer of feelings from father to humanity, which in the psychosis did not seem a transfer at all but was only an equivalence. Father was the humanity of her childhood. A *realistic* "transference" to humanity from father depends upon giving up her father as the dominant love object for the love of humanity—or, better, what Binswanger would call "caring." Insofar as that is a real caring and not an equivalence or translation into childhood language, she does indeed act in humanity and for humanity; we no longer speak of transference but of sublimation. How is this healthy shift of feelings achieved?

Binswanger starts from Charcot and Janet: A critical part of the illness process is dissociation of mental elements away from integrated function. Further, he understands, thanks to Freud's teaching, that this dissociative process is not a passive one—that is, not a falling apart without pressure—but an active *pushing apart* of mental elements due to conflict, strain, tension among them. Therefore, and now we come to what is innovative about existential technique, the therapist must place himself within the split world of the patient and gain the allegiance of the dissociated elements (not just an alliance with the "normal personality") for the purpose of reuniting the patient. Nothing short of this entering the patient's world, feeling with all elements of the patient's personality, will make such a reunion possible; how can *intellectual* insight march against the dynamic forces of conflict? As Laing particularly has emphasized [7], this reuniting may require more change in the "normal personality," and in the family structure around that personality, than it does in the supposedly sick, dissociated parts of the patient! These last two existential steps need still more explication.

I have already discussed "entering the patient's world." I hope that this entering or meeting is sharply enough contrasted with psychoanalytic "drawing out" of the patient's world so that no confusion between the two exists. Granted that Freud recommended for the analytic third ear a "free-floating," unstructured, receptive listening to match the patient's free associating. This was something like Minkowski's "two melodies." However, the analytic attention was a *listening*, an experiencing of *verbal content* in the search for infantile themes. The patient was to bring this verbal content to the doctor, place it within the doctor's world; Freud did not move his place of business to the patient's living room (at first Freud's patients visited *his* living room). More importantly, there was not the active seeking out of the experienced, felt life of the patient, no great empathic twisting and turning into the patient's world. Freud wanted to understand, to penetrate the most hidden reaches of the patient's motivation, but he did not want to *experience* those motivations, himself feeling them, the two, doctor and patient, living in the patient's world. No, psychoanalysis sought and seeks to dissect free from the personality the neurotic formations, throw onto them the most pitiless possible light, and then, hand in hand with the patient's mature ego, wear away their power. Everywhere the goal is to bring the emotional under the rule of the rational; where the id is, there shall the ego be.

Existential analysis, too, sought a kind of free-floating attention—at least the freedom from rigid ideas, expectations, diagnoses that defined the "psychological-phenomenological reduction." The existential doctor was to listen, understand, like the psychoanalyst, but then, some freedom to listen having been achieved, fresh technical elements appeared. Minkowski, having stayed with the patient and endured his abrasive demands, did not reduce them to an interpretation or postpone their discussion until a later hour. He grasped the patient's world, shook it, moved closer rather than farther away; every effort was being made to retain "contact." This was painful; it was emotionally explosive; there was constantly the danger of the patient's extruding the doctor (as there had been of the doctor's extruding the patient). From the beginning it might have been that Minkowski was not "sincere," that he did not want to stay with the patient but would use only whatever closeness he had to the patient to categorize him, call him sick, express any hatred he had of what he saw in him, the whole justified by a sensible dislike of mental illness. Existential technique *could* become an excuse for emotional license in the patient's presence, just as analytic technique could fall into the excessively neutral, aloof, passive hands of some therapists. However, the *ideals* of both schools were as clear as they were different. Psychoanalysis was to keep on asking of its students: Are you really listening? The comparable question in existential analysis was, Do you really want to be where the patient is?

Minkowski discovered that abandoning the objective, neutral position of descriptive and psychoanalytic psychiatry sometimes resulted not in clinical disaster but in the patient's *improvement.* The delusions fell away and contact occurred, if only for a moment. Later existential case reports extended this beachhead. We catch glimpses of a technique aimed at *retaining* contact. Because the existential therapist tries to stay with the patient, he must be willing to "encounter" or confront aspects of the patient not so comfortably assimilated. This "encounter" produces feelings in the therapist, who must then decide whether to "be himself" or preserve his professional objectivity. Plainly, Minkowski attempted to preserve his objectivity, but he also wanted to remain with the patient and understand; so the explosion was only postponed. By then, however, the therapist had earned the right to express his own, personal responses, or, more accurately, these responses were no longer personal. Then the patient felt, "This man has tried to understand me; his anger is not personal; I must look to myself for its cause." At the point of intersection of the therapist's getting where the patient is and of staying there must occur these explosions, each of which signals a

meeting of feelings. The resolution of these conflictual meet-
ings means continued contact, therefore a later explosion, and,
through the series of explosions, change. As Binswanger
wrote, a relationship is defined as a human contact in which
two people change, and psychotherapy is a *professional* relationship.

It is not easy to exaggerate the amount of discipline required by this technique. More is being asked of the therapists than perhaps even by the laborious technique of psychoanalysis or by the demand for quickness and dexterity made
by Sullivanian methods. Minkowski was in the farthest position from being a "wild analyst." Quite the contrary, he was
obviously embarrassed by the emotional tumult caused in
him by this staying with the patient. One can wonder whether
he did not, like Freud, at this point contemplate abandoning
"the line" of his scientific development, as in fact Joseph
Breuer had. Minkowski seems barely willing to tell us what
he said and did, probably because he was trying to retain the
familiar, traditional medical objectivity even while he was,
largely inadvertently, starting down a fresh path. Perhaps it
was this very conflict of styles that made possible the new development in the first place, for the objective, disciplined,
patient-centered approach of the great medical tradition is also
a necessary part of existential technique, which permits the
abandonment of that objectivity only, as it were, at the last
minute, after the therapist is strained to be objective but cannot.

Some contemporary psychoanalysts and many existential
psychiatrists, like Laing and Szasz [8], emphasize that the
series of explosions should result not so much in maturation
of the dissociated libidinal elements (as psychoanalysis had
originally emphasized) as in change in the ego which had
dissociated those elements. Further, if that ego is to gain more
tolerance and flexibility, the patient's social context must

change. Laing and Szasz met everywhere families and society making mature development impossible and therefore extended their therapeutic net outward. Once securely within the patient's world, therapists discover that the world of surrounding others takes on an unsettling morbidity; the others too must change. Of course, the existential analysis of the relatives must result in understanding *their* worlds as well, after a fresh series of explosions; there can be in the end no one person to blame. What we seek, as Binswanger wrote, is a loving and caring world which is in constant process of creation out of all those attempts to understand, all those encounters and explosions. In the best of possible worlds these processes will go on spontaneously. However, we mean by sickness that world or those parts of the world for which professional assistance is required; then in place of spontaneity we find psychoanalysis, the phenomenological reduction, "being and staying with the patient," and the new willingness to accept a place for emotion in the treatment [9].

5

INTERPERSONAL (SOCIAL) PSYCHIATRY

NONE OF THE SCHOOLS developed in absolute isolation from the others. The term *interpersonal (social) psychiatry* refers to the collection and analysis of social phenomena related to mental problems largely to the exclusion of other phenomena, but such a schematization will be useful only if it organizes our thinking productively, allows us not to lose sight of important elements, and does not itself give birth to a fresh exclusiveness. Sullivan contributed so much to interpersonal psychiatry that we often refer to it as Sullivanian psychiatry, but his thinking sprang from psychoanalytic ideas and experience, and he had a clear grasp of the traditional objective diagnoses. Meyer, precisely because he *had* experienced both the values and the limitations of ob-

jective, diagnostic psychiatry, likewise emphasized many contributors to disease states, including biological, psychological,
and social, and such concepts as reaction, adjustment, habit
deterioration, and chains of events; perhaps because of this
breadth of view he was the foremost critic of objective psychiatry in his time. Moreover, part of the interest in presenting interpersonal psychiatry is the opportunity such a presentation offers to contrast the methods and facts of the other
schools. Such methods and facts are sometimes close, sometimes even overlapping, and sometimes far removed.

There is no obvious *starting point* for what I have called
elsewhere the movement outward [1]. Greek medicine
grasped the main idea of social psychiatry without doubt, as
indicated by its including disappointments, on the one hand,
and satisfactions, on the other, among the phenomena that
set the womb to wandering or lured it home to rest. These
disappointments and satisfactions depend on significant others, even if the "others" referred to by Plato are semen and
phallus and seemingly independent of particular lover or person. The Greek concept recognized that phenomena of sickness could be affected by social events. Recognition of a great
many other social components of disease states preceded the
point at which I have chosen to break in on the movement
outward. A clear example is the recognition of the relationship between depression and the loss of objects or goals, a recognition which is as old as the hills. The starting point I *do*
take, with Meyer and Sullivan, is open to the further protest
that such contemporaries as Bleuler and Wernicke made observations about social factors almost of as much importance
as Meyer's. Moreover, this passing nod to other figures ignores
Janet, whose concept of social functions could have been the
point of departure instead of the one chosen. Finally, Freudian
psychopathology is everywhere shot through with considerations of social factors, despite Freud's fundamental bias, so

heavily shared with Kraepelin, for intra-individual concepts such as instincts and energies.

I begin with Meyer and Sullivan because they pointed the way to *system* and *method* [2]. In order for psychiatric observations or aperçus—such as we find abundantly in Shakespeare —to become part of *systematic* psychiatry, with all its overtones of boredom and heavy-handedness, there need to be developed methods for eliciting the observations and then ideas to connect them. We can ask that observations or insights be granted a new seriousness when we know how to produce them reasonably predictably and also have communicable ideas about the observations' meanings. Meyer not only had a clear interest in social facts that could be related to mental illness but also developed methods for eliciting them (thanks partly to his wife), and he elaborated concepts, notably that of habit deterioration, for relating the facts to one another and to the symptomatic phenomena. To an even greater extent, Sullivan made social phenomena his field of interest. He developed a subtle and complex method, participant observation, to elicit and alter social phenomena in the interview, then set forth an elaborate theoretical structure to explain what he observed [3].

Students and colleagues loved to watch Meyer interview and then hear him discuss a patient. His quiet humanity, thoroughness, and perhaps above all his practical concern for the next steps to be taken made the interviews and discussions memorable. They felt he was "just what the doctor ordered," particularly because many other doctors had not known *what* to order. Quite in a different vein, Sullivan was equally masterful. This man, in many other circumstances aloof and biting, found a comradeship and practical working alliance with patients—the more distant and bizarre the better, seemingly. One looked up to find the "pathology" suddenly gone. He is alleged to have said, "No one is schizophrenic when he talks to me." Although we can hope he was not that vainglorious, there was a measure of truth to the claim.

Despite these gifts for patient contact and understanding, neither Meyer nor Sullivan left behind impressive case accounts. One is treated to the familiar lists of symptoms and signs, disconnected family events, dubiously reliable details from childhood—the whole jerry-built apparatus of case recording. Missing in most of their cases is any hint of the narrative gift Freud had, or Kraepelin's capacity for vivid description, or the sense of another human touched and felt that we get from Minkowski and Binswanger. It will be necessary, therefore, to collect bits of case material from Meyer and Sullivan to sustain the empirical base of these discussions.

The principal reason is not the literary limitations of the two men. Sullivan, anyway, had lyrical moments of a high order, especially when he was discussing preadolescence. But the material both want us to consider is no longer *case* material; they ask us to attend to the clinical *situation* of which the patient is only a part, often not the most complicated part. With Meyer and Sullivan the observer's focus is suddenly widened; he is asked to step back or change his focal setting to a remarkable degree. Meanwhile the old case methods are slow to change. Presenters detail chief complaints, current illnesses, past and family histories, the litany of historical categories that Meyer himself was so instrumental in making routine and that, in their time, *did* represent an expansion of the data thought significant. Henry James had perhaps the greatest *literary* gift for such descriptions, but no one has taught us how to describe clinical situations systematically, how to prevent undue emphasis from falling on the patient alone, how to present him as neither responsible nor the victim. Sullivan could grasp clinical situations but he could not describe them (the same handicap has retarded the development of the closely related group therapy movement). We have therefore to use bits and pieces and reach for some synthesis of our own.

ADOLF MEYER

Here is one of Meyer's briefer and less routine case reports, beginning with a typically Germanic sentence and then marching straight through to the treatment, not once pausing for a speculative flight of explanation. Watch him get right down to business and stay there.

We should have to refer further to those cases in which, as a rule, definite strings of development appear in a person, either originally with difficulties of make-up, or transformed or made unresistive through progressively deteriorating habits of adjustment.

. . . A bright young woman . . . went through nine months of a catatonic attack with a delirious episode, negativism, refusal of food, retention of saliva, stereotyped attitudes, echolalia, grimacing, etc.; improved at the end of nine months, went home almost well, but in a few months became sleepless, harped bitterly about fantastic ill-treatment at the first hospital to which she had been taken, again refused food, complained of pain in the left shoulder, improved slowly at the hospital, was again better and might have gone home if the circumstances had permitted; then got worse again and says now she has no touch with her real environment; her mind dwells on the old story of ill-treatment and she hears remarks on it; she is made to suffer here for another woman; she had refused work for months out of a feeling of aversion and disappointment when transferred to a ward for more chronic patients, but even here was again found at work and much more affable after a review of her situation. Yet this woman is, through fate and the development of her make-up, relegated to the ranks of disappointments of treatment. (She could not leave the hospital.)

Good informants saw nothing peculiar in her and called her efficient, practical, not dreamy. On closer inquiry she was described as very scrupulous about the feelings of others, and equally sensitive to slights, proud of her appearance and reputation, so prudish that she would never undress in the presence of her sister and unusually sensitive about references to sexual matters. She had times when she wanted to be alone and felt nervous and complained of weakness and stomach troubles. Her father had died insane; and a brother (one of five) had had epileptic insanity. The patient herself complains that she *never* was practical; she was a great reader and her sister tells us of a huge scrapbook of poetry. From 1905–07 she stayed away from confession. A young woman against whom her sister had warned her introduced a man to her concerning whom she first spoke with aversion, but who evidently fascinated her under a decided conflict. She was much mortified because she found out that he was a divorced Protestant and he left her after having hurt her shoulder by lifting her up playfully, and after borrowing some money. This was followed by another blunder and conflict; although deeply averse to divorces, the patient helped a young woman get evidence for a divorce from a supposed bigamist, worked all her spare time and found out in the end that there had not been any marriage at all. This was followed by her moving to another city; there the conflict preyed on her, and a depression came on which rapidly led to a catatonic climax, without the slightest attempt at rapport on the part of the patient or physician, until she was transferred to another hospital and finally discharged after an illness of nine months. The pain in the shoulder which had recurred when she came to us disappeared after an electrical examination of the really existing slight atrophy. The details of the development and the reminiscences from the first hospital were then gone into, but evidently not traced completely to a balance or to the fundamental sore points. The circumstances of her family and the crowding of the hospital necessitated compromises to which she reacted unfavorably several times after a certain level was reached; she relapsed and got out of touch with her real environment. She says distinctly—"my mind is always away from here." Yet the adjustments in changing the mere rumination into open discussion and giving space for direct and concrete interests has an unmistakable influence on the patient [4, II, p. 449].

Meyer gives another case report and summarizes this way:

These sketches must suffice. They should show that they deal with developments far from being inconceivable as chains of faulty mental adjustment and far from demanding artificial explanations by specially invented poisons, and a clamoring for invented "things back of it all," if at least we acknowledge the long time and mass of doings and their kind [4, II, p. 450].

". . . the long time and mass of doings and their kind." Not a Germanism now, but words flat, successive, turgid, even as the patient's life had become. The successive points of the case reports are clear despite these opening and closing sentences which are like slag heaps with the whole mass of points piled one on top of the other. How often the doctors begin to sound like the patients, or is it the other way round?

"Good informants saw nothing peculiar in her and called her efficient, practical, not dreamy," in contrast to what "closer inquiry" revealed in the way of impracticality, repeated blunders, and what she said of herself, that she *"never* was practical." The "objective" report, by "good informants" was not to be trusted, Meyer is saying; we have to reach a "historical perspective" and we have to do what the psychoanalysts were doing at this same time: move behind appearances. Social psychiatry was to retain a special interest in this error of the "good informants." It was one of the countless pieces of evidence that people can learn to play social games and give the appearance of good adjustments while, in fact, their lives are crumbling about them. Indeed it became possible to detect personalities largely given over to creating *appearances* of one kind or another, perhaps of loving others, or working hard, and so forth, while the bulk of their interests lay elsewhere— the "as if" personality. Here again psychiatry gradually penetrated behind appearances, in the case of the movement outward discovering that behind the first-given, readily perceived social events lay processes that were as far removed from everyday consciousness as the repressed *intrapsychic* material was from consciousness. As another example, the "healthy family" of many early case reports of dementia praecox gave way to a fresh question: Who is the sicker one, patient or parent?

How was this penetration to the previously unknown *social* reality achieved? First it was necessary for Meyer to specify the *area* under investigation, essentially where the facts of relevance lay. "Much is gained," he wrote, "by the frank recognition that man is fundamentally a social being" [5, pp. 6–7] and only subordinately a biological, instinctual, or value-making being. The first order of business in any investigation of fresh cases is "a sizing up of the situation"—not the symptoms or the personality, but the "situation." "Become thoroughly acquainted," he wrote, "with at least all the facts known by the lay environment before interviewing the patient" [4, III, p. 239]. Just as Jaspers had specified inner experience as the area of investigation for phenomenology, so here Meyer puts down social phenomena as his first interest. Thus, too, as Minkowski had moved in and stayed with the patients, so Meyer helped send social workers into patients' homes (one of the first was Mrs. Meyer), seeking not inner experience but outer circumstances [6].

He insisted that homely details, as well as social disasters, played a part in mental illness. This was the despised *psychiatrie de concierge*. "A young woman against whom her sister had warned her introduced a man to her concerning whom she first spoke with aversion, but who evidently fascinated her under a decided conflict. She was much mortified because she found out that he was a divorced Protestant and he left her after having hurt her shoulder by lifting her up playfully, and after borrowing some money." There is another blunder with a similarly mortifying end. Perhaps it was all due to "schizophrenia," a weak will, poor brain, or even persisting love of her father which made her idealize men and then be hurt, but so much for "things back of it all," Meyer is saying. The mass of social doings is explanation enough for her slide downhill even to depression and dementia. Certainly there must be reasons why she coped so poorly, why she was so poorly *adapted* to life, but here Meyer puts between such "ultimate" explanations and the symptoms and signs events that make the symptoms and signs understandable. Against the claims of psychoanalysis, Jaspers had protested that all the talk in the world about Oedipus complexes, fixations, penis envy, or whatever, would not explain the *form* the illnesses took. It would not explain why, when, and to what degree one patient became psychotic and another depressed. At this juncture Meyer put a vital piece into the vast picture puzzle of psychopathology. Study only the everyday doings, and undoings, of the patients and we are left wondering, Why were they not mad years before? Although each of us likes to think we suffer, there are those who suffer more—so much more, indeed, that madness would seem to be a veritable godsend.

For Freud, social realities or "events" were like photographic developing fluid, bringing to visibility drives and conflicts otherwise concealed. Katharina looked in the window to see her father making love to her cousin and drew back dizzy, giddy, unable to breathe [7]. Common sense says the sight was shock enough. Freud rejected common sense and insisted the sight was traumatic because of memories and interests Katharina had had long before the sight. The father, years earlier, had made advances to Katharina. Freud told the patient, "You thought: 'Now he's doing with her what he wanted to do with me that night and those other times.' That was what you were disgusted at because you remembered the feeling when you woke up in the night and felt his body" [7]. Nor did Freud mention the *jealous* feelings that might have been aroused or Katharina's *own* wishes for her father. But the point was clear: Circumstances only trigger forces running apart from circumstances and within the individual.

Meyer now and then expressed respect for, but more often made light of, these forces "back of it all" and, like most critics of psychoanalysis, he seldom applied the method able to expose them. Moreover, he made light of what Freud had discovered because he was so busy collecting information of quite a different sort. How busy he was! From Kankakee to Worcester, to New York, to Johns Hopkins, he left behind a trial of elaborately detailed records and of associates and students laying down still more detailed reports. What he meant by a full record was an extraordinary range of facts under numerous headings, from evidences of infantile sex life ("rhythmic movements, self-excitement") to the more familiar area of relatives' personalities and illnesses [4, III, p. 228]. So critical did he feel were these details that he urged clinic workers to determine the number of cases they admitted to their clinics by the number of records they could complete! In addition, Meyer was urging that psychiatric work be extended deeper and deeper into the community! Hence the continuing agonized conflict of those professionals bent on helping everyone.

The details were to be organized into a life chart. Each detail was dated and placed in the appropriate year space of what looked like a rocket or time capsule starting at birth and shooting into the future [8]. The goal was a sense of relationship and trajectory, but few of the details held together, and one feels as scattered reading Meyer's life charts as reading Kraepelin's symptom lists. There is a dearth of ideas to hold the many facts together; one hears almost exclusively about habit from Meyer and about will from Kraepelin. Meyer also shared Kraepelin's concern for objectivity although he applied this objectivity to patients' histories. They had the same primary interest in the patient's course, despite Meyer's interest in society, as well as a dedication to the active examination. This hard work of finding out what actually happened in the patient's external life stood in the sharpest possible contrast to the evolving psychoanalytic technique, that of waiting for the patient to tell us. The *methods* of Meyer and Kraepelin were active; their *thinking* was almost passive. Psychoanalysis shows the reverse.

As indicated before, the implication of Freud's work was that social events—"realities"—were only precipitating agents; the real power lay elsewhere. The force of Meyer's work was the opposite: If the doctors would only leave their hospitals and consulting rooms and get out into the world, they would discover "facts not found in hospitals" that, in this way too, would make madness not only understandable but seemingly inevitable.

The study of fantasy uncovered surprising, often shocking, ideas and images. Even today these ideas and images meet disbelief from the great bulk of those at least middle-aged; the name of Freud still suggests more scandal than science. Young people feel less this way; they took Freud in with their Beatles and their Spock. It is still too soon, however, for the late fruits of *Meyer's* concern and method to be accepted by either young or old. We hear about battered and murdered children and families in which the murder is "soul murder." The actual facts of average family life are only now emerging. The trip that Meyer began, as earnestly as Freud began his boundingly, ended with the discovery of facts no one predicted. Today neither the inner world of fantasy and hidden wishes nor the outer world of family and other institutions bears any resemblance to the descriptions of 70 years ago.

Once having grasped the difficulties of the patients' circumstances and the limits on their ability to cope, Meyer made his boldest move. Perhaps chronic daydreaming, poetry writing, and impractical blundering pass without sharp transition into autism, delusion formation, and dementia. Unable to conquer the world, in fact repeatedly defeated and humiliated by it, patients draw back more and more into their inner worlds and finally into dementia. Here Meyer joined the mainstream of psychiatric thought, which had moved from Bleuler's emphasis on autism as *a* fundamental process in schizophrenia to Freud's making "withdrawal" *the* fundamental process in what he called the "narcissistic neuroses" and perhaps dementia praecox. The patients were not only split internally but split from the world. At the same time, by suggesting a relationship among habit, situation, and pathology, Meyer pointed forward to the later concept of "vicious circle," self-fulfilling prophecy, and feedback.

Bad "habits" or modes of "adjustment" (Meyer, a close friend of John Dewey and an admirer of William James, took up the psychological concepts of the day) plus bad situations equal the disease processes. Observation of the social phenomena, the patient groping in the world and the situations of that groping, explains enough to make unnecessary a search for intrapsychic or intracellular factors. The official Adolf Meyer of later years would disown such a narrow statement and take up every school's contribution in the spirit of pluralism that he shared with William James. Clearly, at his *innovative* period Meyer was trying to show the power of social data to explain. This was a psychiatry of social experience in its concern with habits and the external shaping world, a crude behaviorism.

Meyer was also at pains to show the power of social interventions to *improve*, "but even here [she] was again found at work and much more affable after a review of her situation." "The details of the development and the reminiscences from the first hospital were then gone into, but evidently not traced completely to a balance or to the fundamental sore points," or else she would have been improved still more. Such is his faith in the effects of reaching a "balance" between the conflicting elements and in airing out the "fundamental sore points." "She relapsed and got out of touch with her real environment. . . . Yet the adjustments in changing the mere rumination into open discussion and giving space for direct and concrete interests has an unmistakable influence on the patient." What a rich variety of therapeutic processes are thrown down before us, as if each were immediately understandable or the whole somehow clear and definite! As always with Meyer, his actions are described modestly. The appeal is made to common sense, which *does* carry the day because frank discussion, airing sore points, "giving space for direct and concrete interests" seem such obviously good ideas.

What are these "fundamental sore points"? He means painful experiences and relationships never sufficiently "gotten over" but shut out of consciousness, avoided in conversation, and needing a physician to probe and drain in order to bring about "unmistakable" relief. He does not tell us how this "talking treatment" worked. Was relief due to sharing past misery with another, abreacting its "repressed" emotional charge, or the result of close contact with reality, "direct and concrete interests," the replacement of daydreaming by a "wholesome" contact with life? The common denominator seems a *social* one, that is, sharing with another what was hitherto private (Meyer complains that no "rapport" was established during a previous hospitalization), and thus moving into the world, again in contrast to the indrawn and private. The emphasis was on practical success in mastering life's problems of work and love because the illness had been a maladjustment to life, an inadequate or substitutive or partial *reaction* to life.

Note how the doctor's approach to the patient was to reflect these matter-of-fact, direct, practical solutions. Not only was the physician to be thoroughly informed before he saw the patient (phenomenologically expanded, perhaps exploded!); he was to cultivate certain attitudes and postures taken over from the objective school. Rather than prepare himself to meet the patient's world of feelings or to remain analytically aloof and receptive, Meyer's physician was to assume an attitude of "helpfulness" and "respect"; he was to avoid both sentimental and withdrawn attitudes. Clearly, a familiar picture of the physician was being sought, reminiscent of the sentimental portraits once so common in doctor's offices: The physician stands by, slightly apart, concerned and even a little moved, but basically the captain whom death and disease cannot dismay. Even the cheerful, almost lighthearted brilliance of that other great Hopkins physician, William Osler, is a little shadowed by Meyer's example; sobriety, almost shyness, permeates Meyer's descriptions.

"Business-like," practical, the doctor was also to be "spontaneous" and "natural." "The direct examination aims to bring the patient as rapidly as possible into the most natural and intelligent rapport with the physician, and in the most natural way . . ." [4, III, p. 243]. Here all the "natural" *difficulties* are put aside in the name of the natural and intelligent and spontaneous. Meyer seldom, if ever, gives us a sense of what might systematically obstruct the work and call for special methods; there is a consistent appeal to "commonsense" views, perhaps his favorite word. We have to ask ourselves how a relationship could remain "natural" that was searching out memories of the patient's rhythmic infantile sexual behavior!

Finally, if a practical adjustment to real life is desirable, there might well be desirable changes also in what is to be adjusted to. The patient need no longer be the sole subject of treatment; the treatment should be directed at the *environment to be adjusted to,* by whatever means available, be it social service, family therapy, political change, or a thousand other forms. Meyer was faithful to these clinical hunches, so different from the working hypotheses of descriptive, psychoanalytic, and existential psychiatry which all applied primarily, or even exclusively, to the person designated as sick. Meyer was the principal moving force in the community hygiene movement in the United States. He worked for outpatient clinics and health districts, with responsible local facilities aimed at the *whole* community, and he worked with policemen, ministers, and schoolteachers, all of whom were to leave behind their narrow interest in crime, evil, and ignorance for this vision of a wholesome communal life. His early statements are rendered simpleminded and ingenuous, although he was far from either of these, once we grasp how subtle, powerful, and essentially mysterious were the forces with which he proposed to wrestle, forces that the discoveries of social psychiatry later illuminated (the transformation of the habit concept, for example, into the concept of self-fulfilling prophecies). The fact is, he gave America its particular native vision of psychiatric work, a vision powerful enough to bend into a social form all the important schools—descriptive, psychoanalytic, and existential—as they were taken up into American psychiatry.

This triumph of the *psychiatrie de concierge* reflects new perceptions never limited to psychiatry. What we observe is part of a general movement of thought, an ever widening representation of reality. Hear Auerbach's account of the revolution in the *drama* from Greek to Shakespearean times; the words could be Meyer's.

[In classic drama] To whatever else may have happened to him during his life, so long as it is not part of the prehistory of the present conflict, to what we call his "milieu," little attention is given, and apart from age, sex, social status, and references to his general type of temperament, we learn nothing about his normal existence. The essence of his personality is revealed and evolves exclusively within the particular tragic action; everything else is omitted. All this is based upon the way in which antique drama arose and on its technical requirements. Freedom of movement, which it reached only very slowly, is much less, even in Euripides, than in the modern drama. In particular, the above-mentioned strict limitation to the given tragic conflict is based upon the fact that the subjects of antique tragedy are almost exclusively taken from the national mythology, in a few cases from national history. These were sacred subjects and the events and personages involved were known to the audience. The "milieu" too was known, and furthermore it was almost always approximately the same. Hence there was no reason to describe its special character and special atmosphere. Euripides challenged the tradition by introducing new interpretations, both of action and character, into the traditional material. But this can hardly be compared with the multiplicity of subject matter, the freedom of invention and presentation which distinguish the Elizabethan and the modern drama generally. What with the great variety of subject matter and the considerable freedom of movement of the Elizabethan theater, we are in each instance given the particular atmosphere, the situation, and the prehistory of the characters. The course of events on the stage is not rigidly restricted to the course of events of the tragic conflict but covers conversations, scenes, characters, which the action as such does not necessarily require. Thus we are given a great deal of "supplementary information" about the principal personages; we are enabled to form an idea of their normal lives and particular characters apart from the complication in which they are caught at the moment [9].*

Substitute present illness for "prehistory of the present conflict," habits and relationships for "normal existence," psychosis for "tragic action," and accepted diagnoses for "national mythology," and we see a parallel opening up of the facts thought relevant to the main events. We can thus place Meyer's achievement, and many other achievements discussed in this book, squarely within the developments Auerbach details. These are the development of a broader and broader perception of reality, the gradual admission of a greater variety

* From *Mimesis: The Representation of Reality in Western Literature,* by Erich Auerbach, translated by Willard R. Trask (copyright © 1953 by Princeton University Press; Princeton Paperback, 1968). Reprinted by permission of Princeton University Press.

of classes and types of people and events of life, both inward and outward, into what can be accepted as the truly real, or, for the problem of the present book, the gradual admission of factors hitherto unrelated to mental illness into an understanding of it. All the developments subsumed here under the schools constitute only divisions or phases of this broadening perception of the significant reality for understanding pathological human nature.

So here again art precedes medicine, just as science fiction and fictional science precede real science, which perhaps means no more than that we are able sometimes to make systematic and lawful what at first were free, imaginative hopes and hunches.

HARRY STACK SULLIVAN

Harry Stack Sullivan is the most original figure in American psychiatry, the only American to help found a major school. He stares past us now, two decades after his death, through those nearsighted Joycean Irish eyes, half participating and half observing, his own man to the last. We will have to answer the high European contempt for his *psychiatrie de concierge* to take full pride in him, but pride we should take in this great American contributor to the mainstream of psychiatric advance.

He made two outstanding contributions. He demonstrated the effect that changes in the immediate social field have on symptoms, an effect that has since been shown to result not only from two-person situations but also from families, hospitals, and perhaps society and culture as a whole. In addition, he gave hints on how to manage the social field so as to provide optimal effects on symptoms, hints which can be drawn forward into a systematic method or technique. The only other figure to make both types of contributions to psychiatry so single-handedly was Freud, although someday the same claim may be advanced for Pavlov or Skinner.

And he made his contributions walking on one leg. At least twice acutely psychotic himself, he never gained the spontaneity, receptiveness, and capacity for intimacy his own interpersonal school worked to achieve for others. A trenchant teacher, a man legendary in his own lifetime, he remained sealed within the projections he was so adept at recognizing and correcting in others. How often psychiatric investigators are subject to this condition! Perhaps all investigators are. The searcher starts at home, on the familiar ground of his own conflicts and disappointments, in Sullivan's case with psychosis and personal isolation, working outward and forward to a greater freedom and power, at least for others.

Happily his writings fell into the hands of devoted literary executors who worked and reworked his lectures. We seldom know how much we read is Sullivan, how much Helen Perry and others, or the ideas of Patrick Mullahy. That is a small price for the reward.

The step from Meyer to Sullivan is short but decisive. If the patient adapts by his illness to the world, what would happen to the illness if the world adapted to the patient? [10]. Sullivan attempts to explore just that.

Here is vintage Sullivan, in both style and method. Note his interest in concealment—not the concealment of deeprunning anatomical or familial fantasies at this stage, but deceptions born of everyday transactions with real and familiar figures.

The psychiatrist, the interviewer, plays a very active role in introducing interrogations, not to show that he is skeptical, but literally to make sure that he knows what he is being told. Few things do the patient more good in the way of getting toward his more or less clearly formulated desire to benefit from the investigation than this very care on the part of the interviewer to discover exactly what is meant. Almost every time one asks, "Well, do you mean so and so?" the patient is a little clearer on what he does mean. And what a relief it is to him to discover that his true meaning is anything but what he at first says, and that he is at long last uncovering some conventional self-deception that he has been pulling on himself for years [11, p. 21].*

Sullivan does not take for granted that he understands what the patient means, as Meyer tended to; neither does he discount verbal material, as Kraepelin did (and skeptical as Sullivan is), nor does he let the verbal material emerge freely, as in analytic work. From the start he involves himself actively with what he assumes will be distorted communications. Note how directly he speaks out and then separates himself obliquely from other figures in the patient's life.

Let me illustrate this last by telling you of a young man who had been clearly sinking into a schizophrenic illness for several months and who was referred to me by a colleague. Among the amazing things I extracted from this poor citizen was that, to his amazement and chagrin, he spent a good deal of his time in the kitchen with his mother making dirty cracks at her, saying either obscure or actually bitter and critical things to her. He thought he must be crazy, because he was the only child and his mother, so he said, was perfect. As a matter of fact, he had two perfect parents. They had done everything short of carrying him around on a pillow. And now he had broken down just because he was engaged in a couple of full-time courses at one of our best universities. In other words, he was a bright boy, and had very healthy ambitions which represented the realization of the very fine training that he had been given by these excellent parents. I undertook to discover what was so surprising to him about this business of his hostile remarks to his mother, and he made it quite clear that the

* Reprinted from *The Psychiatric Interview* by Harry Stack Sullivan, M.D. Edited by Helen Swick Perry and Mary Ladd Gawel. By permission of W. W. Norton & Company, Inc. Copyright 1954 by The William Alanson White Psychiatric Foundation. All other quotes in this chapter with a citation to Note 11 are from the same source and are quoted with permission.

surprising thing was that she had never done him any harm, and had actually enfolded him in every kind of good. To all this I thought, "Oh yeah? It doesn't sound so to me. It doesn't make sense. Maybe you have overlooked something."

By that time I was actually able to say something like this: "I have a vague feeling that some people might doubt the utility to you of the care with which your parents, and particularly your mother, saw to it that you didn't learn how to dance, or play games, or otherwise engage in the frivolous social life of people of your age." And I was delighted to see the schizophrenic young man give me a sharp look. Although he was seated where I didn't have to look directly at him, I could see that. And I said, "Or was that an unmitigated blessing?" There was a long pause, and then he opined that when he was young he might have been sore about it [11, pp. 21–22].

He is also one of the very, very few psychiatric writers who can be funny on purpose [12].

Anyone who has dealt long with people even moderately schizophrenic knows how much Sullivan has already accomplished in these few moments. Such patients are characteristically terrified of criticizing their parents, even of thinking thoughts that might seem critical of them. Sullivan not only has managed to keep in the patient's mind a thought critical of the parents but has been able to make the patient reasonably comfortable in expressing it. This is a feat more or less the equivalent of removing an appendix without anesthesia.

We want to understand how this is possible, that is, to understand the method of interpersonal psychiatry. But note first how he stays with what he has gained and then puts it in perspective. Note, too, as with Meyer's case, the good results of a "more direct approach."

I guessed that that wasn't the whole story—that he was still sore about it, and with very good reason. Then I inquired if he had felt any disadvantage in college from the lack of these social skills with which his colleagues whiled away their evenings, and so on. He recalled that he had often noticed his defects in that field, and that he regretted them. With this improvement in intelligence, we were able to glean more of what the mother had actually done and said to discourage his impulse to develop social techniques. At the end of an hour and a half devoted more or less entirely to this subject, I was able to say, "Well, now, is it really so curious that you're being unpleasant to your mother?" And he thought that perhaps it wasn't.

A couple of days later the family telephoned to say that he was greatly benefited by his interview with me. As a matter of fact, he unquestionably was. But the benefit—and this is perhaps part of why I tell the story—arose from the discovery that a performance of his, which was deeply distressing to him because it seemed irrational and entirely unjust, became reasonably justified by a change in his awareness of his past and of his relationship with the present victim of his behavior. Thus the feeling was erased that he was crazy, that only a madman would be doing this—and, believe me, it is no help to anybody's peace of mind to feel that he is mad. His peace of mind was enhanced to the extent that it was no longer necessary for him to feel chagrin, contempt for himself and all sorts of dim religious impiety; but on the other hand he could feel, as I attempted to suggest in our initial interview, that there wasn't anything different in his behavior from practically anybody else's except the accents in the patterns of its manifestation. As he was able to comprehend that the repulsive, queer, strange, mystifying, chagrining, horrifying aspects of his experience reflected defects in his memory and understanding concerning its origins, the necessity to manifest the behavior appeared to diminish, which actually meant that competing processes were free to appear, and that the partitioning of his life was to some degree broken down. The outwardly meaningless, psychotic attacks on his mother did not give him the satisfaction that came from asking her more directly why in the devil she had never let him learn to play bridge. With the substitution of the possibility of a more direct approach, the psychotic material disappeared and he was better [11, pp. 22–23].

Sullivan had reached a sore point, aired it out, and suggested that substitution of clear practical questions to the mother for the previous kitchen-badgering of her. We do not learn that the patient actually asked his mother about his upbringing or what she answered if he did. Many parents need more help in answering sensible questions from their children than the children need in order to question them. What we can learn from this example is something about Sullivan's method of surfacing the sore points.

"I have a vague feeling that some people might doubt the utility to you of the care with which your parents, and particularly your mother, saw to it that you didn't learn how to dance, or play games, or otherwise engage in the frivolous social life of people of your age." This is a translation of his earlier, unspoken thought "Oh yeah? It doesn't sound so to me." The spoken version starts out with a lie—Sullivan's feeling was not vague—displaces responsibility for what Sullivan is thinking onto "some people," and ends with an accusation against the parents. In short, he is being fey, roundabout, and finally disrespectful, but for all that *systematic*. Here is another example:

. . . However, during an interview one may learn that a person is married, and if one is feeling very mildly satirical, one can say, "And doubtless happily?" If the answer is "Yes," that "Yes" can have anything in the way of implication from a dirge to a paean of supreme joy. It may indicate that the "Yes" means "No," or anything in between [11, p. 8].

Sullivan wants to discover the actual marital condition. The technique is *provocative*, rather than confrontational, analytic, or examinational. Compare his "doubtless happily?" with the earlier "unmitigated blessing?"

Here is another example, which should put us still closer to the common denominators of this method.

. . . In paranoid states there is the utmost secrecy about all sorts of things which, so far as I know, are of no interest to anybody but the patient. The psychiatrist, in trying to get at various things that he needs to know, may bump into these areas of secrecy; in such circumstances he may say, for example, "Am I to understand the difficulty that you have with this troublesome neighbor of yours without any information at all about it?" At this the patient may glare for a while, being in somewhat of a dilemma, because, as far as he is concerned, the psychiatrist really should be able to do just that; yet it does sound rather peculiar when put that way [11, p. 33].

The paranoid patient expected Sullivan to be able to read his mind because he feels everything about him is of great interest to others and because he has projected onto Sullivan his knowledge of himself; thereupon, Sullivan challenges both the grandiosity and the projection. Like Meyer he wants to know the specific details of the patient's experience that make his feelings about the neighbor understandable, but he knows that commonsense direct questions about that experience will come to grief on the patient's psychosis. So the inquiry must be put "that way."

"Am I to understand the difficulty that you have with this troublesome neighbor of yours without any information at all about it?" "And doubtless happily?" "Was that an unmitigated blessing?" "I have a vague feeling that some people might doubt the utility, etc." I will maintain that in all these instances Sullivan is first challenging the patient's assumptions or projections about Sullivan, the interviewer, and secondly doing so without making the patient aware of his remarkable assumptions.

He challenges the assumption that he, Sullivan, can read the patient's mind, the assumption that all marriages are bliss, and that all mothers are angels. In no case, however, does he directly assert, as we are so often tempted to do, that the patient is crazy enough to believe any of these things; at worst he offers the patient the chance to extricate himself immediately from such a position. In short, he separates himself sharply from the patient's assumptions while subjecting the patient to the least possible humiliation for making those assumptions. Again we have to think of painless dentistry or surgery.

Nor are these gimmicks. Both rest on fundamental discoveries about interpersonal situations, specifically Sullivan's knowledge of what goes wrong in interviews and most extravagantly wrong in contacts with psychotic people: The patient is afraid, makes wrong assumptions; then the doctor does not correct those assumptions and may, in fact, deepen them.

Psychotic people are particularly prone to this sequence because they are more withdrawn than others and project more, especially hostile thoughts and feelings. Psychotic people are least "in the world," to use existential language. In psychoanalytic language, they lack object cathexes and meet only their "hostile introjects" thrown out on the world. Such are actually each school's definitions of psychosis.

But in fact, few or none of us, psychotic or otherwise, make the happy assumption that the psychiatrist will love or even like us.

The real facts of the interview situation might be expressed: "If I tell the doctor the truth, he won't think well of me." Or, "Well, I must put a good face on that; otherwise I might make a bad impression." Or again, "My God! If I do things like that, of course he won't authorize my employment." All of these covert operations show an attempt on the part of the interviewee to read the interviewer's mind. A great many of them form defects in the process of communication, for all of them spring from a dreadfully troublesome and significant question in the mind of the interviewee: "What will he think?" The complex products which the interviewer gets from the interviewee arise from the latter's attempt to avoid even the faintest sign of an unfavorable answer to that question in his mind [11, p. 98].

It is easy to pass over these statements as if they were self-evident, widely accepted and appreciated, or, on the other hand, exaggerated. The fact is that before Sullivan they had been given no systematic place in psychiatric, psychological, or medical work. The objective school, for example, assumes that the illness is one thing and the person another and that we can talk rationally to the person about the illness. Psychoanalysis makes a similar assumption that normal and neurotic persons enter social and professional situations without the self-centered fears, the narcissistic preoccupations to which Sullivan alludes. In contrast, Sullivan takes a "realistic" view of the hostile and dependent currents prevalent in social life. At least it is realistic by the light of the present writer's experience, as well as by that of the most experienced epidemiologists of mental illness [13]. Earlier Freud had taken a similarly "realistic" view of the sexual fantasies and motivations endemic to psychic life. Establishment people were no readier to credit his discoveries than they are Sullivan's.

So much for the interviewee's problems. What is the interviewer to do about them? It is easier to start by describing what he should *not* do about them.

Were any one of us to be interviewed about a significant aspect of our living by a person who gave us no clues as to what he thought and how we were doing, I think we would be reduced to mutism within a matter of minutes. Our uncertainty would be frightful, and we would simply be too acutely anxious to go on. In short, none of us feel that safe, and we won't feel that safe until the social order has greatly improved in its utility for living. The interviewer actually gives signs by tonal gestures, by physical gestures, and by verbal statements, which can be, and are, interpreted and misinterpreted by the interviewee. The skill in interviewing lies in not doing this in the wrong way [11, p. 103].

Again psychotic people offer the extreme situation. Not only are they farther into their own heads than most of us, but they also tend to make other people more uncomfortable or downright hostile than most humans, thereby fulfilling the patient's worst prophecies. The psychotic patient regularly gives us opportunities to hate or disdain him quite spontaneously, opportunities which, if cultivated, confirm not only his assumptions but ours. This hostile interaction between psychotic patient and doctor and its potential for escalation is Sullivan's premier example of the "field of data" of his school, but he observed that such processes color every social interaction to some degree.

If inadvertently encouraging the other person's psychotic assumptions constitutes the "wrong way," how does one set about the "right way"? "Part of the interviewer's development of skill comes from observing, more or less automatically, what is *probably* the case with respect to the interviewee's feeling about the interviewer's attitude." [11, p. 113]. The language here is simple, almost informal. There is little technical vocabulary to help us through what are essentially technical matters. The sentence makes use of only two technical terms, *interviewee* and *interviewer*, and these confuse rather than clarify, for in fact the whole thrust of Sullivan's discoveries is away from a sharp separation of roles. He writes elsewhere that both parties interview each other, so that the terms *interviewee* and *interviewer* represent holdovers from the old objective psychiatry in which this separation of roles was assumed.

The critical expression is *observing one person's feelings about another's attitudes*. This is a truly *social situation* statement. It should be contrasted to the objective-descriptive account of feelings in the same way one might contrast observation of a fixed, stained cross section of a heart muscle with what that muscle looks like during an experiment on cardiac contraction. In the one case the material is in final form, to be looked on as an object. In the experimental situation the muscle is only part of the observational field, which includes the experimenter's manipulations as well.

By using the term *feelings*, rather than, say, *ideas*, Sullivan conveys that the patient's reactions are not articulated, not fully conscious, and are also very powerful; he is referring to essentially unconscious, visceral processes. These are, however, affected by the surrounding real world, in particular by the *attitude* of the interviewer. This term, too, is chosen with care. Note that he does not say *feelings* of the interviewer. *Attitude* suggests something more objective, something to be reacted to, something seen from outside. It means less feeling than the form of the feelings and ideas of the interviewer. Note, too, that he makes no assumption that the feelings of the patient are not appropriate. Sullivan is neutral as to the part reality and fantasy are playing in this interaction; he holds open the possibility that the patient's feelings are simply a response to the real attitudes of the interviewer (a contemporary Sullivanian, Harold Searles, has explored this possibility extensively). Nor does Sullivan imply that the interviewer's attitude might not be a function of the *patient's* attitude!

These remarks only set the stage for the interviewer's observation and participation. Again we need to ask, what is the "right way" to participate in this system? So far only a general answer has been given: that one wants to correct misunderstandings but not humiliate the misunderstander. This could be generalized still further into: one wants to learn and teach lovingly. A little more specifically, Sullivan has made it a point to challenge any false assumption he observes that the patient makes about him (the patient's "feelings" about his "attitudes"), in order to avoid confusion in the interview (and, of course, with the later, broader purpose of preparing for corrections of misunderstandings that may color the patient's whole life). Also we have observed that he avoids humiliating the patient, by making use of indirection, by giving the responsibility for his ideas to others, and by offering possibilities rather than insistences so that the patient can skip away if Sullivan's remarks prove too threatening.

Sullivan had learned from Bleuler and Freud that withdrawal was perhaps the fundamental process in psychosis. He had learned from Freud that this drawing back from the world was followed by a strange reaching out; the patient found all about him his own preoccupations, fears, aggressions, and loves. Sullivan's contemporary, Paul Federn, suggested that the *boundary* between ourselves and the world had been broken in psychosis so that the person going mad flowed out onto the world as through a broken dam.

Sullivan saw more clearly than Freud that the projection process is *unconscious*. In psychoanalytic language, projection takes place in an unconscious part of the ego. Not only is the machinery behind the projection silent, but so is the symptomatic result. The hysterical patient often knows his leg is paralyzed or his arm numb, but projection goes on in silence; it is like those messages sent in wartime which are too secret to be revealed even to their bearers. The person projecting believes he sees the world as it is. A critical part of Sullivan's contribution is that he emphasized how common and yet how little recognized this projection process is. The transference does not develop just in the treatment. It does not take long to develop. Transference occurs every day with everyone (and therefore deserves a new name, parataxis) and comes ready-made into every human situation. We can say that Sullivan broke the seal of silence on projection.

Breuer had said with Janet that the hysterics suffered from weak egos; hence the flight of part of their thoughts and feelings into the unconscious or onto the world. Federn's boundary defect was only this same weak ego writ into psychosis. Sullivan stayed with Freud's response to Breuer and Janet, and to Federn. Perhaps the ego is weak, but that is not an "explanation"; it invokes a god, if a flawed god, from the machine. What we can observe is conflict, the extrusion of one conflictual psychic element by another. So in hysteria and psychosis, Freud and Sullivan said, incompatible elements are forced in the first case into the body and in the second onto the world.

Now the need for the fresh technique should be still more evident, for what the therapist has to deal with are *unconscious, unacceptable* projections. The patient does not believe he distorts and he will not want to believe it! Hence the extraordinary difficulty of managing projection.

Besides Sullivan's technique, there are two systematic methods for dealing with projections, one an action technique, the other verbal, insight-dependent. The clearest modern example of the first is anaclitic therapy, a treatment aimed at substituting, for example, good nursing experiences for the bad ones the patient may have had. This treatment says to the patient: I will be your mother, but a good mother; I will make up for what you did not receive earlier. (In psychoanalysis the same is called "a corrective emotional experience." It also bears a resemblance to extinction in behavior therapy.) Essentially, the projection is accepted by the doctor, but direct attempts are made to change its emotional coloring.

Secondly, psychoanalysis attempts to deal with projections through *interpretation*; the patient's attention is called to the transference distortions. The psychoanalyst wants the patient to understand what he, the patient, is doing. The matter of stopping what he is doing, it is hoped, will follow on that understanding. It may, however, be achieved only through repeated interpretations or fall away subsequently as the wishes and experiences related to the distortion are brought to consciousness and abreacted. Indeed, analysts have little interest in the rapid resolution of projections, for only by allowing the the little projections (transferences) to flower into that larger projective system, the transference neurosis, can the neurosis be fully surfaced and then worked over. In short, analysis encourages rather than prevents projections, and then, when the projections are to be dealt with, the goal is consciousness of them, not primarily their disappearance.

The Sullivanian technique stands in the clearest possible contrast to this method of analytic transference interpretation. *Awareness* of the projections may even be avoided and their rapid *reduction* or *elimination* sought. Recall now the first intervention of Sullivan quoted: "I have a vague feeling that some people might doubt the utility to you of the care with which your parents, particularly your mother, saw to it that you didn't learn how to dance, or play games, or otherwise engage in the frivolous social life of people your age." Sullivan does not point out to the patient his assumption that the parents are perfect, or the patient's further assumption that he, Sullivan, accepts them as perfect, too. (The patient assumes everyone regards them as perfect.) Sullivan does not say, "You think your parents are *perfect*," or "I don't think your parents *are* perfect." Instead he raises questions about these issues in the patient's mind and takes a neutral position on the issues himself (hence, "some people"). At the same time that he is helping the patient gain distance on his delusional assumptions, Sullivan is disengaging himself from those delusional assumptions.

This is not a matter of directness versus indirectness or awkwardness versus tact, although the result of Sullivan's method is often indirectness and frequently tact. He was just as likely to seem blunt or even savage, especially in contrast to the cautious interventions characteristic of many psychotherapeutic efforts. When he did seem blunt, it was because he felt he had cleared the interpersonal field of projections sufficiently to have the patient take his remarks at face value.

So Sullivan's advice to the therapist is: First, determine what the patient is assuming (projecting), what his "feelings" are about your "attitudes." Then do something that makes the assumption more difficult. Above all, do not say or do anything that makes the assumption easier for the patient.

Sullivan is not attempting, at this point, to go behind the patient's projections to the hidden needs or past experiences which make those projections more fully explicable. The first job is to deal with their occurrence in the present. The doctor's assumption must be that they are still necessary, not only because the old needs are still present, but because the patient is still creating the old situations (self-fulfilling prophecies), and the doctor is very likely to help him continue that re-creation. Sullivan's implication is that, first, projections are unconscious and their basis is unacceptable in consciousness to the patient, and, second, we must deal with the real current world that renders them invulnerable to a purely historical approach. Therefore, insofar as the real current world, including the doctor, is playing into the patient's projections, the doctor must dissociate himself from that world if he is to help the patient gain perspective on his projections.

Finally, undermining the patient's false assumption requires *force*. A purely intellectual understanding of their inappropriateness must prove inadequate before the dynamic forces maintaining the projections. Sullivan's patient *needed* to believe his mother was perfect; he was not likely to surrender that belief in the absence of another opposing need at least equally powerful; hence the final part of Sullivan's technique. He must discover and have the patient share with him a felt injury that contradicts the parent's perfection. "I inquired if he had felt any disadvantage in college from the lack of these social skills with which his colleagues whiled away their evenings, and so on. He recalled that he had often noticed his defects in that field, and that he regretted them." Out of this sprang the patient's willingness to consider his mother less than perfect.

Not only does the past felt injury drive home a fresh perception of the parents against the old false assumption; that fresh perception is necessary in order to feel the old injury! As a boy the patient had "regretted" his inability to dance. He had not then blamed his parents but may well have blamed himself. This incident, probably augmented by many others, served to form the patient's sense of himself as awkward, odd, and even crazy. If he had been able to blame the parents, he might have seen *them* as crazy. To bring back into consciousness such painful times is difficult; one's being fights against reexperiencing the pain (as well as defends the ideal parental image). It is for this reason that behavior therapists introduce the phobic stimulus very gradually and, in the technique of reciprocal inhibition, reduce anxiety by having the patient eat, be medicated, or share the experience with a comfortable person. Sullivan's method accomplishes the same purpose in a different way. Remembering regrets and past humiliations will be hard or even intolerable if the patient is left, at the same time, with the conviction that *he* is to blame and that it is *he* who is crazy. However, if in the process of remembering his pain he is partly freed of blame for it, and, with that, freed of his conviction of being mad, the pain can be faced. Thus the disruption of the projection and the airing out of the old wound go on together, each necessary to the other.

Modern psychoanalysis also grasps this point, as is demonstrated in the statement that analysis of memories, drives, and the "id" must go on *pari passu* with analysis of the ego [14] or mechanisms of defense, of which projection is one. On the other hand, psychoanalysis *seeks* the transference neurosis and must therefore accept Sullivanian techniques gingerly.

Meyer's goals are now reached from a fresh direction with the airing of the old wound and the freeing up of the old projections, and space is given for "direct and concrete interests" and action. Perhaps it became possible for the boy to confront his parents constructively; we know it was at least possible for him to feel better about himself. Granted the base line of schizophrenia, this is a great gain.

The misunderstandings, projections, and parataxes Sullivan found so rife in human communication demand the active, repeated interventions which are the signature of interpersonal technique, he argued. The social situation must be phenomenologically reduced, to use existential language, freed of those parataxes that identify illness. This "reduction" *does* affect illness, for symptoms are not "static characteristics of a thing." It is more accurate to ask, "How does Mr. A act with Mr. B?" "What goes on in the situation integrated between A and B?" [15, p. 37] than to accept the old fixed view of symptoms characteristic of the objective schools.

SOCIAL UNDERSTANDING OF HYSTERIA

The role of fantasy in society is so great that we cannot approach it with any thought of doing the subject justice. Some would say society is hardly more than fantasy and that the games played out from day to day take their principal coloring and significance from the private meanings they have for each of us. Even in those rare circumstances in which we perceive each other as we actually are, the *results* of those perceptions are taken up again into our private worlds of fantasy and expectation, the worlds of transference and parataxis, so that in the areas of both perception and conception social events surrender much of their meanings to our inner processes. Paradoxically, while psychoanalysis emphasized the importance of fantasy in mental illness, it spoke of transference as if it were largely a process occurring in treatment and then slowly, while Sullivanian psychiatry saw transferences everywhere but was more optimistic than psychoanalysis about their treatment! Reality could be bent to offset fantasy, especially by that therapeutic maneuver called participant observation.

The modern student of psychology grows up on Freud's accounts of hysteria. We can almost say the modern temper has been shaped by Anna O., and perhaps most of all by Dora, just as an earlier generation studied Janet's Marcelle and Irene and Morton Prince's Miss Beauchamp. It will therefore be valuable to present some of Sullivan's account of hysteria, both by way of contrast to Freud's and because it will serve to illustrate Sullivan's psychological concepts in their simplest form.

Here is the familiar concept dissociation, now making its appearance for interpersonal theory.

I have spoken of the magnificence of the apparatus—the system of dynamisms, of more or less permanently running processes—which is required for the maintenance of dissociation. I have talked about how the dissociated personality has to prepare for almost any conceivable emergency that would startle one into becoming aware of the dissociated system and of how, as a result, one literally has to set up a whole group of special awarenesses, special alert signals, if you please. Now the clinical entity, hysteria, shows almost in caricature how that is done. Thus, although the hysteric dynamism is very much simpler than the dissociative dynamism (as in schizophrenia), it is extremely illuminating for the theory of dissociation [16, p. 203]).*

"The hysteric," Sullivan goes on, "might be said in principle to be a person who has a happy thought as to a way by which

* Reprinted from *Clinical Studies in Psychiatry* by Harry Stack Sullivan, M.D. Edited by Helen Swick Perry, Mary Ladd Gawel, and Martha Gibbon. By permission of W. W. Norton & Company, Inc. Copyright © 1956 by The William Alanson White Psychiatric Foundation. All other quotes in this chapter with a citation to Note 16 are from the same source and are quoted with permission.

he can be respectable even though not living up to his standards."

In the hysteric, you see that the whole achievement of the dynamism employed is to prevent the environing people from recognizing and being able to prove the existence of the impulses which are behind the hysteric facade—or, for my purposes, which are dissociated. In the great dissociative processes (schizophrenia, for example), on the other hand, there is no awareness at any level of the evaluation that other people might place on the dissociated system. That is all blotted out in the readjustment within the self-system which gives security by virtue of the dissociation. In the hysteric the self-system is so sketchy that as soon as the other person hits on a fairly well-aimed guess as to what the dissociated impulse is, the whole thing shifts. In other words, one particular self-against-impulse process may be abandoned and a new one developed. Thus, hysteria is very much simpler than dissociation in its fully developed form; but it is immensely interesting as a diagram [16, p. 204].

To illustrate how the hysteric dynamism comes into operation, let us say that a man with a strong hysterical predisposition has married, perhaps for money, and that his wife, thanks to his rather dramatic and exaggerated way of doing and saying things, cannot long remain in doubt that there was a very practical consideration in this marriage and cannot completely blind herself to a certain lack of importance that she has in her husband's eyes. So she begins to get even. She may, for example, like someone I recently saw, develop a never-failing vaginismus, so that there is no more intercourse for him. And he will not ruminate on whether this vaginismus that is cutting off his satisfaction is directed against him, for the very simple reason that if you view interpersonal phenomena with that degree of objectivity, you can't use an hysterical process to get rid of your own troubles. So he won't consider that; but he will suffer terribly from privation and will go to rather extravagant lengths to overcome the vaginismus that is depriving him of satisfaction, the lengths being characterized by a certain rather theatrical attention to detail rather than deep scrutiny of his wife. But he fails again and again. Then one night, when he is worn out, and perhaps has had a precocious ejaculation in his newest adventure in practical psychotherapy, he has the idea, "My

God, this thing is driving me crazy," and goes to sleep [16, pp. 204–205].

"This thing is driving me crazy" is the "happy thought" which leads to the symptoms. The patient thereupon wakes up early in the morning and has a dramatic attack of some kind. The wife is frightened, medical people appear, and we have a case of hysteria.

The account is remarkable, perhaps because of its piquancy and the emphasis on here-and-now, but Sullivan moves quickly to even less familiar ground. The freshness of his observations springs from studying the patient as someone-in-relation-to-others.

He notices that the patient, for all his understandable annoyance about the vaginismus, is a remarkably self-centered man. He does not, for example, allow himself to consider that vaginismus might be a sign of the wife's annoyance with *him*. The patient's own suffering in this sad domestic tangle is almost the only thing that concerns him. From the beginning of their marriage his behavior suggested to the wife her small importance in his eyes. Now once again the wife is relegated to being an onlooker at the husband's dramatic doings.

To our surprise Sullivan presents hysterical people as in one sense extraordinarily *less* realistic than schizophrenic people. The latter are deeply absorbed in fantasies, but their fantasies are a constant re-creation of glorious and dismal possibilities of living in the service of compensating or warning about actual events ahead. Sullivan hypothesizes that schizophrenic people have always had to live with hostile and dangerous parents and have therefore developed a supreme alertness to external reality; their delusions are responses to that very alertness. The delusions are both reparative and preparative measures, to expand the psychoanalytic formulation. On the other hand, Sullivan hypothesizes that hysterical people have grown their egos at the knees of people remarkably self-absorbed, dramatic, self-important. The hysteria-learning child receives neither warmth nor coldness. He learns to live in fantasies for their own sake, not now as defenses against the world. Thus when schizophrenic people say they are great, no one, least of all themselves, believes it. But hysterical people really believe they are great, or, as Sullivan puts it, of great "personal individuality" [17, p. 221], and the world often believes it with them.

We are now very close to the work of Wilhelm Reich and the whole study of "ego psychology." I have chosen to present this aspect of modern psychiatry through Sullivan's words not only because of his remarkable contributions to it but because he refused to consider the development of the ego (for which he often used the word *personality*) apart from the development of relations with other people. "For all I know every human being has as many personalities as he has interpersonal relations" [17, p. 221]. I doubt that this 'societizing' is the whole truth, but it is enough of the truth to make his observations and ideas strikingly useful.

We are also close to the psychoanalytic concept of narcissism and to the negative of existential "being-in-the-world." Both these ideas include, among much else, the self-absorption and self-centeredness Sullivan is putting at the center of hysteria. I write *close to* because both the psychoanalytic and existential concepts imply some element of withdrawal from the world into the self, while hysterical self-centeredness is experienced as very much "in the world." The patients seem at first glance "real." Certainly they interest us, and they establish relationships easily, more easily than any other neurotic or psychotic group. From the vantage point of interpersonal analysis, however, we are asked to concentrate attention on the *dramatic* and *theatrical* aspects of these hysterical relationships. The patients themselves alert us to this necessity out of their own experience; they often tell us they have no friends and little love, despite all the dramatic attention paid to them. As Sullivan said, it is "pseudo-living." What is the meaning of this hysterical drama or pseudo-living?

Psychoanalysis has given its own convincing answer. The meaning is oedipal, an old family drama enacted and reenacted with a frequency and intensity of repetition that suggests a fresh principle, the repetition compulsion. Furthermore, the more persistently and closely we study hysterical patients, the more fragments appear from a still earlier time of life. We see repeated elements from the relationship with mother, such as oral dependence, unrealistic thinking, and primitive rage; hence the modern concept of oral or primitive hysteria.

Existential psychiatry, studying the hysterical drama from within, notes the "embodiedness" of hysterical phenomena—how life is experienced through the body—and understands that this is not a free outgoing or ongoing bodily experience but one locked in repeated, tic-like patterns that show the hand of the past. The patient will not give up the early concrete bodily experience of life and will not be drawn fully into life.

Descriptive psychiatry also has *its* way of identifying these patients, who have the look of people who are looked at.

From the standpoint of interpersonal psychiatry none of these phenomena is central; they may not even be reported by Sullivanians (so great is psychiatric insularity!). Instead attention is called to the relationship between actor and audience in the hysterical drama. Hysterical drama is remarkable for its vividness, simplicity, attractiveness, and above all for our willingness, even eagerness, to participate. Psychoanalysis alerted us to the countertransference opportunities so invitingly presented by the hysterical encounter. Sullivan pressed this lesson home with the following result: It was possible to see that the hysteric had mobilized his whole circle—sometimes whole communities—into the enactment of his fantasies, so that hysteria often "broke out" in epidemic form, with fierce reprisals.

The self-centeredness of hysterical people expresses the same capacity. Hysterical people are able to center their social world in themselves; they can draw into their drama those about them. Here is the essence of what we mean by saying someone is dramatic or theatrical. Our cooperative response allows the trait not only to become vivid but to continue and to grow beyond being a transient accent. Hysterical narcissism is therefore not so much a drawing away from the world as a drawing of the world into the hysterical self. We do not readily notice the withdrawal because we gladly accompany the patients into it!

Thus it is that hysteria keeps changing. The descriptions of one epoch are unrecognizable in the next. The same role played again and again loses verisimilitude, and the audience its interest. Hysteria being recognized is no longer hysteria, in Sullivan's special language: "In the hysteric the self-system is so sketchy that as soon as the other person hits on a fairly well-aimed guess as to what the dissociated impulse is, the whole thing shifts. In other words, one particular self-against-impulse process may be abandoned and a new one developed" [16, p. 204]. As the painfully gained medical knowledge of hysteria spreads, fresh symptoms must develop, to command fresh sympathy and interest, so that relatives and friends can be drawn without skepticism into the game.

I hope these sentences of mine do not deride hysteria as do many of Sullivan's sentences about hysteria, which are in such striking contrast to his writings about schizophrenia. As the illusions the hysterical dramatist creates are pierced, disillusionment follows, and with it irritation, even fury. Having been taken in, we want to throw the patients out—our response also to psychopathic people as we learn the depth and breadth of their malfeasances. But we have no more right to curse the hysteric than we have to curse the playwright when the play is done. Because the hysteric also gives pleasure with the deception, our chagrin is mean.

How much more therapeutic for both patient and doctor to congratulate the actress, take off their costumes, and begin serious work. But see, even in that "innocent" description, how sexual analogies flower and we are drawn back again into the old seductive relationship. Still we do need to "penetrate" behind the deception and help the hysterical person give up this exciting "pseudo-living."

SOCIOLOGICAL PSYCHIATRY

Sullivan's discomfort with hysteria was probably a discomfort with sex. He told a student that hysterical patients seldom kept their appointments with him [18]. Certainly he was never more lyrical than in his descriptions of *pre*adolescent life; where else but from personal experience and a sharp sense of his own limitations could such moving melancholy lines as these come?

[In preadolescence] a new form of participation develops, in part from sympathy and understanding, in part from awe at the newly expanded world. The preadolescent evolves the practice of *collaboration,* a valid functional activity as a person in a personal situation. This is a great step forward from cooperation—I play according to the rules of the game, to preserve *my* prestige and feeling of superiority and merit. When we collaborate, it is a matter of *we.* The achievement is no longer a personal success; it is a group performance—no more the leader's than the led.

In this brief phase of preadolescence, the world as known gains depth of meaning from the new appraisal of the people who compose it. The world as rumored is a wonderful place; the quest of Sir Lancelot rises from the mists of faëry to all but a pattern of life to be lived. Experiences reported from excursions away from home carry a coloring of friendly wonder. The future is constructed in relatively noble terms by the reveries that prepare for tomorrow and that assuage disappointment, take the humdrum out of monotonous tasks.

The imaginary people of preadolescent fantasy may seem to us insubstantial; the imaginery play of the preadolescent may seem but old romatic folklore crudely adjusted to the spirit of the times. The illusions that transmute his companions—if they be illusions—may seem to us but certain of an early end, a disillusionment. But whatever his people, real, illusory or frankly imagined, may be, they are not mean. Whatever his daydreams with his chum, whatever his private fantasies, they are not base. And as to his valuations of others; here we may take pause and reflect that it may be we who see "as through a glass, darkly."

These young folk are grossly inexperienced. They are often grossly misinformed as to the motives that are prominent in adult life around them. But I surmise that after the measure of their experience, they see remarkably clearly. Also, I believe that for a great majority of our people, preadolescence is the nearest that they come to untroubled human life—that from then on the stresses of life distort them to inferior caricatures of what they might have been [15, pp. 26–27].*

So much of wisdom and so much of Sullivan speaks to us from these lines! The careful study of large populations has shown that the majority of our people do fall far short of "untroubled human life." And Sullivan himself had difficulty in collaborating, as he wrote, rather than cooperating. His principal contribution to administrative institutional psychiatry, which was his creation of the ward milieu program at Sheppard and Enoch Pratt in the late 1920s, seems to have been his first true group experience, the closest working and sharing of ideals with others that he had experienced up to then, in this case with staff and patients, all male. Just as we suspect

---

* Reprinted from *Conceptions of Modern Psychiatry* by Harry Stack Sullivan, M.D. By permission of W. W. Norton & Company, Inc. Copyright 1940, 1945, 1947, 1953 by The William Alanson White Psychiatric Foundation. All other quotes in this chapter with a citation to Note 15 are from the same source and are quoted with permission.

that this was a new reality for Sullivan, so was it meant to be a new reality for the patients, thus to carry them past their earlier life experiences.

However easy it is to see the limitations set to Sullivan's work by his own psychology, how easy it is as well to see the fresh ground he broke! The institutional structure of psychiatry has been for centuries medieval, despotic, at best paternalistic, a monarchy not yet even "constitutional." Pinel's description of the Governor of the Asylum de Bicetre, whom he greatly admired, gives this away immediately. "His firmness is immovable, his courage cool and unshrinking. As to his physical properties, he is manly and well proportioned. His arms are exceedingly strong. When he speaks in anger or displeasure, his countenance expresses great decision and intrepidity, and his voice is that of thunder" [19, pp. 107–108]. Terror, manipulation, and deceit had regular places in treatment, as they still do. Here are two anecdotes from Rush's text, a foremost manual of practice through much of the nineteenth century.

I attended a young man in the year 1806, who cherished an obstinate hypochondriac belief, after his recovery from the autumnal fever, that he should die, and felt at the same time a great dread of death. I assured him over and over that he was in no danger, but without being able to inspire him with the least expectation of life. In one of my visits to him, I asked him, upon entering his room, how he was; "very bad," said he, and repeated his belief that he should soon die. His nurse, who sat by him, added, that he had fixed upon an hour in the approaching night as the time for his dissolution. After pausing a few moments, I asked him if I should send a joiner to measure him for his coffin. This question instantly gave a new current to his feelings, and from that time he recovered rapidly; nor did he ever mention an apprehension of dying to me, in any of my subsequent visits to him [20, pp. 111–112].

A physician, formerly of this city, used to divert his friends, by relating the history of a cure which had been performed of a patient in this form of madness, who believed himself to be a plant. One of his companions, who favoured his delusion, persuaded him he could not thrive without being watered, and while he made the patient believe, for some time, he was pouring water from the spout of a tea-pot, discharged his urine upon his head. The remedy in this case was resentment & mortification [20, p. 110].

The partial substitution by the end of the nineteenth century of medical for religious and moral attitudes in administration did not alter the pattern of authoritarianism. Medicine brought with it, if anything, more titles, classes of personnel, and uniforms, and a greater degree of hierarchy. Patients were, if anything, brought lower in the social order of the hospitals, and the authority of the medical superintendents was unquestionable. One still meets in the state hospitals and the schools for the retarded in the United States degrees of central authority rarely present elsewhere in society.

I mention these features of psychiatric administration (themselves so much a part of the objective psychiatric schools, whether descriptive or psychoanalytic) by way of contrast to what Sullivan introduced. Undoubtedly the contrast is not so stark as one could suggest by juxtaposing the Governor of the Bicetre and Harry Stack Sullivan, for many of the moral treatment era leaders, for example, were as psychologically skilled as they were religiously motivated, and Sullivan could also throw his weight around. But the Sheppard–Enoch Pratt ward pioneered on several fronts.

Sullivan struck toward a *democratization* of mental hospital life—less hierarchy and less authority [21]. He was no pal to his staff or doctors and attendants but he spent much time with them, both socially and as their teacher. Just as he did not want force, fear, and deceit used in the relationships with patients, so he desired that relationships between staff members be as free of these as possible. The goal was a "school" for personality growth, rather than custodianship of personality failures, and the best teachers in that school, he early decided, were those *like the patient*—those who, for example, had had schizophrenic episodes and experienced a favorable outcome. The central element was some equality of experience leading to a feeling of being with, or sympathy for, the patient. (We can contrast this with the existential interest in something more inward and empathic.) It is true that doors were often locked and women kept away (like cures like, the homeopathic principle), although not so far away as they are kept in many mental hospitals and especially prisons. An approach was being made to the egalitarian ideal that would reach its climax in the English mental hospitals of Maxwell Jones [22] and R. D. Laing.

More original (for religious orders have sometimes ordered hospital life along egalitarian lines) were the results of Sullivan's *scientific* interest in the ward. It was a sociological laboratory. Recording equipment was introduced, the better to study interactions; the practical manipulator Sullivan was adept at wiring rooms so that the recording could be done elsewhere and the patient left unaware, at least presumably [23]. Other efforts were being made to observe and record social phenomena and to study the effects of environmental changes, particularly on pathological phenomena.

Of course Sullivan did not unaidedly discover that the actions and attitudes of the observer affect the observed. Bleuler made the point charmingly:

"How much is twice two?" may be a good question but under other circumstances it may suggest to the patient another question, viz., whether the physician is crazy. A test of the sense of pain with needle pricks is something entirely different if the patient is distracted or not, if one dashes at him with the instrument, or first begs him to indicate whether he notices the prick, etc. In short, in these matters one must have some practice and above all native tact and comprehension of the situation and the consequences, otherwise all special directions and details are useless [24, p. 185].

Add to this Wernicke's mention of his surprise at demented patients' *casual* display of knowledge the examiner had searched for in vain by systematic and directive means. These limitations on the power of the traditional objective methods were well known and implied the need for observations of the *context*, "the situation and the consequences," in which pathological phenomena manifested themselves.

To my knowledge, however, Sullivan was the first to create a clinical setting specifically directed at making such social observations, the first to replace the individual examinational and the free associative by systematic sociological methods. The two principal discoveries that resulted, both already suggested in the sociological literature, concern the intercommunication of pathological affects and of pathological ideas. Setting these down will clarify the specific method of the interpersonal school from another perspective.

Meyer had suggested that symptoms were pathological reactions to social and other circumstances. For the next 50 years the words *reaction* and *reaction type* occurred prominently in psychiatric terminology. Characteristic or frequent reactions he called habits. Meyer, together with Muncie and Campbell [25], suggested further that pathological phenomena were attempts at *adjustment* to surrounding circumstances. The idea of an active adaptive function of the symptom was added to the simpler concept of reaction. (Psychoanalysis brought together the same ideas of reaction, habit, and adjustment in the concept of the mechanisms of defense.) Then, as the study of family, institution, and society at large gained momentum, it became possible to ask and answer the question, Adjustment *to what?* The individual might have limited or primitive capacities for adjustment but also extraordinary difficult situations to adjust to. One could not take for granted that the bulk of the pathology lay in either the individual or society. But the most striking result of Sullivan's work was a still further step: Pathology might not lie in either place but in the processes of interaction between them!

The prototypic observation comes from the sociology of crowds. Affects are contagious. By whatever mechanism, strong feelings in one excite strong feelings in others, which in turn may excite even more the source of feeling. In addition, feelings excite the *same* feelings, with the exception that reactive affects may occur, that is, anxiety or anger against the feelings aroused.

To use an example from Sullivanian sociopathology, anxiety on the mother's part elicits anxiety in the child. Similarly, anxiety in either patient or therapist flows to the other, as do anger, affectionate feelings, and the rest [26]. Hence the importance of the feelings surrounding the patient and the patient's learning the results of his own moods. Here are being described powerful upward and downward spirals—fear, for example, breeding fear; friendliness, friendliness (in the language of popular culture, the power of negative and positive feeling and thinking).

Not only are pathological affects intercommunicated, but so are pathological ideas. Hobbes had written that prophecy is itself a great cause of what happens. Experimental studies confirm this comment. We observe powerful effects of expectation on learning, recall, and judgments of others, the so-called self-fulfilling prophecies. This idea, in turn, has a *sociological* counterpart in the idea of vicious circles or negative feedbacks: My expectations shape you, who may in turn confirm or deepen those expectations. Thus paranoid people typically anger others (partly through the contagion of affects just mentioned) and excite reprisals which confirm the paranoid expectations. The result is a "chronification" of symptoms and syndromes. These *active* processes of symptom maintenance make significant change difficult.

Circular pathological processes are everywhere. This patient's obsessional hesitation makes her dull; rejected because of her dullness, she is still more hesitant. Or each party to a relationship discovers something negative about the other early in the relationship; it serves as an excuse, entitlement, or even good reason not to change what the other has discovered and resents, no matter how obviously abrasive. Of course there are also corrective processes, but in view of those that are pathological, we should lose any surprise we have at the frequency and chronicity of much mental illness.

Another sociopathological process has broad implications for hospital, family, and perhaps institutional life in general. This was discovered at Chestnut Lodge, a private mental hospital where Sullivan himself taught. Stanton and Schwartz described the effects of staff disagreements on patients' symptoms; covert disagreements between staff members appeared to deepen illnesses [27]. The intermediate mechanisms between the staff disagreements and the appearance of symptoms are not clear. Perhaps the patients are double-bound—that is, given conflicting signals, which do not admit of a "normal" solution—and symptoms result. In any case, social conflicts relate to symptoms and represent the sociopathological equivalent of what psychoanalysis has contributed to psychopathology. Conflict, especially unconscious conflict, whether intrapsychic or social, constitutes perhaps the main process of symptom formation!

First Meyer, then Sullivan, and next Adelaide Johnson discovered that psychotic delusions and hallucinations were often barely disguised reproductions of actual family experiences. As far back as 1917 [28], Meyer had suggested that catatonia might be a *favorable* adaptation, an improvement over prepsychotic rigidities and a response to an at least difficult world. Later sociopathy was shown to spring from social circumstances, the first mental illness to be thus understood so convincingly. In the experimental laboratory, Harlow and his associates have been able to produce catatonic-like phenomena and sexual aberrations by manipulating the maternal environment of monkeys; monkeys at least can drive each other mad. In short, the *psychiatrie de concierge* has graduated into a full-fledged psychiatric school.

The shift was away from a patient-centered pathology to a society-centered one in the case of social or interpersonal psychiatry, and to an attempted obliteration of subject-object and patient-doctor distinctions in the case of existentialism. The resulting positions stand in clear contrast to both objective schools of descriptive and psychoanalytic psychiatry. One cannot imagine developments more divisive or ones throwing practitioners into sharper dilemmas as to how, in fact, they should practice [29].

II

MAIN CURRENTS OF PSYCHIATRIC DEVELOPMENT

Creating a new theory is not like destroying an old barn and erecting a skyscraper in its place. It is rather like climbing a mountain, gaining new and wider views, discovering unexpected connections. . . . But the point from which we started out still exists, although it appears smaller and forms a tiny part of our broad view.

Albert Einstein

THE CONTRIBUTIONS of the various schools may seem to be unrelated and even contradictory unless one considers the difference in the times, the methods used, and the focus of the observations. Moreover, the innovators of these schools developed their own language, even inventing new vocabularies. The impression of chaos is reinforced by their claims of etiological significance: Schizophrenia must be a metabolic disease; every neurosis is the consequence of sexual repression; psychopathology results from and produces disturbed interpersonal relations. Thus these investigators laid their own foundations for being misunderstood. My present effort to delineate the distinct schools may strengthen the appearance of chaos, this spectacle of a psychiatry riding off in every direction at once.

Nevertheless, all the schools contribute to the main currents in the scientific growth of psychiatry. Chapter 6 sketches temporal development, by which I mean the shift of psychiatric concern from the present only, to include also the past and future, and subsequently, the division of whole lifetimes into distinct phases—infancy, childhood, adolescence, etc.— and the emergence of developmental concepts that relate the phases. In Chapter 7 the tenet of distinct, seemingly unrelated causes reveals itself to be, in actual fact, sequential processes: dissociation, then repression, introjection, and others, as well as physiological and sociological processes. Chapter 8 deals with psychiatry's advance in its relationship to the patient. At first, the patient is a distant alien object, whether hated or revered. He is gradually approached, taken out of holes in the ground and prisons, put in hospitals that are little better than prisons, studied more and feared less. Doctors spend more and more time with their patients. Psychoanalysis lengthens this contact, then itself lengthens. Existential analysis almost merges the lives of doctor and patient; indeed, the doctor gives up part of his interest in relating to people as patients.

The results of practice are measured by our concept of health, and all these heretofore mentioned developments re-shape psychiatric ideals, as revealed in Chapter 9. Madness is at first the grossest disturbance, and most people seem well. Bit by bit illness appears everywhere, and the normal or ideal person becomes the exception. At the same time, the standards of judgment are refined; more and more subtle degradations from full health are observed; we begin to have as many standards or levels of psychological health as we do measures of physical health. Surprisingly, the great schools converge in their ideals, or goals of treatment, which are easily translated back and forth.

6

TEMPORAL DEVELOPMENT

C ASE REPORTS were once mere *vignettes,* brief
sketches shading off into an undisclosed past and future. The reader had no sense of events *unfolding;*
events *occurred* and were left floating in time and space. We
can speak of a real temporal fragmentation and isolation. The
following sentences from Pinel catch the reader's interest for
a moment, but that interest, like the patient himself, soon
recedes, and ends, as the description does, in uneasy quiet.
Something turbulent, without meaning, has passed by, what
Pinel called "a perfect image of chaos." We can hold our
attention only with difficulty to an experience so little understood.

He came up to me, looked at me, and overwhelmed me with a torrent of words, without order or connection. In a moment he turned to another person, whom in his turn he deafened with his unmeaning babble or threatened with an evanescent look of anger; but, as incapable of determined and continued excitement of the feelings as of a just connection of ideas, his emotions were of a momentary effervescence, which was immediately succeeded by a calm. If he went into a room he quickly displaced or overturned the furniture, without manifesting any direct intention. Scarcely could one look off, before he would be at a considerable distance, exercising his versatile mobility in some other way. He was quiet only when food was presented to him. He rested, even at night, but for a few moments [1, pp. 163–164].

We are told nothing about the patient beyond these striking present phenomena.

The past was entered not only because it was past, and therefore germane to the present, but because it contained some part of the present in largely unchanged form. Watch Pinel now as he follows almost fixed phenomena over a great stretch of time.

An only son of a weak and indulgent mother, was encouraged in the gratification of every caprice and passion, of which an untutored and violent temper was susceptible. The impetuosity of his disposition increased with his years. The money with which he was lavishly supplied, removed every obstacle to his wild desires. Every instance of opposition or resistance roused him to acts of fury. He assaulted his adversary with the audacity of a savage; sought to reign by force, and was perpetually embroiled in disputes and quarrels. If a dog, a horse, or any other animal offended him, he instantly put it to death. If ever he went to a fete or any other public meeting, he was sure to excite such tumults and quarrels, as terminated in actual pugilistic encounters, and he generally left the scene with a bloody nose. This wayward youth, however, when unmoved by passions, possessed a perfectly sound judgment. When he came of age, he succeeded to the possession of an extensive domain. He proved himself fully competent to the management of his estate, as well as to the discharge of his relative duties; and he even distinguished himself by acts of beneficence and compassion. Wounds, law-suits, and pecuniary compensations, were generally the consequences of his unhappy propensity to quarrel. But an act of notoriety put an end to his career of violence. Enraged at a woman who had used offensive language to him, he precipitated her into a well. Prosecution commenced against him, and on the deposition of a great many witnesses, who gave evidence to his furious deportment, he was condemned to perpetual confinement at Bicetre [1, p. 115].

The economy of detail of these early accounts is striking. It it as if everything were explained by knowing the patient hallucinated, was incoherent, or had a fierce temper! And perhaps it did seem so, once these frightening behaviors were observed; at least the observer might not be ready to take in much else for a while. It is true that hysterical and many depressed patients were known in greater detail, but the outstanding fact is how sparse these early reports were, as if the whole picture could be painted with one stroke.

Gradually the present and the past filled up with more and more details. Investigators adapted to the darkness of mad people and could see more. At first details were noticed simply because they were there, without any sense of meaning or connection. One picks up a great deal in the hope of finding something valuable and then, having no understanding of what is important, can put nothing down. The result is a crowded, static, but at the same time eye-darting landscape, reminiscent of Bosch or Brueghel. Here is an illustration from Pinel's great student Esquirol, who took psychiatry several steps forward but still faced mainly chaos.

A woman, about 58 years of age, of a strong constitution and sanguine temperament, had become a mother by M. R., at whose house she lived as door-tender. This was a source of deep mortification to her. She afterwards experienced gastro-intestinal affections, and became a bigot. The events of the revolution, concurred, with the cessation of the catamenia, to produce an attack of mania. She was brought to the Salpêtrière where she passed many years. In stature she was small, her neck thick and short, her mind strong, and she was of a very full habit. There was something mysterious in the expression of her countenance, and she complained of pains at the epigastrium, which was sensitive to the touch. She had copious eructations, and was often affected with dysmenorrhoea. Habitually calm, she occupied herself in sewing. They called her in the hospital the *Mother of the Church,* because she constantly talked on the subject of religion. She attributes her sufferings to the wickedness of Pontius Pilate, . . . (the father of her child). This infamous wretch has taken up his abode in her bowels. She sees him there, and every time that she meets me, she beseeches me to expel him. She believes also, that she has in her belly all the personages named in the New Testament, and sometimes even those of the whole Bible. She often says to me, "I can hold out no longer; when will the peace of the church come!" If her pains are exasperated, she repeats to me with imperturbable coolness, "Today the crucifixion of Jesus Christ takes place; I hear the blows of the hammer with which the nails are driven." She believes that the popes hold their council in her bowels. Nothing can dissipate illusions so strange [2, pp. 114–115].

Our minds connect the employer-father of her illegitimate pregnancy, her Motherhood of the Church, the hallucinatory personages she harbored, and the threatened parturition, but to even the extraordinary Esquirol such connections would have seemed as strange as the illusions themselves.

Perhaps we should think of temporal development more microscopically, as involving all the moment-to-moment events and the emerging connections between them, which slowly reduce the chaos. Sometimes these connecting ideas are hardly conscious, yet we sense meaning in the descriptions. No one better represents this phase of temporal development than Emil Kraepelin, for his descriptions encompass vast masses of detail (indeed, individual case examples are often lost sight of). We are left with an awareness of unity difficult to validate by specific connecting ideas, as in fact it remained for

Bleuler and Freud to supply; but with Kraepelin there is this growing sense of connection. Here is one of his descriptions of a patient, not unlike the first one from Pinel.

. . . You see a servant-girl, aged twenty-four, upon whose features and frame traces of great emaciation can be plainly seen. In spite of this, the patient is in continual movement, going a few steps forwards, and then back again; she plaits her hair only to unloose it the next minute. On attempting to stop her movement, we meet with unexpectedly strong resistance; if I place myself in front of her with my arms spread out in order to stop her, if she cannot push me on one side, she suddenly turns and slips through under my arms, so as to continue her way. If one takes firm hold of her, she distorts her usually rigid, expressionless features with deplorable weeping, that only ceases so soon as one lets her have her own way. We notice besides that she holds a crushed piece of bread spasmodically clasped in the fingers of the left hand, which she absolutely will not allow to be forced from her. The patient does not trouble in the least about her surroundings so long as you leave her alone. If you prick her in the forehead with a needle, she scarcely winces or turns away, and leaves the needle quietly sticking there without letting it disturb her restless, beast-of-prey-like wandering backwards and forwards. To questions she answers almost nothing, at the most shaking her head. But from time to time she wails: "O dear God! O dear God! O dear mother! O dear mother!" always repeating uniformly the same phrases. If you try to grasp her hand she draws it away very suddenly, and at last, if she can no longer avoid you, begins to roll it up in her apron. Orders are of no use; on the contrary she resists in everything you try to do with her. But when she quickly hides her hand if one speaks of taking away the bread, it becomes evident that she understands what is happening around her [3, pp. 30–31].

This description begins to flow. Kraepelin has sufficiently mastered the case details to connect them, largely by contrasts or contradictions. Seemingly senseless and demented, yet the patient "understands what is happening around her." Emaciated, she moves constantly. Kraepelin intervenes and finds her strongly resistant. At other times she is passive; pricked on the forehead, she scarcely winces and leaves the needle sticking there. The description is held together by this tension of opposites, as if her mind were a needle swinging between magnetic poles.

Kraepelin grasped this fact of deep psychological contradictions, of sharp mental shifts from moment to moment or year to year. Each of the two great pathological entities, schizophrenia and manic-depressive psychosis, that he more than anyone established, rests on observed contrasts. The schizophrenic patients were most remarkable not so much for their bizarre ideas and postures as for the presence of such bizarre phenomena in people otherwise oriented and intelligent. The contrast was between the most bizarre of delusions and an often clear or superior intelligence. How like the *idiots savants* who know the day of the week June 15, 1999, falls on but cannot make change! Mental life is capable of extraordinary specializations and contradictions.

Similarly, the concept of manic-depressive psychosis rests on a play of opposites. Mania and depression had been noted to follow each other closely and repeatedly. The French school described all sorts of variations—mania followed by depression with or without free intervals, several depressions and then a manic attack, etc.—and Kraepelin collected the whole into his concept of maniacal-depressive insanity. Mania and depression *are* opposites. The manic person's mood, thoughts, and actions are all elevated and speeded while the depressed person's are lowered and slowed, so that again striking antitheses emerge close together in mental life. We see a point of connection made out of the very clarity of difference!

I stress this concept of related opposites because it became and persisted as one of the principal ideas by which phenomena could be connected over time. Rush had observed that many patients going mad became the opposite of what they had been like before. There are cases, he wrote, "in which

persons of exemplary piety and purity of character utter pro-
fane, or impious, or indelicate language, and behave in other
respects contrary to their moral habits" [4]. Except for noting
that acute illnesses might also be the *exaggeration* of personal
characteristics present before and that the ideas of the sick
person related to events apparently precipitant, Rush had
literally no other psychological concepts by which dissimilar
phenomena could be connected.

The various traits and personalities taken up by hysterical
patients in fugues and somnambulisms are among the most
dramatic contrasts in all psychiatry, contrasts that Janet loved
to illustrate:

> A man of thirty-two, Sm., presents a still more singular case. He
> usually remains in bed, for both his legs are paralyzed. In the mid-
> dle of the night he rises slowly, jumps lightly out of bed—for the
> paralysis we have just spoken of has quite vanished—takes his
> pillow and hugs it. We know by his countenance and by his words
> that he mistakes this pillow for his child, and that he believes he
> is saving his child from the hands of his mother-in-law. Then,
> bearing that weight, he tries to slip out of the room, opens the
> door, and runs out through the court-yard; climbing along the
> gutter, he gets to the housetop, carrying his pillow and running all
> about the buildings of the hospital with marvelous agility. One
> must take great care to catch him, and use all sorts of cautions to
> get him down, for he wakes with a stupefied air, and as soon as he
> is awake, both his legs are paralyzed again, and he must be carried
> to his bed. He does not understand what you are speaking about,
> and cannot comprehend how it happens that people were obliged
> to go to the top of the house in order to look for a poor man who
> has been paralyzed in his bed for months [5, pp. 28–29].

Paralysis on the one hand, "marvelous agility" on the other.
Janet had the same explanation Kraepelin took over from
Wernicke and Bleuler: personality is capable of "dissociating"
into parts. (But how little the word *dissociation* illuminates
the *degree* of contrast!) These hysterical patients might not

fall in ruins like the schizophrenic ones, but their "mental weakness" led to conflicting, contradictory traits and personalities, and Janet left the matter there.

So did Kraepelin. He made no effort to *resolve* the contradictions. He did not, for example, suggest that mania and depression might be related, one as "defense" against the other, a later hypothesis of connection. Although he accepted Wernicke's and Bleuler's concept of a dissociating process, he did not take the additional step Bleuler took, toward an "ambivalent" process, a deep-running *clash* of opposites, which Freud was to make his central engine of mental illness.

EVOLUTION IN PSYCHIATRY

As we have seen already, it was in hysterical cases that the first successful efforts were made to connect events over time by principles other than contrast and similarity. Charcot's pathogenic sequence in hysteria and its hypothetical disease process connected heterogeneous phenomena up to then considered separately. Freud extended the pathogenic sequences far backward in time, uncovered types of phenomena, notably evidences of sexual wishes, that caused as much conflict within the profession as they did within the patients, and then expanded Charcot's insight into a theory of normal and pathological developments. The idea of *evolution* had entered psychiatry, as it had earlier entered biology and geology; progression and regression related changes over time. True, the power of Freud's ideas reduced complex phenomena too quickly to a few elements, so that whole human lives, even whole families, seemed simply illustrations of the Oedipus complex or the repetition compulsion. In these cases the psychoanalytic armies had outrun their sources of supply—even if for a moment everything had seemed theirs—and would have to fall back on more modest frontiers. But temporal development had entered its maturity.

Movement outside the present required access to the past and the future, which one might liken to a great darkness through which the present travels like a tiny light. The past was illuminated first by recollections, then by repeated examinations over time, hypnosis, free associations, more and more intimate interactions with patients, relatives, and friends, as well as by comparing notes among the relatives. Still more recently children have been observed from birth on, so that the patient's past could be open to all the methods of studying the present. Entering the future required, most of all, stable communities and unchanging commitment. The patients needed to remain available and trust the investigators enough to go on talking. Some patients could be followed because they were in institutions, but then no one knew what was illness and what was hospital; many institutions have been such as to drive strong men mad. Records must be well kept, and patient, long-lived investigators must want to read them. Because all these conditions existed for them, it was possible for German and Scandinavian workers to do the most thorough longitudinal studies, while the British stayed behind their hedges and the Americans were forever moving.

Perhaps we have gone too far already in the presentation of temporal development without making clear the different methods in use at every step. Of course, we seldom know what the original investigators actually did—how they looked or how much they talked, whether they touched the patients or listened for long periods. Like a surveyor reconstructing land points, I can only infer from descriptions of what they saw where they must have stood. We have seen how the various school methods were gradually refined and even, I suppose, occasionally practiced as they were preached. From today's record-and-method-conscious age will come transcripts, tapes, and movies, to do for psychological investigators what was once done for politicians and poets, breathing tinnily for all time. No matter how difficult it may be to do so, we must continue to reconstruct the different methods or the reader will infer a homogeneity or simplicity of approaches when, in fact, by the time of Charcot, psychiatry had begun to break into well-demarcated schools with their own special methods.

Charcot stood at a critical intersection of modern psychiatry not only because he commanded, simultaneously, neurological *and* psychological ideas but because he both observed and listened. This is no easy feat. Nature says, If you want to know me, pat your head and rub your stomach, and psychopathological nature adds, Do it while the neighbors look on and the children laugh. The *observer* looks, searches, pokes, and disappears suddenly down alleys to follow footprints. He must be active, watchful, a great visualizer, with an eye for detail. The *listener,* on the other hand, attends, but quietly, lest he disrupt or divert the emerging scene. Details must be *brought* to the listener, as Sherlock Holmes, the observer, brought lines of fact to his listening brother Mycroft. If I watch too closely, the listener says, my wary quarry will feel watched and disappear, so I must be hardly there, a subtle presence able to pick up slight vibrations but not so intrusive as to disturb them. Psychiatrists, therefore, observe *or* listen, think *or* feel, seek objectivity *or* closeness, neutrality *or* partisanship, in keeping with the demands of their school allegiances.

CONTRIBUTIONS OF THE SCHOOLS

The schools, then, contribute to temporal development separately. Psychoanalysis is centrally concerned with infancy and childhood and seeks to reconstruct the individual's past. Meyer studied his patients' lives from their beginnings but did not give a dominant influence to childhood, nor did he have much faith in predictions about the future from the disease model. On the contemporary scene, Erikson unites psychoanalytic and Meyerian themes, emphasizing both childhood and successive adaptational tasks. It is an irony of psychiatric history that a psychiatrist of adults, Freud, laid out a valuable developmental scheme for children, while a psychoanalyst of children, Erikson, laid out the scheme for adults [6]. Psychiatrists just cannot mind their own business!

Existential psychiatry, attempting to be and stay where the patient is, immerses the investigator in the felt experience and decision needs of the patient. It seems, therefore, present-bound but in fact aims for a complex relationship to time, using the past, living in the present, maintaining movement into the future.

With Kahlbaum and Kraepelin a deep-running prognostic interest entered descriptive psychiatry. Patients were followed up over several decades, and much came to depend on the longevity of the investigator. The course of diseases over time meant, in the beginning, little more than the course of the signs and symptoms noted first in the present, as I have illustrated earlier. The past was not listened to because it was past. Thus diseases were partly named by the times of life in which they occurred—for example, involutional melancholia and dementia praecox. Gradually more and more phenomena besides symptoms and signs came to comprise psychiatric data, until it was necessary to speak of clinical biographies or pathographies. And genetic studies extended still further psychiatry's temporal commitments: disease states were to be traced back through the generations. But throughout, objective-descriptive psychiatry looked to the past and future only insofar as they contained the illness.

The changing status of the present in the development of objective-descriptive psychiatry is nicely illustrated by psychiatric prognosticating. When the idea of typical disease courses had been established, signs were sought for each disease course. At first the present was searched: What in the examination foretells the future? There appears to be no limit to what people can hope for in this crystal gazing, but the actual fruits have been few. *Past* behavior, what the patient has been able to do socially and vocationally, the duration of the illness, whatever appears to have precipitated the illness—these give the most secure guides. Once the present is understood as a moment in time against the long stretches of the past and future, we should lose any expectation of its telling us much.

Psychoanalysis has concerned itself centrally with the influence of the past on the present—the influence of the past as primitive but persistent wishes or instincts and the past as memories, old attachments, what experience has left behind in the nervous system, on present thought, actions, feelings. It is less interested in the impact of the present on the present, and least of all in the influence of the future on the present, the impact of expectation, goals, ideals, the existential world-as-becoming. Psychoanalysis seeks the fullest possible *reconstruction* of the past, in the sense of clarifying both persistent wishes and the structure of the past as it was experienced. Again, by way of contrast, in psychoanalysis the present is not seen as actively and continuously reconstructing the past except as it distorts a real fixed past; there is a static element to the past of psychoanalysis which allies this school with objective-descriptive psychiatry. This fixed past is to be brought forward, so to speak, from the relatively inarticulate or unconscious place it has been put. Every effort to make the reconstructive process more complete also makes it more prolonged, so that psychoanalysis itself becomes part of the patient's past (in some cases one psychoanalysis becomes a major subject matter of the next psychoanalysis) and molds the characteristic reactions of the patient along the very lines of the psychoanalytic reconstructive methodology—specifically, reflectiveness, deliberateness, a new sense of the past. Many features of the psychoanalytic method become part of the patient's intimate prolonged experience. We have here a freeing from the past and the simultaneous part-provision of a new past which is meant to shape the future more happily. The present is, to a large extent, put aside in this construction and reconstruction. Indeed, it is replaced by a fresh concept of moratorium or therapeutic abstinence while the new lines between the past and the future are being laid down. This is only a partial delay or abstinence, however, for a treatment experience takes the place of life experience, a treatment experience which is successful insofar as it gains the intensity of a life experience. The transference neurosis is also a real neurosis and must make difficulties for the analyst nearly comparable to those made for others in the patient's life.

In contrast to the psychoanalytic emphasis on the childhood past and the treatment-experience present, Meyer, Sullivan, and most richly and recently Erikson encourage us to study *successive presents*. They have extended the concept of development beyond childhood (where psychoanalysis, like the Jesuits, left it) into adolescence, through adulthood, into middle age, to the very end of life. These successive presents, with their particular tasks and problems, take on an importance psychoanalysis had assigned largely to the childhood past. And because treatment must occur in the midst of one or more of these successive present tasks, it must be in part oriented to the outside present world, not only as the locus of the repetition of the past, as in psychoanalytic reconstruction, but as posing new problems which have no anlagen in the past. (This is Erikson's approach whether he is writing of Gandhi or of the play of a child.) The social psychiatrists and Erikson, who like Sullivan is also a psychoanalyst, direct attention both outward and backward, with necessary strain on the clinical decision of when to emphasize one or the other.

Erikson writes eloquently of the moratorium periods of life. He gives us an understanding of the treatment situation, however, which sharply restricts the analytic moratorium, for life goes on. This worker also challenges what Freud himself had already challenged, the possibility of psychotherapeutic termination: Adult life, being developmental, successive, novel, not simply a residue of childhood, must offer opportunities for neurotic and psychotic solutions ended only by death.

Freud saw some periods of life as containing more development than others, especially childhood; the process of change is not continuous. But as usual, he had an alternative way of conceptualizing this: Perhaps it was as accurate to say that a fresh process of change—that is, decay—speeded up during the course of life as it was to say that processes of growth slowed down. Phenomenology has pointed out this speeding up of the subjective experience of time. Certainly we speed up in the rate of losing things, whether our hair or our friends! Freud made no decision between these alternatives.

Even the Freudian and Eriksonian extension of the temporal developmental interest of psychiatry to death does not, however, close out the contributions of the schools. Existential psychiatry throws new light on temporal development, but from the standpoint of the *present-future,* words I use to refer to the continuous flow into the future, the time of existential psychiatry.

The successive presents of Meyer and Sullivan, as well as of Erikson, are challenged by existential psychiatry as too schematic, as freezing real time into intellectual categories and making impossible the solution of the very problems or tasks described. The same or even harsher criticism had already fallen on psychoanalysis, with its relatively static past, and would fall on any school not grasping this existential present-future. Our attitude toward the future, Binswanger wrote, shapes both the present and the past; what we remember, how we reconstruct the past, is shaped by our relationship to the future. A host of fresh problems entered psychiatry with this interest, notably the problems centering on values, of both therapist and patient, because values concern future directions and goals.

History is constantly being created. This is not to say it is undetermined, but a principal determinant of what happens is the "decision quality of human existence." The past as a determinant of the present and future ignores this present-decision quality, existential psychiatry says, and throws both the investigative and treatment emphases of psychiatry too much into the past.

Here Freud, that great archeologist of the dead hand of the past, stands beside Binswanger and Minkowski, who would move men into the future. Each deals delicately with the other, Binswanger respecting that the past clings and Freud writing of the battle of life-forces against repetition and death; and Freud's fear that our values, however nobly proclaimed, reflect old issues and urges matching Binswanger's fear that the study of the past will become an end in itself and freeze us and the past together.

Meanwhile, the Eriksonian psychiatry of successive presents puts between the psychiatry of the past and that of the future a continually changing panorama which neither the past nor the future exhausts. At once schematic and developmental, like psychoanalysis, it insists on a flowing, never altogether repetitive, endlessly novel human experience, being in these ways like existential psychiatry. Thus each school illuminates a part of time, gives its attention to one part to the neglect of others, but the total result is a great spreading out or differentiation of the concept of lifetimes. It would be as easy now to write a "special psychiatry" of *life periods* as it has been to use the established categories of the disease states [7]. Grant that middle age has not yet attracted its investigators, despite the rich psychopathology of paranoia and depression characteristic of that period, and that between middle and old age lies a period so far even unnamed. Nor is the study of any one time ever completed. Human life evolves. The character of adolescence changes, and adolescence is prolonged. There are vastly more old people, who live longer. In addition, fresh understanding of any time throws new light on all the other times. But the point is, psychiatry has impressively strengthened its temporal grasp of human life [8].

7

CAUSES

W E C A N O B S E R V E a comparable development in the understanding of causes. I will describe how psychiatry gradually sharpens and deepens its "etiologies" and how it does so through the method-specific investigations of the different schools, and I will show that the result is a complex, internally dynamic, even contradictory picture that must leave the practical man asking, What is most important; what shall I emphasize now?

BURTON

Let us start with Burton's (1620) synopsis of the causes of melancholy, by which he meant almost all mental illness except mania and dementia [1]. Note the great crowding of details, an encyclopedic quality, as if anything and everything could be a cause. We are hard put to find relationships of any kind among these fragments.

The discussions under each section and subsection are very detailed, as in his description of six kinds of subterranean dev-

BURTON'S SYNOPSIS

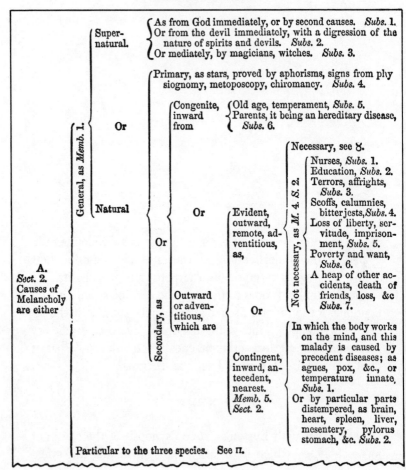

II. Particular causes. Sect. 2. Memb. 5.

Of head Melancholy are, Subs. 3.

Inward
- Innate humour, or from distemperature adust.
- A hot brain, corrupted blood in the brain.
- Excess of venery, or defect.
- Agues, or some precedent disease.
- Fumes arising from the stomach, &c.

or Outward
- Heat of the sun immoderate.
- A blow on the head.
- Overmuch use of hot wines, spices, garlic, onions, hot baths, overmuch waking, &c.
- Idleness, solitariness, or overmuch study, vehement labour, &c.
- Passions, perturbations, &c.

Of hypochondriacal, or windy Melancholy are,

Inward — Default of spleen, belly, bowels, stomach, mesentery, miseraic veins, liver, &c.

or — Months or hemorrhoids stopped, or any other ordinary evacuation.

Outward — Those six non-natural things abused.

Over all the body are, Subs. 5.

Inward — Liver distempered, stopped, over-hot, apt to engender melancholy, temperature innate.

or Outward. — Bad diet, suppression of hemorrhoids, &c., and such evacuations, passions, cares, &c., those six non-natural things abused.

ᵟ Necessary causes, as those six non-natural things, which are, Sect. 2. Memb. 2.

Diet offending in Subs. 3.

Substance
- Bread; coarse and black, &c.
- Drink; thick, thin, sour, &c.
- Water unclean, milk, oil, vinegar, wine, spices, &c.
- Flesh { Parts; heads, feet, entrails, fat, bacon, blood, &c. Kinds, { Beef, pork, venison, hares, goats, pigeons, peacocks, fen-fowl, &c.
- Herbs, Fish, &c. { Of fish; all shell-fish, hard and slimy fish, &c. Of herbs; pulse, cabbage, melons, garlick, onions, &c. All roots, raw fruits, hard and windy meats.

Quality, as in — Preparing, dressing, sharp sauces, salt meats, indurate, soused, fried, broiled, or made dishes, &c.

Quantity
- Disorder in eating, immoderate eating, or at unseasonable times, &c., Subs. 2.
- Custom; delight, appetite, altered, &c., Subs. 3.

Retention and evacuation, Subs. 4. — Costiveness, hot baths, sweating, issues stopped, Venus in excess, or in defect, phlebotomy, purging, &c.

Air; hot, cold, tempestuous, dark, thick, foggy, moorish, &c., Subs. 5.

Exercise, Subs. 6. — Unseasonable, excessive, or defective, of body or mind, solitariness, idleness, a life out of action, &c.

Sleep and waking, unseasonable, inordinate, overmuch, overlittle, &c., Subs. 7.

Memb. 3. Sect. 2. Passions and perturbations of the mind. Subs. 2. With a digression of the force of imagination. Subs. 2., and division of passions into, Subs. 3.

Irascible — Sorrow, cause and symptom, Subs. 4. Fear, cause and symptom, Subs. 5. Shame, repulse, disgrace, &c., Subs. 6. Envy and malice, Subs. 7. Emulation, hatred, faction, desire of revenge, Subs. 8. Anger a cause, Subs. 9. Discontents, cares, miseries, &c., Subs. 10.

or

concupiscible — Vehement desires, ambition, Subs. 11. Covetousness, φιλαργυρίαν, Subs. 12. Love of pleasures, gaming in excess, &c., Subs. 13. Desire of praise, pride, vainglory, &c., Subs. 14. Love of learning, study in excess, with a digression of the misery of scholars, and why the muses are melancholy, Subs. 15.

ils. Yet for all the superstitiousness and partly tongue-in-cheek religiosity, Burton warns against overstating the importance of supernatural and astral causes. There are innumerable "references" to learned authorities (this is a "review"), but the charm of the book lies as much in his thrusting aside these authorities as in their quaint opinions: Burton respects local, immediate, human physical causes, for example, of the melancholy of maids, nurses, and widows.

The several cures of this infirmity, concerning diet, which must be very sparing, phlebotomy, physic, internal, external remedies, are at large in great variety in Rodericus a Castro, Sennertus, and Mercatus, which whoso will, as occasion serves, may make use of. But the best and surest remedy of all, is to see them well placed, and married to good husbands in due time, *hinc illae lachrymae*, that is the primary cause, and this the ready cure, to give them content to their desires.

Some of his distinctions now seem outlandish: head versus windy melancholy, or natural versus supernatural. Others remain in use; inward and adventitious correspond to today's endogenous, exogenous, process, and reactive. Although he suggested a sequential process by the distinction remote versus nearest, the overwhelming impression is of unrelated causes. Burton breaks every rule you make about him, but for the most part he gives arbitrary groupings and almost no clear lines or sequences of events.

BENJAMIN RUSH

Compare Benjamin Rush's (1812) discussion of causes. Here is my summary of his causes of all the "diseases of the mind":

All causes are remote, exciting, or predisposing. Rush quickly combines the first two "inasmuch as they commonly act in concert." They are divided "1, into such as act *directly* upon the body; and 2, such as act indirectly upon the body, through the mind."

In addition, there are certain local brain disorders, brain diseases, insolation (sunstroke), certain odours: "There is a place in Scotland where madness is sometimes induced by the fumes of lead."

There are also "causes which induce madness by acting upon the brain in common with the *whole* body"—for example, gout, dropsy, "the sudden abstraction of the stimulus of distension," as having a baby; "the excessive use of ardent spirits, inordinate sexual desires and gratifications," great pain, extremely hot and cold weather.

Madness can also be induced by corporeal causes acting *sympathetically* on the brain: certain narcotic substances, worms in the alimentary canal, "metastasis" of some other disease to the brain, hysteria ("the morbid commotions in the nervous system are sometimes transferred to the blood-vessels and the brain where they induce transient or chronic madness"—in short, hysterical psychosis).

Certain causes induce intellectual derangement by acting upon the body through the medium of the mind, directly or indirectly, for example, intense study, the imagination ("the great extent and constant exercises of the imagination in poets, accounts for their being occasionally affected with this disease"), joy, anger, fear, delicacy ("a school master went mad after being discovered upon a close-stool by one of his scholars") [2, pp. 30–73].

Rush quotes a physician who himself suffered from melancholy, what Rush calls tristimania: "When no air has blown across my affairs, and no shade observed my sun, then am I most miserable."

In all such cases it would be absurd to suppose the disease existed without a cause. Many diseases take place in the body from causes that are forgotten, or from sympathies with parts of the body that are supposed to be in a healthy state. In like manner, depression of mind may be induced by causes that are forgotten, or by the presence of objects which revive the sensation of distress with which it was at one time associated, but without reviving the cause of it in the memory [2, p. 46].

Intellectual derangement, he wrote, is more common from mental than corporeal causes.

Of 113 patients in the Bicetre Hospital, in France, at one time, Mr. Pinel tells us 34 were from domestic misfortunes, 24 from disappointments in love, 30 from the distressing events of the French Revolution, and 25 from what he calls fanaticism, making in all the original number. I have taken pains to ascertain the proportion of mental and corporeal causes which have operated in producing madness in the Pennsylvania Hospital, but I am sorry to add, my success in the inquiry was less satisfactory than I wished. Its causes were concealed in some instances, and forgotten in others. Of 50 maniacs, the causes of whose disease were discovered by Dr. Moore and his assistant Mr. Jenney, in the month of April 1812, 7 were from disappointments, chiefly in love; 7 from grief; 7 from the loss of property; 5 from erroneous opinions in religion; 2 from jealousy; 1 from terror; 1 from insolation; 1 from an injury to the head; 2 from repelled eruptions; 5 from intemperance; 3 from onanism; 2 from pregnancy; and 1 from fever; making in all 34 from mental, and 16 from corporeal causes [2, pp. 46–47].

Then he lists [3] "all those circumstances in birth, certain peculiarities of the body, age, sex, condition and rank in life, intellect, occupation, climate, state of society," etc., which "*predispose* the body and mind to be acted upon by the remote and exciting causes that have been mentioned." For example:

Dr. Burton, in his *Anatomy of Melancholy*, remarks that children born of parents who are in the decline of life, are more predisposed to one of the forms of partial insanity than children born under contrary circumstances [2, p. 52].

A predisposition to madness is said to be connected with dark coloured hair [2, p. 54].

There is a greater predisposition to madness between 20 and 50. Madness seldom occurs under puberty. Single people are more predisposed to madness than married people. Madness seldom occurs in Spain or Russia (all these claims being supported by numbers) [2, pp. 50–70].

Finally, "the predisposing causes of madness . . . sometimes act with so much force as to induce it without the perceptible cooperation of a remote or exciting cause" [2, p. 73].

Note that astrological and demonological causes have dropped out. The physiological notions are better developed than Burton's, although for Rush every other cause finally acts through disorder of the vascular system (for Pinel it was the gastrointestinal system); hence Rush's profuse, often deadly, bloodletting. More impressive is his reference to experience and numbers; authorities are seldom mentioned unless they have an experience to report.

Also, the faint sequence implied in Burton's remote and nearest has become Rush's remote, exciting, and predisposing causes, a clearer ordering into sequences of events, almost a process. Further, a reciprocal relationship is claimed between Rush's precipitating events, whether remote or exciting, and his predisposing events, so that great strength in one means less strength is needed in the other.

PROCESSES

Once this point had been reached [4]—that is, the recognition that one event may gain in significance from setting in motion another (and not just as a theoretical possibility found in Aristotle, but illustrated by psychopathological events)—advances could occur in two directions: as discoveries of previously hidden relationships among temporally ordered but apparently separate events, or as discoveries of relationships between seemingly separate sequences themselves, for example, between psychological and physical or sociological sequences. These relationships were called processes.

We have already encountered Charcot's hypothesis of a process linking trauma, emotion-fixed ideas, changes in consciousness, and the symptoms. He assumed that the process fermented largely unseen, like the physical processes he had observed in the body, that it required time (hence the *intervalle d'élaboration* or incubation period) and might show itself in unexpected ways. One event did not simply exert an effect on another, like dominoes falling over; this was the point Rush had reached. Events were signs of processes already going on, or events themselves set processes in motion. It became difficult to think of causes at all with that concept's implication of discrete or isolated effects.

Almost from the start students of mental illness had argued the relative importance of physical, psychological, and sociological factors; not everyone had Burton's catholic tastes. The various schools, collecting different types of information, tended to assign etiological significance to whatever each discovered [5]. Thus objective-descriptive psychiatry observed bodily processes, whether catatonic gestures or signs of infection; Kraepelin gave great significance to the first and was ever ready to propose analogies to the second. Psychoanalysis, in contrast, collected fantasy material and therefore assumed that fantasies, especially conflictual fantasies, were critical causes; the processes assumed were psychological (although in Freud's parallelism fantasies were the psychic representatives of biological forces). Interpersonal psychiatry, studying the social matrix of illness, gave society responsibility; its processes were social. (Twentieth-century American work too, whether in social psychiatry, psychoanalysis, or behaviorism, has emphasized the shaping that personality receives from social experience.) Finally, existential psychiatry, studying expectations, values, the "decision quality of human existence," made them the shaping forces; man is free, his decisions form him; the past seems decisive only because, viewed from the present, it is settled, memorial; we forget the unsettled quality it had from moment to moment.

A few great figures, like Burton and Charcot, see across the boundaries. Charcot's sequence included psychic, social, and physical events, and he hypothesized both psychological and physiological processes. He even tried to put them together, in the concept of a "dynamic, functional, cortical lesion." Freud, too, struggled to keep biological and psychological problems together, but his data, unlike Charcot's, were largely psychological.

In short, the method-specific investigations of the schools limit the investigators, as is illustrated by the various meanings given the term *process*, which also illustrate the gradual advance of knowledge.

Kraepelin's *verblodungsprocesse* was only a little less mysterious than the old uterine pathogenic process of the Greeks. It is true that *verblodungsprocesse* had analogies to real physical processes, metabolic or infectious, cretinism or syphilis. On the other hand, it lacked the nice point-by-point relevance hysteria had to the clinical syndrome of the uterine hypothesis: Kraepelin's process had no specific clinical implications, except for prognosis. Wernicke's sejunction and Bleuler's dissociative process were a little step forward. Both suggested that some unknown, perhaps toxic, process might fragment the mind, at the synapses or between large areas of brain function, producing incoherence or a splitting of thought from emotion or from appropriate action; the nature of the process was related to clinical phenomena. Wernicke and Bleuler remained faithful to the objective-descriptive school's expectation that disease processes must be physical, but both picked from Kraepelin's endless symptom lists many of the same psychological phenomena to be fundamental. The physical process had to explain these.

Janet's functional loss or degradation process did for neuroses what Wernicke's and Bleuler's suggestion did for psychoses. Neurotics lacked sufficient energy (life-force or élan vital—all were contemporary notions) to maintain the higher *integrative* function, Janet suggested. Put negatively, neurotics *dissociate,* permitting lower, more primitive functions to emerge. For example, one of the highest human functions, that is, a function requiring integration of many lesser functions, Janet called "the function of the real": our capacity to relate to reality; the negative is Bleuler's autism. Janet found this function disturbed in all mental illness, discretely in hysteria, diffusely in psychasthenia, most severely in the dementias. In short, Janet broadened Charcot's dissociative process to include many new clinical observations and related it to the then popular ideas of energy and evolutionary stages.

Freud, in turn, replaced these general process conceptions (dissociation was being used to explain nearly everything) with less inclusive processes better related to specific clinical events. Thus the depressive-introjective process of *Mourning and Melancholia* connected loss, hallucinatory replacement, self-accusations, and suicide in a time-consuming flow. Freud could have included Charcot's step, the *intervalle d'élaboration,* but at this point processes were assumed to take time. Similarly, the paranoid-projective process connected fantasies of becoming the other sex, rapid displacements, loving and hating feelings toward father, god, doctor, elaborate megalomanic and paranoid delusions, in what remains one of the least understood but most promising conceptions in all psychiatry. As I have detailed in Chapter 3, pathogenic sequences were being discovered and then explained by pathological processes, which Freud pushed farther and farther back in time. This was another step in the series of steps already sketched, from single causes poorly related, to successive causes acting on one another, and then to underlying processes; finally the underlying processes were differentiated and related to more specific events. *Process* was not a word that psychoanalysis took up strongly, but the popular adjective *dynamic* made the same point.

At what time Freud's step is taken depends in part on when the description of the symptom or syndrome is agreed on. Thus the classic American description of psychopathy does not appear until 20 years after Bleuler's description of schizophrenia, and Cleckley's description, like Bleuler's, includes an explanation that we might guess would be the concept dissociation. Thereafter, other investigators, notably Adelaide Johnson, provided more specific processes, for example, defective superego formation, a process which like introjection or projection unites sequential clinical observations.

Specific brain processes related to mental illness also came later into the books. By "brain process related to mental illness" I mean, not tumor formation, infection, toxic processes which can have psychic and social manifestations, but those brain processes in which we are hard put to know which causes what—whether the physical disturbances cause the psychological ones or the other way around; or perhaps both go on in parallel. Some of the first well demarcated of these are the catecholamine brain processes, which stand in some relationship to mania and depression [6].

The discovery of sociopathological processes also came after the discovery of many psychopathological ones. Sullivan's anxiety contagion is a clear sociopathological process. Here is sociologist Talcott Parsons' account of another, the "vicious circle," closely related to "self-fulfilling prophecies."

The presence of such compulsive motivation inevitably distorts the attitudes of an individual in his social relationships. This means that it imposes strains upon those with whom he interacts. In general it may be suggested that most pathological motivation arises out of vicious circles of deepening ambivalence. An individual, say a child, is subjected to such strain by the compulsive motivation of adults. As a defense against this he himself develops a complementary pattern of compulsive motivation, and the two continue, unless the process is checked, to "work on each other" [7].

"Compulsive motivation" might, in turn, be understood through some psychological process, thereby establishing a little-understood relationship between psychic and social processes. At present we do no more than assume that the two processes reinforce each other; the result is what we can call a continuity or "chronification" process, which may well account for the bulk of human suffering. Such a conception, however, resembles the outmoded dissociation idea and awaits differentiation into clinically specific sequences and processes.

Also, various midbrain, endocrine, and other physical phenomena have been related to social events, feelings, and fantasies, so that an elaborate relationship among processes must be assumed. The old simplicities, nature and nurture, mind and body, give way to social, psychic, and physical events connected by more and more specific relationships.

The result is that today the most-read workers, Erikson and Laing, give little sense of coming down anywhere. Everything is referred to something else. Specific causes, forces, even relationships dissolve in fields of force, the so-called systems theory or transactional analysis. If anything is blamed, it is society, which turns out to mean almost everything and nothing. The various schools agree that internal, social, and physical forces act in concert, but little progress has been made in weighing their impacts. Once much was oedipal; now it is oedipal or oral or both; a friendly but vague fluidity prevails. At first a blow on the head seemed to explain everything. Then there was talk of emotional blows, and finally of shaping events and relationships, often undramatic, repeated, unnoticed. On the internal side, there was "defective constitution or anlage," then specific observations on the premorbid personality and body type, and more recently some understanding of how character develops, as well as of genetic factors. With these last steps, of understanding the little blows and the development of character, there is a convergence:

The little blows in part form the character, and the character invites certain little blows. But except for some concordance rates in twin studies of schizophrenia and effective predictions from family structure to delinquency, every factor seems worth something, yet no one knows how much.

If process conceptions of cause give few quantitative measures, they at least hold out the hope that whatever precedes must be more important. There is a great searching after the First Cause.

Thus paranoia was initially a disease of "false ideas." The symptoms were the cause. Then, preceding these "false ideas," a general autistic tendency was found, a splitting off or withdrawal from the world, and in addition a deterioration of habits. Still earlier, unconscious conflict between social standards and perverse wishes weakened the potential patient's grasp on the world and contributed directly to the delusions. Earlier yet, Schreber's father was found actually torture-training the future judge to produce both a rigid conscience and unfulfilled yearning toward the father. And perhaps even earlier, there were family disharmonies, peculiar patterns of communication, chromosomal aberrations. Which is the cause?

Every fresh element discovered in a sequence stirs up the hope of its being the First Cause. Bleuler took cognitive *or* affective elements to be primary. The patients had a thought disorder or a disturbance of affect—a clear line back to the old faculty psychology [8]. And when Freud's patients told him of being seduced early in life or of having incomplete sexual experiences, he, too, made these causes. When the actuality of the seductions fell under suspicion and the incomplete orgasms did not seem the start of neuroses, another temptation appeared: to regard fantasies of seduction as causal, or whatever just preceded the sexual failure. Rush had blamed a catatonic patient's illness on selling his farm. At a later time, the patient's body type, premorbid personality, fury, fantasies of death would be mentioned. Thus as sequences are discovered bit by bit, each bit has its moment of etiological glory.

Even genetics fails us. Some have tried to make of genetics a modern form of predestination: Life is only the unfolding of the chromosomes. But in fact "behavior is never wholly inherited or wholly acquired, but always *developed* under the combined influences of hereditary and environmental factors" [9]. Genetic differences in behavior do not all appear early in development, later to be modified by experience. Instead, genetic differences may themselves develop under the influence of environmental factors and not be observable until late in life. So much for First Causes.

POINTS OF INTERVENTION

Still we want to know what is most fundamental, or at least where we can intervene most effectively.

In the passage that follows, Binswanger contrasts existential explanations of a phobia with psychoanalytic ones [10].

We should, therefore, not explain the emergence of the phobia by an overly strong "pre-oedipal" tie to the mother, but rather realize that such overly strong filial tie is only possible in the presence of a world design exclusively based on connectedness, cohesiveness, continuity. . . . Everything is supposed to stay as it was before. If, however, something new does happen and continuity is disrupted, it can only result in catastrophe, panic, anxiety attack. . . . The inner or existential maturation and the time orientation toward the future are replaced by a preponderance of the past, of "already-having-been-in." . . . It is this type of temporal orientation that permits the element of *suddenness* to assume such enormous significance; because suddenness is the time-quality that explodes continuity, hacks it and chops it to pieces [11].*

In contrast, "the world of the healthy" has greatly varied contextures of "references and compounds of circumstances." "If it is threatened in one region, other regions will emerge and offer a foothold. . . . Phobia is always an attempt at safeguarding a restricted, impoverished 'world,' whereas anxiety expresses the loss of such a safeguard."

No single impulse, however conflictual, no single loss, could have pathological consequences, Binswanger is arguing, unless the person's "world design"—what we can also call his expectations of the world—makes such a conflict or loss unbearable. Pathological events cannot be reduced to a few elements alone, for these elements, many of them experienced by everyone, derive their significance from the general attitudes, expectations, "world design" of the patient. Thus some bear terrible hardships with equanimity while others cry over raindrops.

Almost all the schools have a word or words for such infantile expectations of painless continuity: Psychoanalysis speaks of the narcissistic orientation; interpersonal psychiatry, of self-centeredness. Only objective-descriptive psychiatry eschews altogether such holistic concepts, and only existential psychiatry puts them at the center of its explanations. These are differences in figure or ground emphasis, with existential psychiatry emphasizing the ground of existence, others the figure, while we have to accept that neither figure nor ground can exist apart from each other; indeed each can become the other, as in familiar optical illusions.

* Excerpted from Chapter VIII, "Insanity as Life-Historical Phenomenon and as Mental Disease: The Case of Ilse" by Ludwig Binswanger in *Existence: A New Dimension in Psychiatry and Psychology,* edited by Rollo May, Ernest Angel and Henri F. Ellenberger. Copyright © 1958 by Basic Books, Inc., publishers, New York.

Clinically we can say, *Vive les différences,* despite all the frustration aroused in those who want clear, single causes. Instead of one, we have now two, three, or more causes, which provide that many more points of intervention.

Hints are available toward a "whole" psychiatry. The objective-descriptive school identifies the illness, analysis tells much about its development and emergence, social psychiatry about the outer conditions of illness, and the existential school about patients' basic attitudes which make illness possible. Without any sense of completeness—indeed, wondering whether completeness is even possible in this ongoing world—we can recognize lines, relationships, processes which make psychiatric causes sometimes even clear.

8

RELATIONSHIP TO THE PATIENTS

OTH TEMPORAL and causal developments require
extraordinary changes of psychiatric scene and attitude.
First to be overcome are the terrorizing and chaotic conditions of hospitals and clinics, which disconcert both patients
and observers. Even when the patients have been taken out of
dungeons and chains, the crowding, noise, screaming, starva-
tion, and death make scientific observation almost impossible.
Pinel did his work not only under these conditions but with
additional pressure from the revolution going on around him
in Paris. On the other hand, no small amount of the "libera-
tion" of mental patients was the work of revolutionary mobs
roaming through the Bicetre. And when a simple clearing and
ordering of hospital conditions had been achieved, there was

the fresh problem of the *artificial* conditions under which patients were observed and the corrosive effects of long incarceration on the subjects of observation. Awareness of *hospitalism* as a disease in itself in turn favored a movement back to community resources and the freeing up of the whole hospital apparatus so expensively created to overcome the old chaos [1].

There are suggestions of a change in the relationship between doctor and patient running parallel to these institutional changes. The "authority of the doctor" and the "patient as a person" are two nodal points. Doctors have a great stake in their authority, and patients support this authority for their own reasons, especially during life-and-death crises. One result is that doctor and patient condition each other. The different psychiatric schools take up sharply different attitudes toward this conditioning, but the trend may be away from at least simpleminded authoritativeness, and perhaps away from seeing patients as objects and toward seeing them as persons. Although relating to people as persons is rare in any human circumstance, the following developments suggest a trend: Awareness of the effects of the doctor's behavior on the patient, apart from any planned treatment of the patient, has turned psychiatrists in on themselves, to the point that they get more treatment than many a patient. Still more recently, doctors have become aware of the patients' effects on them. O sanctum sanctorum! Further, existential writers suggest the concept that the "patient" should disappear altogether; it is a midpoint between object and person too long occupied.

These summary comments need filling out.

GROWTH OF UNDERSTANDING

What caused the early symptoms and cases to be brought together, as Janet suggested, was partly the astonishment, chagrin, fear, and confusion they inspired in the observers. At each stage of the work fresh fears are encountered—fears of sexual thoughts and feelings, anger, the actual facts of family life; psychiatry repeats and repeats the struggle general medicine underwent when it established human dissection as respectable. And when organic illnesses and neuroses became intelligible and were split off, the difficulty of understanding and empathizing with the psychoses continued to stand as the main phenomenon uniting them. Even as late as the time of Bleuler and Jaspers, the words *incomprehensible* and *unintelligible* recur again and again to describe psychotic patients. Later, much that had seemed dangerous or fatal came to seem familiar, safe—indeed, favorable. We can contrast Minkowski's comfort in the presence of insanity after spending two months living with a psychotic person to Esquirol's, and Sullivan's sympathy with catatonia to Kraepelin's objectivity. Instance after instance of this change in attitude toward psychopathological facts could be cited.

Before the time of Pinel and Rush, patients were dangerous sinners whose deviltry must be expunged by the most ruthless methods available. Such was the work of the Inquisition, and long afterward. Or the patients were revered, worshiped, looked to for guidance or revelation. Techniques for recognizing mental disorders, especially for recognizing that seductive creature hysteria, commanded a high premium and reached surprising subtlety; we have seen that some are still used in modern neurology. The patient, once recognized, was put apart, banished, sometimes killed. We can observe a similar pattern in the social relationships of children who call each other crazy, or nowadays "mental," as a means of demeaning and isolating the different individual and of projecting feared parts of themselves. The same practice persists in medical diagnosis when patients are called schizophrenic or neurotic, as if they were only schizophrenic or only neurotic rather than having a touch of this or a serious case of that.

A change appears to have occurred at the turn of the eighteenth into the nineteenth century, as exemplified by the attitudes of Pinel, Rush, and several others. Moral treatment came to rival moral outrage [2]. Paternalism, friendly manipulations, efforts to reform rather than expel were prominent in the accounts of treatment. Of course patients still endured ruthless acts done in the name of theories of disease. Rush purged and bled countless patients of all kinds as a result of his vascular theory, and we can suspect that moral outrage was persisting and being disguised by the medical "explanations." But it *was* disguised, and the ostensible attitudes and occasional institutional practices were those of kindness and caring.

The moral treatment era can be recognized by its paternalism. The patient was a dangerous or childlike object to be manipulated by the wise doctor [3]. The latter knew best; he must influence and reform; he must substitute good ideas for evil ones and good habits for dissolute ones. Trickery on the doctor's part was accepted if it resulted in diagnosis or cure. The bland, self-satisfied way even such a shy figure as Pinel speaks of fooling patients and manipulating their ideas rather shocks the modern mind, which at least pretends a great respect for individual dignity and self-determination. But we can understand Pinel's or Rush's attitudes if we realize that they saw the patients as inferior objects requiring reform, not as partners in a therapeutic enterprise.

The movement from hypnosis to a free associative method illustrates the same development. The hypnotized patient is an object to be manipulated by the hypnotist, a child in the operator's hands. On closer study it appears that much hypnotic behavior is *simulated;* many subjects "go along" with the hypnotist, are not really helpless at all, and may even play tricks of their own on the apparently omnipotent doctor. But that is only a further illustration of the *object relations* between operator and subject; each stands a little apart and manipulates the other.

Freud gave up hypnosis not only because many subjects resisted it but because the very act of hypnotizing prematurely shaped the relationship and its verbal productions. He wanted the patient to cooperate spontaneously; the associations were to be *free*. Of course his seeking free associations seldom by itself produced them. In a larger sense freedom was the goal of the whole treatment and could not be expected at the start. The important point is that Freud was taking a step away from objectification and manipulation and toward a relationship between persons.

Further steps have been taken since. On the contemporary scene, many therapists seek to establish in the patient's mind a separation of the neurotic, childlike, or sick portion of the individual from observing ego, healthy self, or adult development, as various schools term it. A working alliance is sought between the doctor and his patient's observing self. These serve as equal partners in a joint venture. Authoritarianism on the doctor's part is then a sign of discomfort with the patient and no longer a right conferred on the physician by long training and accumulated knowledge. Existential workers seek a still more egalitarian position: The doctor must obliterate all differences from the patient, accept the possibility that he, the doctor, may be sicker than the patient, and avoid even thinking about the patient as a patient, because that might objectify and distance him. Therapists must merge their mental lives with those of the sufferers. This process may end, however, in an artificial, condescending sociability or a mystic communing, and the two parties have to draw back awhile.

Recent studies have suggested that class, economic, and educational levels make large contributions to the diagnosis and treatment mental patients receive [4]. It is not yet clear whether differences among the *illnesses* of different groups account for the discrepancies, or differences among the responses of the doctors who diagnose and treat the various class or educational groups. Perhaps some other factor is at work. What does come clear is the contemporary awareness of the issue. Class differences are considered in the planning of scientific studies and not permitted to influence the results silently.

But this consideration requires that patients be seen apart from their class or group. If we abstract the feature of poverty, we are on the way to imagining that the patient might be something else, perhaps a person. Contrast this response with the attitude of even so great an observer of human nature as Balzac. Many of Balzac's peasants are simply *poor men*. Similarly Rush did not believe poor people had the same "sensibility" as the rich; they presented less surface for reaction to the outside world, remained preoccupied with present labor and physical suffering, and had neither the concern with the past and future nor the sensibility to mental experience that he believed brought on psychiatric disease. Rush also expressed the opposite attitude, again determined by class considerations: He felt occasionally puzzled that a patient could fall ill in view of his good education and superior breeding. The implication was that upper-class experience should *protect* against psychiatric disease. We observe some portion of an individual being put in place of the whole person, and our reactions are determined by our feelings for the portion. The result is an *objectification* of the person. Thus it is common to speak, usually in a hostile mood, of individuals being neurotic, or lower class, or to assign them some racial designation that is used to "sum up" people.

A related development occurred with respect to therapeutic goals. One early goal was *catharsis*, the discharge of hitherto pent-up feelings. Gradually one hears less of this and more of the need for *emotional contact with others*. The goal is no longer a discharge of feeling removed from the object of feeling but an emotional *relationship*. The doctor can no longer simply stand back and observe. Early in this development, the object of feeling was not thought of great importance; the patient would *transfer* his unconscious misunderstandings onto anyone who sat still long enough to receive them. But lately *particular* features of the resulting transference neuroses have become apparent, the individual character of each therapeutic relationship. This makes it impossible for some people to work fruitfully together but may be the very reason others can. Now the doctor counts himself successful not chiefly if he produces an emotional explosion but if the patient *feels* toward the therapist and then in his everyday relationships along a broader range of response. And the issue arises, Can the patient long feel toward me if I am neutral toward him? Thus we observe a development from objectless expression, to expression toward any object, to a cultivation of individualities in the therapeutic encounter.

At first the patient stood alone. He was diseased, or a symptom appeared which was equated with disease. Later it became difficult to separate the patient's disorder from his family's or society's, and the symptom from a host of other phenomena. As long as society isolates mad people, medical descriptions reflect the isolation, but then patients and phenomena come into relationship with one another and with the world around.

COMING INTO RELATIONSHIP

"Coming into relationship" means more than a static addition. We now enter a problem difficult to articulate. Even clinical illustrations, which should make the point clear, may not do so. It will help to separate out two different effects of "coming into relationship."

First, the significance of a symptom will be determined by

the company it keeps. That is a point almost everyone has come to accept, and it has large implications. Little or nothing is then *pathognomonic*. Little or nothing can stand alone for a particular disease. Here is an example from Kraepelin: "The probability of considerable improvement becomes more remote insofar as those peculiarities develop which are in the foreground of the large number of conclusively incurable cases. Among these is the loss of good natured responsiveness with comprehension preserved. . . ." *Not* the loss of good-natured responsiveness alone, but with *comprehension preserved*. The same phenomenon in a clouded sensorium with turbulent affect has clinical implications that almost entitle us to use the word *opposite*, so different are the diagnostic and prognostic results. Psychotic symptoms in an emotional, confused patient, what at first glance appears obvious, thoroughgoing madness, mean a high probability for the disappearance of the madness, while the quiet, clear patients should make our blood run cold.

The failure of single elements to be pathognomonic, their replacement by groups of elements, results in composite portraits which are necessarily vague at the edges. Syndromes share symptoms, which have radically different meanings from one syndrome to the next. But here the representation of edge, center, and overlapping circles is misleading, with its implication of inviolate, pathognomonic centers. Instead we must allow our circles different sizes and realize that the edges of some will contain the centers of others. Then there is no portion of any one entity that may not be in some other.

The search for absolutely definitive elements, for portions of each circle that are not overlapped by others, goes forward anyway, perhaps to some eventual success. The great imitative and adaptive proclivities of humans make complete success unlikely. Fresh ways of going mad will be copied and used for different purposes, to the confusion of taxonomists. What we must grasp is both the lure of the pathognomonic (Freud wrote *never* and *always* in sentence after sentence, indicating his desire that some phenomena be able to stand by themselves, whatever their surroundings) and its having gradually lost ground. Every fresh area of investigation has reawakened hope (nowadays, that in family interactions we will find something uniquely schizophrenic), but the result has been transitional phenomena and events which gain at least part of their meaning from their surroundings. One outcome is that "relating to the patient as if the patient were a disease" becomes increasingly difficult.

Coming into relationship also means that symptoms are found to be relative and tentative *in themselves*. Not only do they change meaning in different contexts; they themselves change. Here is a discovery that succinctly contains both the therapeutic hope and the scientific despair of psychiatry.

Bleuler wrote, "Whoever does not show the physician any deeper feeling in the course of a protracted examination is no mere neurotic." Bleuler's fundamental, for which we can substitute pathognomonic, symptom of *affective flatness* or lack of "deeper feeling" is to be noted *in context*. The implication is that it may disappear in a protracted examination or be missed in a short one. We are not here concerned with a *change of meaning* but with the *disappearance of the phenomenon itself*. Suddenly the length of the examination and the behavior of the physician become of great importance. Both increased scientific complexity and the hope of therapeutic gain follow.

Sullivan made the extreme claim along this line. Perhaps almost everything strange, bizarre, dissociated, flat, the whole diagnostic armory would fall away if the interviews were lengthened sufficiently and the physicians modified their behavior this way or that. Now we lose the distinction between diagnosis and treatment. Interviews carried on long enough become treatment; only a trial of treatment can uncover the diagnosis. Instead of textbooks on diagnosis and prognosis

the generation after Sullivan read manuals of psychotherapeutic technique by Sullivan himself, Fromm-Reichmann,
Hill, Berne, and many others. There is no longer a patient and
a doctor at one moment of time but a patient-doctor system
over time. Diagnosis rests not alone on the psychological phenomena but as much on the operations performed to elicit and
test them. The hysterical patient becomes, to some extent, that
patient we understand with relative ease and have certain feelings about. The schizophrenic is the patient who remains unintelligible and out of empathic reach longer than the others.
The doctor's individual style must be scrutinized. His degree
of aloofness, sensitivity to this topic or that, convictions of right
or wrong—his ways of approaching the patient—will affect
what the patient present psychologically. The impact on psychiatric education is to give still more prominence to treating
the *doctor* and to supervisory experiences. The student psychiatrist's operations must be minutely reviewed, not only because therapeutic skill is being sought but because an awareness of the importance of the doctor's actions has entered every
phase of the work; hence psychiatric operationalism. The traditional fixed units give way to relationships which come to
resemble fields of force.

I speak of fields of force because each relationship shapes
the parties to it, whether the relationship is among seemingly
isolated elements within an individual or among individuals
within a group. Everyone observes that so-and-so brings out the
best (or the worst) in this person or that. The repetitive character of much interaction reduces this shaping. We react to
many men as if they were father, uncle, brother; there is vast
psychic inertia. Yet the shaping is never altogether absent. Its
extent, rules of operation, and modes of transmission constitute a major research question in psychiatry. The contemporary study of the degree and types of psychotherapeutic effectiveness is the same question, especially when such issues as

these are raised: what results from liking or disliking the patient, which individuals work fruitfully together, and so on. Contemporary family studies seek the interpersonal or relationship processes that shape individuals from their starts. Sooner or later someone asks, as Sullivan did, whether there is any other issue in *psychiatry*, since the matter of shaping concerns the effect of psyche on psyche, when, who, how, why? We can only be surprised in retrospect at how late the problem came clearly into the books, for with every stage of psychiatric development particular stances of the different observers have been modifying the observed. (Someday the effects of the contemporary self-conscious approach will be studied.) Certainly every psychiatric research stumbles upon the problem, To what extent and in what ways does the investigative relationship change its subjects?

The extreme note is sounded by some existentialists, who regain one of our starting points in the temporal line of development. There is no real past. The past exists only in the present, is re-created at each moment by the present. Everything seemingly outside the current field of force is actually dissolved in it. We cannot dismiss this radical subjectivity so easily as many would like. *To some unknown extent* the present person *is* continually reworking and remaking his memories, his structure, his very cells.

Similarly, the existential impatience with subject-object distinctions questions the whole concept "relationship with the patient." Existentialism argues that insofar as we apprehend the "object" at all, the subject disappears. Insofar as we are "where the patient is," we cannot think any more of a "relationship," which suggests lines connecting two separate objects. Instead one attempts to reach the other, to live a little while in his or her life; something is left in each of the other (perhaps these residua of contact can be called the relationship), but as long as the two parties stand only in "relationship" to each other, we have more an impression of distance than of closeness. The extent of this contact or encounter, Binswanger suggested, is measured by the extent to which both parties change, but that implies more than a relationship between separate objects. Hence the existential use of such words as *contact* or *encounter* or *meeting*. Hence, also, the existential impatience with psychiatry's study of the subject, its great *self*-consciousness. Any self-consciousness holds the subject away from the object. Existential writers appear to seek the "savage mind" of Lévi-Strauss, which lives in nature, does not see itself as separate from nature or observing nature, and is utterly without consciousness, at least according to some of his descriptions [5]. The whole painfully arrived-at account of the self and its impediments to development and relationship, which forms so much of the history of Western thought, is disdained by existentialism as a false path. Just as Minkowski and Binswanger give a fresh sense of time and return temporal development to its beginnings, so Lévi-Strauss, like Rousseau, asks for a less sophisticated, unselfconscious relationship to one another. But now we approach the subject of psychiatric ideals.

9

PSYCHIATRIC IDEALS

THE APPARENTLY PHILOSOPHICAL matter of ideals is in fact practical first and last. Ideals set in motion therapeutic activity, because people want to be without pain or live longer, and they set what limits to medical enterprise are not set by the plain disappearance of disease. These limits keep changing. The ideals of reducing suffering and death have been joined by the ideal of a fuller life. Health is now not merely the absence of illness but a perhaps infinitely widening conception of new possibilities. When the normal meant the average, we were all bound to one another. When the psychiatrically average man was found to be sicker than expected, the average and ideal denotations of *normal* clashed. Today the normal means more and more the ideal. There are

263

norms that almost no one reaches, yet we use the term *normal* because these remain ideals for many. One result is an extraordinary gap between the haves and the have-nots among psychiatric patients. The first get almost unlimited periods and intensities of treatment, especially in psychoanalytic and existential work. The others are barely aware of any need for treatment, which is just as well because they could not secure it. Thus the ideals of both patients and professionals have widespread practical consequences.

I will indicate the principal changes in psychiatric ideals by reviewing the ideals of the various schools. Since, particularly in respect to this matter, the schools have refined their separate vocabularies, it will be necessary to translate each ideal into the language of the other. The result will be perhaps surprising extents of agreement, as well as provocative disagreements. We can then enter the final chapters with some sense of what the practical aims of psychiatric work are.

CHANGING IDEALS

When, as with Rush, the whole illness consisted of an illusion, and illusion meant the grossest perceptual distortion, crazy people were rare. Diagnosis of Kraepelin's dementia praecox required several clear-cut symptoms present for some time and then a downhill course; most of us could breathe easy. But as soon as a *process* of illness defined the disease— for example, dissociation—it became easier to think of degrees of illness; the schizophrenia concept therefore took in many more patients than did the dementia praecox one [1]. Indeed setting any limits to schizophrenia became difficult, for who has not been dissociated now and then? As another example, beginning students often diagnose hysteria if the conversion of a complex into a somatic symptom seems present. This diagnosis produces many false-positives, which using the Greek syndromic definition prevents. Such is regularly the effect of moving between symptomatic or syndromic definitions and process ones.

The understanding of pathophysiological processes similarly enlarged the patient group in general medicine. It became possible to diagnose early cases, subclinical cases, even those who had had the illness years before, all of which was impossible when the definition of illness was tied to clear-cut symptoms.

The discovery of physiological, psychological, and sociological disease processes moved treatment efforts away from symptom removal and against these processes. Epidemiological investigations made the shift still more pressing because studies of whole populations revealed 75 or 80 percent to have symptoms. Symptom removal was thus an obvious practical impossibility; what treatment there was must be set against the processes leading to sickness. Even the behaviorists, who seemed eager to mount a fresh effort against symptoms, began to concern themselves more and more with attitudes, habitual patterns, and approaches to life [2].

Physiological processes have been the hardest to find. Antipsychotic drugs are still used largely symptomatically although we can guess that their actions must be more profound. Psychological processes have been the easiest to find but very difficult to change, so that psychoanalytic treatment has lengthened in keeping with the number of pathological processes discoverable and their resistance to change. The discovery of social disease processes, in turn, set psychiatry against society. The family, hospitals, society at large, the medical profession itself must be studied and reformed. Here the principal figure has been Thomas Szasz.

The psychoanalytical and social psychiatric developments produced two fresh ideals. The earlier analytic ideal, of genital character, came to seem narrow, too specific; the recent literature stresses more the growth of *persons*. For its part, social psychiatry has had no single term for its ideal. Certainly the spontaneity, intimacy, and receptiveness hoped for in the social experience of individuals would need other terms to describe institutional health. But the goal of institutional maturation has entered psychiatry.

Ideals must be constantly redefined, not only as new disease processes are discovered but as the old ideals are in part attained. There is no doubt that the worst back-ward cases have largely disappeared, at least from among new cases in the United States; practitioners also have reported fewer and fewer symptom neuroses. By definition, ideals must lie beyond us. Certainly both the new psychoanalytic and the social psychiatric ideals seem distant indeed.

Many times psychoanalysis has been attacked for its ideals and the consequent prolongation of the treatment. Perhaps the patients were being coddled. Is analysis a refuge for rich bored people who have nothing better to do with their time and money? Is analysis merely tinkering with people who need, if anything, less attention and introspection? Maybe I am wrong to speak of ideals at all if the goals may be comfort, retreat, or enriching the doctors.

I doubt that anyone who has practiced among the allegedly idle rich could recognize these descriptions. Since I have always carried on my work both at a public hospital and in private practice, for me the rich and the poor have sat side by side. It is hard to judge who is the unhappier. Certainly epidemiological studies have found more and worse sickness among the poor, and a commercial society terribly handicaps, in particular, the offspring of those not skilled or grasping. But it is also true that the most sensitive epidemiological studies report appalling rates of psychiatric illness in all classes, so the reason for treating the poor is not that the rich are well.

Psychoanalysis, like any complicated, expensive medical

technique, must always defy broad application. The present methods of dealing with kidney and heart disease through transplantation and dialysis are, if anything, more expensive and their uses at least as restricted. We have to ask ourselves whether a technique should not be used because it cannot be used everywhere, and whether such techniques by bringing to reality ideals of development or prolongation of life previously unrecognizable do not provide the motivation and sometimes the detailed knowledge which makes possible the discovery of other methods more broadly applicable.

The discoveries of social psychiatry have also deepened our awareness of illness and perhaps exposed an even seamier side of life than that laid open by psychoanalysis. Indeed social psychiatry is as helpless still to correct the conditions it exposes or to fulfill the ideal it can define as is psychoanalysis. In fact social psychiatry seems to be repeating the unhappy history that psychoanalysis has just recently put behind. The result of Freud's discoveries was public displeasure and contempt. Almost no one wanted to believe what the content of human mental life was really like. Freud was blamed for his discoveries for the same reason the bearers of ill tidings were slain in ancient times: One hopes to do away with the fact by doing away with the informer. Very soon, I predict, social psychiatry will receive the equally fierce displeasure of a society reluctant to confront the actual facts of family and institutional life. Inescapable as are, for example, the implications of the battering and murdering of children by their own parents, every effort will be made to escape them.

And social psychiatry exposes not only the realities of *institutional* life; as I have detailed, Sullivan saw little intimacy or perceptiveness in the average human transaction. People, he claimed, are mostly in their own heads or looking out to see what they wish or fear to see. In technical language average human life is vastly more autistic and projective than had been believed. The implication is that ideals of social health, of intimacy, spontaneity, and perceptiveness, lie much farther off than was formerly assumed.

Existential psychiatry thrusts aside the term *illness*, substituting *the human condition*. Illness is only a category of retrospective understanding. There is no way of knowing, from moment to moment, what will in retrospect prove to be illness. Every effort to define it in an ongoing clinical situation separates doctor and patient and must be phenomenologically reduced. Put differently, the human condition is itself sick and there is no knowing in advance whether the doctor is not sicker than the patient. Existential health—that is, being-in-the world—occurs now and then, perhaps never more than partially. We all draw back in dread from leaving our heads, our private special selves, from putting aside the masks of profession, duty, religion, and ideas. The goal of treatment is *meeting*, being with the other. Doctors exist, Jaspers wrote, because there are people without friends or love. But some doctors are doctors because they too are incapable of friendship and love, so that the patient must experience their treatment as a reinforcement of their fears. In short, illness is too static a conception to be clinically useful because we cannot know at any moment who is sick (the final death of the pathognomonic!). The apparently sick act may prove of decisive healthiness. All we can do is involve ourselves as fully as possible in understanding the patient. If Ilse had persuaded her father by burning her arm, we would be less likely to call the burning sick and more likely to call it heroic. In unlivable human situations crises occur which require extraordinary actions. These are sick only in the sense that they are part of sick human situations; blame is possible only when someone is not understood. Thus social psychiatry makes us very critical of parents—but from the standpoint of the children. Existential psychiatry asks us to put aside all this "blaming."

The result is life-historical purposes which may miscarry so that the person is thrown out of the world, into patienthood. The hope is that the doctor can return the patient to the world. But all that is retrospective. It may be that the patient returns the doctor to the world. No one can decide in advance.

UNITY OF IDEALS

Surprisingly, these philosophical comments give us psychiatric ideals not so remote from the concepts of the other schools. Existentialists speak of being-in-the-world; the interpersonal school, of true or mature object relations; and psychoanalysis, of genitality. Perhaps the same phenomenon is being described on philosophical, social, and biological planes. True existence means freedom from the bondage of the past and the capacity to involve ourselves fully with others. True object relations mean commitments to others "for themselves"; people are not merely to be manipulated, loved as mirrors of our traits, or used to satisfy our own desires. By genitality, psychoanalysis means escape from fixations and distortions of the past and a concern with others that is not just a concern with ourselves. The *pregenital* is whatever appears through the lens of the primitive unconscious, which magnifies good things into divine and magic gifts or bad news into the devil's work. Then no one can be met for what he is: A gesture brings back the loved or hated father and a tone of voice old fears and their defenses. The past triggers the putting on of masks, and we withdraw from true existence into the masks of the past. Relating to others "for themselves" means dropping masks. Relating to others for themselves means intimacy, receptiveness, spontaneity, because "being where someone else is" means intimacy with him, receptiveness to what he gives, spontaneity in response. And what is this forbidding "genitality" but closeness, give-and-take, the putting aside of oral incorporation, anal retentiveness, phallic aggressiveness?

Are not these separate descriptions largely efforts to depict the same ideals as viewed from the special vantage point of each school? The psychoanalytic concern with fantasy and the possible biological phenomena fantasy may express leads to a concentration on primitive, premature fantasy and the construction of a biological ideal, genitality. Its features, of creativity, receptiveness, and being in contact at the same time, remind us of the ideals of the social school, spontaneity, receptivity, intimacy, or, in the typical holistic summary of existential psychiatry, being-in-the-world. All seek to escape the autistic, the manipulative, the exclusively passive or aggressive, a goal which reminds us that medical descriptive psychiatry, the symptomatic school, has defined similar ideals by negation. For example, Janet's functionalism, so faithful to the facultative concepts of descriptive psychiatry, concerns itself with the functions of the real, the energy of synthesis, higher and lower functions, all pointing to ideal capacities of the individual for organization and integration leading to the familiar ideal in-the-worldness. Thus the biological, social, existential, and symptomatic descriptions leave us on common ground.

DIVERGENT IDEALS

Unfortunately this happy union of viewpoints does not stay happy or united very long. Differences and conflicts remain even after allowance has been made for the separate vocabularies and areas of observation.

The social psychiatric ideals is of the individual in society, yet we cannot speak any more of the individual or of personality because social psychiatry raises the question, Is there any personality apart from social roles? Indeed, as Sullivan asks, is there a continuous personality at all? What is left of us when social roles are stripped away? Is personhood perhaps only the name for the whole man in the good society, the two built up bit by bit from social roles and functions?

The existential ideal of obliterating subject-object distinctions carries us still farther from the ideal of individuality and personhood. Here is an aborigine speaking, quoted by a sophisticated existentialist, attacking man's self-conscious separation from nature: "Why should I live in a house? A white man puts up four walls to keep the weather out, knocks holes in the walls to let the weather in, covers the holes up with glass to keep the weather out, and then shoves the windows up to let the weather in. He doesn't know what he wants" [3].

Being in society may mean only the assumption of anti-natural and social masks. Man should seek, existentialism argues, the fullest possible immersion in nature and other men. The social "relationships" advocated by social psychiatry still do not carry us far enough from the prideful individuality fostered by Western ideals.

Psychoanalysis responds to social psychiatry, arguing that this being in society forgets the biological man, predicates a degree of sublimation of conflict unattainable by man, and destroys freedom in the name of social conformity. Freud insisted that no matter how many social institutions were reformed or how thoroughly, basic conflicts must remain between the individual and society. Therefore social psychiatric ideals, for all their contemporary reformist bent, must inevitably enslave individuals to social norms.

Psychoanalysis responds to existential psychiatry that the latter posits a "tenuous identity through intensely engaged relationships" [4]. The existential ideal has even been characterized by analytic writers as psychotic, as obliterating the necessary boundary line between the individual and the external world. Existential writers have been attacked for advocating a kind of "clinching." The battered individuals in the world hold on to each other in desperation until they are ready to return to their individuality. In this criticism, too, psychoanalysis remains faithful to its metaphor of life as conflict, and its ideal of rationality, man's one guide among the conflicting forces [5].

Finally, the objective-descriptive school places the ideal in the nonsymptomatic. Leave the person, nature, and society alone, behaviorists and many medical psychologists argue. Take care of the symptoms, and the illnesses will take care of themselves. The endless conflicts of psychoanalytic, existential, and social psychiatry, they assert, have arisen largely because psychiatry has lost its footing apart from the disease concept.

But what is a symptom, the other schools ask? Are there not social diseases, that is, collections of knowledge about disorders in society and between the individuals in society that can be approached as medical diseases can? Traditional symptomatology makes convenient the recognition of cures. It allows behaviorists to argue, for example, that the symptomatic cures they achieve do not result in fresh symptoms. But to what extent do their studies include sufficient accounts of the patients' life experiences, their social interaction, their inner experience in general, to let them decide that the illness has indeed disappeared so completely?

In turn, does not psychoanalysis favor a great flowering of individuality, of self-concern, of pride, which opens it to the criticisms of existential and social psychiatry? How many patients have been rendered even more intolerable because by completing psychoanalysis they have reached a contemporary state of perfection? The very length and expense of the work foster a sense of its importance and an investment in the belief in one's improvement. The result must sometimes be a great buttressing, not of health, but of unresolved disease elements and the sending out into the world of people whose individuality—perhaps we should even use the term *narcissism*—has been immeasurably strengthened.

Yet social psychiatry also offers no final resting place. The analytic criticism seems apt. Does anyone really believe that the conflicts between the individual and society can be finally resolved? Have we not passed far enough beyond the old Marxist hopes to see the intrinsic antagonism not only among individuals and nations but between the individual and society?

And what should we say to the savage mind satirizing man's house-constructing propensities?—perhaps that the extraordinary selection process that produced aborigines hardy enough to survive sleeping naked on the freezing tundra is no touchstone for the ideal but simply a surrender to nature rather than a union with nature and the turning away from all the conquests over pain and disease, however dearly paid for, in the development of Western culture. Man may open and shut his windows or build new windows and cover over old ones, but so too does nature change and man may justly seek in a dangerous and unpredictable universe some points of safety and individuality that he can call his own.

•

We have to ask ourselves, Is there one place, one ideal, to measure our efforts by in a pluralistic universe? This question has particular importance for us as we resume the discussion of clinical methods, which generate specific types of data that are suited for only limited objectives and themselves shape the medical enterprise quite apart from any purposes we may have for it.

TOWARD A PLURALISTIC
PSYCHIATRY

Steady advance implies the exact determi-
nation of every previous step.
                              Georges Sarton

10

TECHNOLOGY OF THE SCHOOLS

How are we to understand the development of psychiatry? Should we acknowledge separate developments leading to a fragmented result? Or do the schools emerge one from the other, so that we can speak of a progressive, although admittedly pluralistic, psychiatry? The *methods* appear distinct, as I will now demonstrate in detail. So do the even more varied medical and surgical methods, so that the physician or the surgeon may be delayed but need not be immobilized. Today, however, each psychiatric school disdains the others' methods, castigates them as old-fashioned, superficial, impractical, or of only limited, occasional usefulness. The new man coming on the psychiatric scene is hawked at like a circus-goer and wanders where his fancy, his temperament, or the allure of his teachers leads him. Medicine, on the other hand, compels a more objective, patient-centered, less personal and idiosyncratic standard for decisions.

I shall begin by presenting the school methods as separate developments with their own distinct areas of observation, vocabularies, goals, and technologies. Later will come the question, What should the investigator or the therapist do?

It will be easier for therapists reading these descriptions to recognize what others do rather than what they themselves do, for actual practice is a mixture of methods that "feel right," and most of us take a bright view of what we do. Whether these mixtures are much different from the pharmacological mixtures and tonics of nineteenth-century medicine, however, we can only speculate.

OBJECTIVE-DESCRIPTIVE PSYCHIATRY

The examination and history constitute the products of examining and history-taking, which are the two principal methods of the objective-descriptive school. The occurrence of such well-demarcated *products* (often called case material), emerging at distinct, prearranged points in time, is characteristic of this school. It serves as a major source of attraction to students liking orderly, methodical, concretely productive lines of work. They are not made to feel helpless when this procedure is used; there is always something else to do! Further, the resulting materials can be shared with others and reviewed periodically, with increments of learning. The doctor is master, and his mastery is objective, communal, rewarding. It is also clear that this productiveness serves as both an attraction and a source of tension to patients. Although the patients reveal themselves privately, they know the revelations will be brought into the professional community and shared, and may even become permanently available in a record library or the "literature," the most secure immortality that medicine provides. Inevitably there is conflict between the "privacy" and the "community," because patients at once fear to be known and are glad their problems are reviewed by others. This last is particularly the case if a patient sees himself as "having an illness" and wants to do more than conceal it or remain the private concern of one doctor alone. Bringing the illness into a professional community can be as great a comfort as entering an efficient hospital or home.

Other points of attraction and tension spring from a second feature of this objective method. Examination and history are both elaborately *categorical* [1]. The student or practitioner is to make observations within categories of appearance, behavior, mood, and insight and to collect bits of history that are "present," "past," familial, vocational, sexual, etc. Presumably everything belongs somewhere. There is a nice pigeonholing satisfaction, a refreshing sense of bringing even complex clinical situations under control. The technical goal is thoroughness. Categories are memorized and then patients and *their* memories "looked over" with the categories in mind. The observer's mind is full as he has much to apply and remember; in fact, his mind may fill up so rapidly that he must resort to either note-taking or an electronic method of recording. The fear that something will be overlooked or forgotten (perhaps it has already been forgotten!) produces tension in doctor and patient. The patient experiences this tension in the doctor's watching and searching, which can become a kind of mental "fleecing." Besides, the doctor's scrutiny makes the patient feel doubted, and skepticism of the doctor toward the patient, and eventually of the patient toward himself, is heightened by the purpose of the doctor's examination, which, of course, is to find something wrong. The detective-doctor looks for the criminal disease.

The effect of the categories is also to *limit* the investigation.

Because there are so many points to cover, not much time can be given any one. The doctor finds himself interrupting the patient—and we are made aware of still another characteristic of the method, active intervention. This becomes necessary if the patient is repetitious, keeps adding "noncontributory" details, or presents material that escapes any category, because there will not be enough time to complete the items! Here the desire for *thoroughness* brings with it the danger of *incompleteness,* with resulting tension.

The tension is not easily resolved for at least two reasons. I have emphasized already that no psychopathological finding alone is definitive. Some, and often all the rest, of the examination and history is needed in order to judge the significance of any finding. Therefore, the examination and history must be completed if they are done at all, or it may be wiser to omit them altogether. Unless they can be finished, some very disturbing finding (which is called positive!) may lead either to dangerous panic or to complacency, which the completed examination would obviate. Completing the examination grows more and more difficult, however, and this is a second hindrance to resolving the tension. As psychiatric knowledge increases, there are more observations to make. To the objective-descriptive examination one might add inquiries about the phenomenological categories. For example, how are time, space, and color being experienced? In addition, we may recall how Meyer's already laborious social histories were extended even farther by his effort to include sexual data brought to his attention by the very different psychoanalytic history-taking. The result in both instances is a greatly lengthened examination and history, with still more conflict between the need for thoroughness and the fear of incompleteness.

We will see that each of the great methods generates its own tensions (in psychoanalysis, for example, as a result of silence and waiting) and has its own means of resolving them.

Objective-descriptive psychiatry characteristically resolves its tensions by *testing* (a form of *active intervention*). Broadly speaking, the tests are either diagnostic or therapeutic, although the latter may have diagnostic implications. Here is my account of two diagnostic tests used by Kraepelin:

The observer suspects catatonia, perhaps on the basis of some stiffness of the patient's gait. He therefore lifts the patient's arm and notes how long the arm remains horizontal. A positive result is still only suggestive of catatonia or indicates only a mild degree of catatonia, so one makes a further test. The patient is told to stick out his tongue. He does this and the observer drives a pin into the tongue. If the patient leaves his tongue out, or if he puts it back out on request, particularly after a second pricking, etc., one diagnoses greater and greater degrees of automatic obedience. Carried far enough, the procedure produces negativism, the opposite of automatic obedience, but also a catatonic sign.

Plainly, such a test must decisively affect the relationship between doctor and patient. It is also apparent that the procedure excludes, at least temporarily and perhaps indefinitely, the use of the other schools' methods. The patient would not now engage in free-association (if he could talk at all!), his paranoid projections would have been amply confirmed, to the point of preventing participant observation, and the possibility of "meeting" would have become more than remote.

In emphasizing the activity of the objective-descriptive methods, I do not mean to imply that the methods of the other schools are not also active. Certainly the methods of social psychiatry are very active. Psychoanalysis, which emphasizes the doctor's listening and pulling back, quite literally out of sight, elaborately structures the clinical situation and lays down rules for the patient's behavior that surpass in detail and restrictiveness those of any other school except perhaps objective-descriptive psychiatry. Even existential methods, while putting the therapist inside the patient's world and quite literally at its mercy, require vigorous confrontation of the patient often to get and by all means to stay where the patient is. I think that what distinguishes the activity of the objective-descriptive school is not so much its degree as its direction.

Its activity is directed at the illness seen as part of the patient but not part of the same class of things as patient and doctor. This distinction explains the ruthlessness of some objective-descriptive interventions, whether Kraepelin's pinpricking or, at the most extreme, lobotomy and electric shock. These pitiless acts are not directed at the patient but at the illness, which is seen as sharply separate. Ruthlessness then becomes a virtue and demonstrates the intensity of the doctor's concern for the patient. We see the same phenomenon in the treatment of cancer. Genuinely violent surgical and pharmacological procedures are used, with widespread acceptance. Particularly with such a cancer as leukemia, the pharmacotherapists experience the same difficulty objective-descriptive psychiatry has in separating illness from patient. The leukemic cells may prove only a little more sensitive to the treatment than do the normal cells.

Not only does the objective-descriptive psychiatrist himself actively observe and attack the illness but he expects the patient to join him in this observation and attack, unless the patient is "actively" psychotic or comatose [2]. The patient is expected to "cooperate." This assumption, along with their common objectivity, allies descriptive psychiatry and psychoanalysis. The analyst forms an alliance with the "mature ego," which then helps the analyst surface and dispose of the infantile formation, conceived of as a foreign body like infection or cancer. Perhaps the ego proves more distorted or even corrupted by the illness than was hoped. Still the whole process of cure in psychoanalysis rests on this alliance with at least a partially mature ego. So, in general medicine and in objective-descriptive psychiatry, cooperation is essential. If the patient does not take the medicine, little can be done except make it sweeter, make it last longer, or hope he comes round.

If the patient does come round, he is quickly enlisted in extensive activity. For example, it is characteristic of this school at present to use questionnaires, checklists, and elaborate forms for self-scrutiny, again *categorized*, so that results among large numbers of patients can be compared. The familiar outcome is *objective products*. Their volume may become so large that again mechanical means are needed, not now for recording but for manipulating the results mathematically. Hence computer technology.

Note the sharpness of the subject-object split: Doctors observe patients, and patients are to observe themselves as objects, and in order to render the observations more objective, something is placed between observer and observed. This is minimally a desk or note-pad. The desk keeps a safe distance between doctor and patient; it also indicates the doctor's knowledge and authority. The note-pad reduces subjective errors of memory. What comes between doctor and patient, however, may be much more elaborate, often a form, or instruments for testing and observation. Moreover, for every concrete object placed between doctor and patient, there are many more abstract objects. The doctor is thinking about the patient all the while and accumulating ideas of which the patient can have only vague suspicions. The doctor's mental products and the effort to order and understand them may grow so great that he must stop observing. This is an *intellectually heavy* method. (In contrast, existential psychiatry provides an *emotionally heavy* method.)

The treatment methods of objective-descriptive psychiatry also exemplify this dominant activity of the school. The psychological side is dealt with by education, persuasion, and manipulation of the patient. Here, too, belongs hypnosis, with its attempted control of the patient: An apparently passive subject answers questions, remembers on command, feels or does not feel, and seemingly takes suggestions which persist post-hypnotically. On the physical side, objective-descriptive therapists use drugs, electricity, and surgery as part of the objective attack on illness.

The newest treatment method closely related to objective-descriptive psychiatry is behavior therapy, which nicely illustrates the features of the school. The behavior therapist examines the patient and obtains a detailed history. Heavy emphasis falls on finding particular symptoms to be removed. A conditioning or deconditioning procedure and schedule are determined and agreed on with the patient, who must cooperate. The doctor is active in repeatedly bringing various stimuli or reinforcers to the patient's attention. No particular emotional bond is sought with the patient beyond a cooperation-facilitating rapport. Certainly the doctor does not expect to interact with the patient as part of the treatment proper, nor does the doctor expect to be shaped or even influenced by the patient. The behavior therapy doctor has knowledge and a powerful method. The patient is expected to stand still while he receives the benefit of this as if it were an injection or an operation. Everything mystic, inner, unique, emotional, and subjective is eschewed. Furthermore, treatment is restricted to the patient, the sick person; family and society are not assumed to participate. The model is an experiment, with its features of repetition, testing, control, and the subject as an object.

•

Kraepelin's tests for catatonia also illustrate the characteristics by which the objective-descriptive method is named. The method is *objective,* first because it treats the patient as if he were a "physical," "tangible" object to be observed from "outside," and second because the method attempts to be "unbiased," "dispassionate," the opposite of subjective. (In fact, all the quoted words are synonyms for or analogous to "objective.") The objectivity of the method allies it closely with physical science, which alliance is its largest source of prestige (like having a prince in the family). All the other schools' methods have been attacked as unscientific.

Psychoanalysis is also an objective school; that is, psychoanalysts collect the free associative products and consider them dispassionately. Elaborate efforts are made to establish the objectivity of the analyst. Analysis of the analyst, for example, is required and is meant to reduce distorting "countertransference" biases; the analyst should be able to hear and respond to the patient's verbal content without emotion. (Note the assumption that emotion must be particularly distorting.) Indeed, psychoanalysis is, in this respect, more objective than objective-descriptive psychiatry. For example, Freud attempted to restrict himself to the "humble art of psychology." He refused to involve himself emotionally with Dora. Objective-descriptive psychiatrists, on the other hand, have usually not hesitated to "persuade" patients, to exhort them, to use their authority as doctors. They may have regarded these persuasions as "objective," but we know from psychoanalytic observations that resorts to exhortation and authority are often emotionally determined, the result, for example, of the doctor's countertransference "rescue fantasies."

What psychoanalysis gains in objectivity, by an almost ascetic restraint on the analyst's part, it loses, however, to the objective-descriptive psychiatry in regard to the type of data each collects. Mental content must seem a more subjective type of data than the observations of gesture, handwriting, appearance, and behavior, or the patient as a physical object viewed from without, that comprise objective-descriptive data. We have noted that Kraepelin liked to weigh patients and to follow the course of their weights over time. Here was an objective measure. Kraepelin did not concern himself that the very process of repeatedly weighing someone might serve to interest the patient in his weight and perhaps affect his eating—and consequently the weight itself. The weighing process was seen as objective, that is, revealing but not affecting what it attempted to measure.

Again psychoanalysis is more faithful to the ideal of objectivity. Psychoanalysts are exquisitely aware of how their interventions affect the flow of the patient's material; indeed, this sensitivity to the effect of the doctor explains in part the relatively parsimonious interventions of the analytic doctor. Also, as I mentioned, psychoanalysts study the ways in which the patient's material affects the analysts, still in an attempt to remain objective.

•

The person as a patient and the patient as a site of disease, to be investigated and tested dispassionately, actively, and thoroughly—these are the central features of the objective-descriptive method [3]. The doctor places himself opposite the patient, with something between the two that will objectify the examination. Knowledge of the patient as a diseased person is actively accumulated (from a paranoid point of view, the patient is asked to testify against himself), and when a diagnostic decision has been reached, active steps are taken to reduce or expunge the disease. Patients are expected to cooperate, not to resent being seen as diseased, and even to thank the doctor for attacking their diseases. Insight is critical because by insight is meant the capacity of the patient to see himself as diseased. Difficulties arise when this insight is missing, as well as whenever disease and person are not easily separated and when the disease does not seem precisely limited to the patient alone.

Such is the approach doctors and nurses learn in their training. It has scored mighty victories against disease of many kinds, both physical and social. Particularly when the disease concept is under such heavy attack in psychiatry, it may be worth paying tribute to an approach which at least saves us from the indefinite or furtive concept of mental illness of the newer schools of social and existential psychiatry. In these schools we may all be sick—or perhaps none of us!

PSYCHOANALYSIS

The development of psychoanalysis must have been enormously influenced by the climate of objective-descriptive psychiatry, in which it grew and which dominated psychiatry at that time. The intimacy of Freud's data, his case histories seeming more like "novellas" than spare clinical accounts, threw a large burden of subjectivity on the psychoanalysts. As we have noted, the fact that many of the patients were hysterical, which meant at the time "suggestible," laid Freud open to the charge of putting his ideas in their minds. As if this were not dangerous subjectivity enough, transference and countertransference were discovered: It appeared that the patient experienced the treatment subjectively, and the doctor had difficulty being objective about the patient. The very foundation of medical objectivity was being undercut. Yet if psychoanalysis was to remain within the medical and scientific mainstream, it had to develop a method objective enough to offset these difficulties.

Additional pressure came from the German academic tradition of separating science sharply from history and art [4]. The two modes of knowing, *erklären* and *verstehen*, were not of the same order, this tradition maintained. Every attempt to mix them could end only in confusion. Meanwhile, Freud used biological, psychological, physical, and literary language interchangeably. He brought the Oedipus myth over into psychiatric etiology and his ideas of zonal primacy over into artistic interpretation. He proposed to be objective about what many felt were irreducibly subjective matters.

The psychoanalytic method evolved partly as a result of the pressure for objectivity. Hypnosis, it is true, was abandoned for more reasons than this. Freud is charged with not being a good hypnotist and, what is more certain, he found himself able to confirm Bernheim's claim that the material one could collect hypnotically one could also collect without hypnosis. I suspect, too, that hypnosis *embarrassed* Freud. Hypnotic subjects occasionally "go along with" the hypnotist's suggestions while experiencing no subjective change in their mental states and then give up the pretense abruptly. The hypnotist is left holding an empty bag. Freud was not pompous, but he took no pleasure in looking ridiculous, which must be the fate of anyone intoning and making passes at a wide-awake skeptical subject. Each of these reasons for abandoning hypnosis, however, pales beside the problems hypnosis makes for objectivity. Its central purpose is to influence the patient; its aim, to put ideas in patients' minds. (This very capacity of hypnosis made it the appropriate experimental method for confirming Charcot's hypothesis about hysterics.) Putting ideas in patients' minds was exactly what Freud was accused of doing while he himself sought the opposite—to discover what was already there.

Nevertheless, the next step in the development of the analytic method fell under the same charge. By literally pressing thoughts out of his patients' heads, Freud made vivid the purpose of the method: to elicit verbal material otherwise censored or forgotten. However, he did so at the price of touching patients, holding them, involving them in a far more intimate relationship than an objective psychiatry could permit. It is hard to know whether this inveterate cigar smoker, with the inevitable stained fingers, *alienated* through touching them more of his patients than he encouraged to fall in love with him. In any case, head-pressing was abandoned too.

Then associations to dream fragments, emotionally charged words, or slips of the tongue were sought—the method still most often associated with psychoanalysis and a handy device picked up by all the schools. It is an uncovering technique of surprising power. With cooperative patients free to take mental soundings, a broad range of hidden events, memories, and yearnings can be exposed. Even uncooperative or defensive people give up much that is hidden in the slips, preoccupations, and fragments that one can find among the ordered flow. If Freud had contributed nothing else than this technique, he would have secured himself a place in medical history.

However, this method, too, greatly influences the material. Our very interest in a dream shapes what we are given, arouses defenses, or may lead the patient to woo us with more of the same. Freud, therefore, reduced still further the analyst's interventions. The analyst was to move only against *obstacles* to the flow of material (the so-called analysis of the resistances). Otherwise, he was to listen, wait, and let the material emerge.

The couch serves to relax patients, again to reduce resistances. The doctor sits out of sight because realistic present stimuli will shape the mental flow, and spontaneous, unstimulated, inner-not-outer, past-not-present associations are being sought. Silence helps, so offices are quiet. Even the doctor's writing should be unobtrusive; hence silent pens. Perhaps the turning inward will be delayed by seeing other patients; some become prematurely jealous and erect difficult resistances; one solution is to have separate entrances and exits. Of course degrees of all these techniques are conceivable. It is possible to associate while sitting up, although the chair should be relaxing, and more freedom may result if the doctor sits some distance away. Sitting close and staring into each other's faces and eyes must be disconcerting and it will stimulate an early intimacy. Every effort is made to set both parties free to think without distraction.

The result is a superbly objective method, almost surgical. The patient is supine; he cannot see the doctor, who operates on the material. Every effort is made to keep the field free of extraneous influences. Attention is concentrated on the gradually appearing lesion, the infantile transference neurosis. Only two surgical features are plainly missing, anesthesia and scalpels! But the hope is that interpretations will be precise and cutting and the patient strong enough to stand the pain.

Here is a source of tension. The very objectivity of psychoanalysis mobilizes powerful forces which must be difficult to manage by objective methods. By "objective methods" I mean reason, insight, and perspective-giving. The power of the emotional forces set loose in the transference neurosis must tempt the use of persuasion, suggestion, even personal influence and threat, if the forces are to be controlled. But no matter how terrifying the light it has thrown into the depth of human unreason, analysis is committed to objective methods, particularly the rule of reason.

The chief of these objective, rational *treatment* methods is transference interpretation. The analyst points to the patient's misperceiving the analyst: "You are reacting to me as you perceived your father, not as I am." The power of the old feelings toward the father, which had been mobilized by the laborious objective procedure of analysis, is turned back against the father. Once turned, these forces seek out, as it were, the father memories and help reconstruct the past experience with the father. Thus the energy of the transference is bent by the interpretation to a reconstructive purpose, which, however, is being continually undone.

It is undone by the tendency of the transference distortions to return, the so-called repetition compulsion. Even after the transference neurosis has been very extensively made conscious, it resists extinction. With each turning back on the original figures, of the feelings mobilized toward the doctor, only a little energy is drawn off to the reconstruction and freed up from the neurosis. The longer the neurosis has been present, the greater the resistance against remembering, the more laborious this task of "working through." Again there is a comparison to surgery, in which the amount of cellular reaction to any pathological process determines the depth and complexity of the material through which the surgeon must cut. The infantile neurosis, however, must be worn away, not cut, made obvious, called attention to again and again, almost bored to death. During this process the reconstruction of the past proceeds, gains depth and extension [5]. The analysand has the extraordinary experience of levels of awareness: One discovers something known already but now perceived from a fresh angle, more deeply. The familiar can be a surprise, déjà vu now with pleasure, not horror! Language gropes for expressions that will reflect this many-sided experience of reconstructing the past.

The energy of reconstruction appears to come from the deflected neurotic energy. A third stopping point, however, appears between the analyst and the past figures. Present objects outside the treatment are also transferred onto. Indeed, it is often the sad results of these pretreatment transferences (Sullivan's parataxes) that precipitate the treatment in the first place. Or, in reverse, if external objects need and reward the patient's neurotic attachments, encourage or even cling to them, treatment may be stopped cold. Thus "successful" people resist analytic treatment while being almost the only ones who can afford it, for much of what the world means by success is a childlike overestimation and excessive activity in behalf of glittering goals. Such investments resist insight. Being held in the present, energy cannot turn to the past, often until the success has turned to failure. Only then may the present be abandoned for the past.

In the same analytic hour one can see the past being woven out of these three strands, now memories, then thoughts of the doctor, now attachments to present figures, back and forth, while gradually the intricate tapestry of the past appears.

Concern with the past is as central to psychoanalysis as objectivity. Further, this analytic past is to emerge spontaneously. The questioning, categorizing, organizing ego of the objective-descriptive method is set aside as analyst and patient *listen* for the emerging material.

Analytic *passivity* creates tension because both present and past put up obstacles to remembering. Current problems call for attention. Much of the past is painful, and the organism resists reentering it, for the events that analysis has found of most importance for neurosis formation are naturally part of the hurtful past, the past of disappointments and unrequited love. Indeed, Freud discovered sources of disappointment in early life previously unknown. The most obvious are oedipal disappointments and loss of the breast and womb, but there are also castration anxiety, penis envy, and the whole process of surrendering the play of instincts to parents and society. The childhood of psychoanalysis stands at the farthest possible remove from Rousseau's happy savage.

For these reasons remembering must be resisted, and hence the importance of analyzing the resistances. At first they were thought to be largely the products of social shame at exposing childhood fantasies and wishes. Later, transference was seen to play a part in resistance; patients feared the analysts as perhaps parents had been feared. Still later, resistances were seen to spring from character, the complicated, heavy armor of defenses against impulse that all of us have put on in the course of development. The discovery of this character armor placed a great tension on analytic passivity, for the classic teaching, intervene only against the resistances, might in numerous cases mean intervene all the time, so fixed and ubiquitous were many character armors. Plainly the possibilities of tension between listening and intervening have grown enormously.

Neutrality is still another attitude toward the past and is central to the analytic method. Neutrality is thought to favor the fullest possible reconstruction of the past because, by allying himself with any particular wish, person, or attitude, the therapist casts his weight against others and hears only what he wants to hear. Neutrality is also a logical result of analytic objectivity; the analyst does not know what is best for the patient beyond the work of analysis itself. Psychoanalysis is not neutral about psychoanalysis. The values of objectivity, rationality, the fullest possible reconstruction and understanding of the past, the value of the search for hidden meanings—about all these analysis is not neutral. On the other hand, analytic solutions are *dialectic,* for Freud saw no single clear-cut answer to life's difficulties. Society must restrict the play of instinct; instinct defies society; there are conflicts among the instincts themselves; development compels the abandonment of many loved objects. Even the hoped-for sublimations are available to only a few and then not always. Neither emotional or sexual freedom nor the acceptance of social demands offers a solution. There *is* no natural solution. Reason can only mediate among incomplete possibilities of existence and do its best to impose controls. In Freud's words, the goal of treatment is to replace neurotic suffering by normal human misery. Therapeutic neutrality is therefore an expression of this awareness of life's difficulties, of the many, often incompatible, elements with which people must still live. To confusion and conflict analysis brings insight and historical perspective, the lights of reason and clear perception, the unmasking of self-deceptions and of short-term solutions. Because the goal is truth, not goodness or beauty, the light is neutral.

The tragic quality of human life further strains the analyst's objectivity, neutrality, and passivity. How is the analyst to retain these qualities as the patient reexperiences, as fully as possible, the developmental history of abandonment and unrequited love? The very insights of psychoanalysis place a heavy strain on analytic method.

The patient, too, must be neutral, learn to listen for inner voices and feelings, no matter how perverse or surprising. A scientific attitude toward oneself is sought, as it is in the objective-descriptive method, but now a passive, not an active, one. The patient must be able to see himself as an object of investigation, just as the analyst sees him. Part of the treatment is this assumption of a rational, patient-investigative attitude. Analysts write of the "intact" ego of the patient allying itself with the ego of the analyst, the two egos observing and directing the play of instinctual forces within and between them both.

The rational, intellectual cast of analysis is heightened still more by the material's being *verbal*. Visual observation is restricted by the geography of the method. Feelings occur but are to be verbalized, neither wallowed in nor acted on. Indeed, actions are to be as restricted as possible. For many years sexual continence was recommended, and this patient asceticism of the analytic method served to reduce man to his sexual instincts. The goal was to bring the instincts forward in the same way a long period of abstinence from food reduces anyone to being a "hungry person." Then the felt experience of yearnings, with attendant memories and fantasies, is to find words. Life is to be reduced to words or, perhaps better, *raised* to words, so that it can be examined, reviewed, reorganized, and controlled [6]. The treatment process is itself a sublimation, so appropriate to that master of words, Freud.

•

The analysis of humans into biological instincts to be mastered through verbalization and historical perspective, the development of a theory so like chemical and physical theories with their forces, energies, diagrams, and the reduction to fewer and fewer elements—these objective, scientific features of psychoanalysis are easily lost sight of when bits and pieces of the method and theory are picked up and used by the other schools [7]. Today the scientific interest of psychiatry is carried by behaviorist and biological workers, and the humanistic tradition by existential and social psychiatrists. The heydey of psychoanalytic popularity has passed, at least in the United States, and we see a reseparation of the two cultures that psychoanalysis for a little while brought together.

Therefore, on the contemporary scene, fragments of psychoanalysis appear in either the scientific or the humanistic camp of psychiatry. Behaviorists make use of analytic observations and ideas [8]. Neurophysiological investigations of the visceral brain, with its pleasure and rage areas, seem like investigations of the id. On the humanistic side, both existential and social psychiatrists use the free associative method and accept the facts of defenses, transference, and family dynamics. Much of psychoanalysis is translated into social psychiatry by substitution of the term *relationship* for *instincts*. Social psychiatry even advances the analysis of the resistances, as I have discussed and which I will return to. With all this sacking of the analytic city, there is less and less eagerness to persevere in the development of the transference neurosis. If anything, we see increased isolation of the analytic institutes from practice and medicine at large, even as these institutes struggle to preserve the method in its developed form, and there is more and more enthusiasm for entering relationships with patients by means of the methods I will now discuss.

EXISTENTIAL METHOD

We have seen that interpersonal psychiatry arose in part from the need to deal with especially resistant patients. In place of Freud's analysis of the resistances it substituted activity against them. The existential method, too, developed partly as a reaction to several features of psychoanalysis that were seen as limitations, notably its objective, biological, and intellectual casts, as well as to the limitations of objective-descriptive psychiatry, particularly its restriction to externals.

Furthermore, each of the great methods began as an addition to earlier methods. Minkowski's emotional outbursts did not at first mean he sought a steadily emotional or empathic relationship with patients. He quickly returned to observing and directing, as the early Freud did after his trials of free association. Only much later was the existential method, as well as psychoanalysis and participant observation, able to gain a degree of power and internal consistency which made switching back to an earlier method undesirable and difficult. Now we cannot imagine the psychoanalyst or existential therapist stopping the analysis or encounter to take up the objective examination.

I am aware that the available meager descriptions of existential method do not suggest either power or consistency. In fact no part of the present work has been more difficult than the discovery and description of the existential techniques. Indeed, I can be accused of having made an imaginative construction of the existential method that is at least partly a creation of my own. In defense of this, I found no technical literature of existential psychiatry, certainly nothing comparable to the psychoanalytic literature on method or the manuals of interpersonal technique. Existential writers have deliberately avoided such discussions because the whole concept of technique defies existential principles. Everything technical is thought to reduce man to the status of an object, which destroys humanness.

Nevertheless I describe an existential method. I realize that such a method, carrying as it does strong emotional, spontaneous elements, shunning every possibility of prediction, in fact, viewing the unpredictable as an essential feature of experience, seems more the outgrowth of an approach to others conceived of as persons, not objects, than it does a technique in the usual scientific sense. Perhaps my use of the words *technique* and, still worse, *technology* is deliberately provocative. Some will surely experience it that way. I do not want, however, to turn aside from the challenge of those words with all their aura of science, experience, and deliberate methodical power over nature. One hears everywhere that this is a technological age, that technology threatens to enslave us, ruin us—perhaps also to save us. It is certainly no neutral term, and I would perhaps have been wiser to avoid it. I did not because we have no other word for this particular development of psychiatry, the development of its tools. Such terms as *attitude, approach to the patient,* and *stance* only beg the question, and the phrase *point of view* substitutes a perceptual metaphor for detailed understanding of psychiatry's methods. Moreover, it is true that any tool is an embodiment of science and science, at the same time, is the precipitate of our tools.

I have already described how the existential method began with the determination of its area of inquiry, inner experience; reports of this were the first, phenomenological data of existential psychiatry, and the traditional objective examinational securing of these reports collapsed in the absence of willing informants. (Similarly, free association, as opposed to analysis of the resistances, revealed its limitations as soon as Freud left behind his "willing informants"!) Minkowski's being and staying was at first only a literal "thereness"; he lived in the same rooms with the schizophrenic person. A psychic being and staying, on the other hand, required great tolerance and patience and then a technical step that flew in the face of everything objective—seemingly in the face of everything technical, too. Minkowski lost his temper. The result of his outburst fell so far outside the official understanding of schizophrenic psychoses and so far outside objective technology that we are entitled to call it a milestone. Minkowski and the patient came closer. The schizophrenic patient was suddenly depressed. For a moment he dropped his delusions, and, in turn, Minkowski felt close to him; there was no more of the "praecox gefühl." I call this an *implosion,* an explos.on of feeling that brought the two closer because, in response to Minkowski's expression of feeling, the patient expressed feelings in turn and changed, if only temporarily, with the result that the two could come closer. It is difficult to believe that anything else would have made possible their staying together.

I have also detailed how this implosive technique developed into an empathic one, thanks largely to Binswanger. (The parallel development in the psychoanalytic method was from catharsis to working through, again the substitution of a chronic for an acute therapeutic process.) The critical tool is the phenomenological reduction. Between therapist and patient, Binswanger argued, accumulate ideas, prejudices, and diagnoses, the precious knowledge in which students and teachers take such pride. All this must be "put between brackets." Empathy is the state of being where the patient is and therefore feeling what the patient feels. Therapists arrive where the patients are only when they abandon all those contents of their own heads which preceded that arrival and let themselves learn from within the patient's experience.

Here, we might say, is an analysis of the resistances of the *therapist.* However, not only the specific analytically discovered countertransferences of the analyst are to be "worked through," or the projective fantasies that Sullivan found between doctor and patient, but the whole categorizing, reflecting, thinking, investigating attitude of the therapist must be set aside. The patient must not even be thought of as sick! This is the supreme challenge to the medical attitude. It comes almost as an anticlimax when existential writers suggest that we be prepared to discover that the *doctors* may be sick.

Without the phenomenological reduction, Binswanger argued, doctors find in the patients what they expect to find. So many patients want to please that the doctor's ideas become more and more entrenched. Human organisms are too subtly responsive to one another for the safe passage of preformed ideas. Approaching the patient naked allows the patient to feel our openness, to take us in, and above all to teach us. Nature, in Darwin's words, reveals her secrets only to those innocent enough to gain her confidence.

Like the resulting phenomenological knowledge, the therapeutic power of the existential method springs from this being and staying. But the therapeutic power is not the power of education, suggestion, surgery, or injection; nor is it the power of the transference interpretation of the infantile neurosis and analysis of its resistances, now from within the patient's world, vulnerable as the patient then is. To exert that power would be to use the existential method like a Trojan horse—to use it in the service of some preformed conception of the patient's needs. *Being and staying is the goal in itself.* No aspect of the existential method is more difficult than this, to center the effort on being and staying and avoid action, explanation, emotional reassurances, and all the "rational" responses that the patient's desperation must evoke from us. Students learning this technique urgently ask what use it is just being with the patients. To my knowledge, the answer has not been fully formulated in existential writings. Much of what follows is made up of deductions from the existential method together with observations from my own and others' experiences.

Most obviously, being and staying offers companionship at a sufficiently desperate moment in the patient's life to make it telling. Some of the patients appear never to have had their aloneness broken into and meet in the encounter their first experience of the therapeutic power of companionship. Further, because the therapist's being where the patient is means the therapist feels something of what the patient does, much that the patient feels can no longer seem bizarre; companionship in the same feelings represents strong testimony to their naturalness. Binswanger (and Sullivan) understood from experience, especially with psychotic people, that a great part of the demoralizing power of insanity flows from the patient's fear and conviction of being insane, different, alone, and that whatever brings this fear out into the open and destroys it eradicates a considerable part of the demoralizing power of insanity.

It is also true that being and staying, sharing the helplessness of the patient, for example, not attempting to push solutions, to save the patient, or to interpret the situation—all this serves to mobilize the patient's resources. The reasons are not fully clear. Probably we should be most surprised that the patient is not made *more* helpless by the felt helplessness of the therapist, but such is often not the case. Perhaps it is the breakdown of aloneness and the reduction of fear of insanity just mentioned that mobilize resources, or the mobilization may come from putting behind some of the secondary or social gain of psychosis. We know that psychosis is, in part, an effort to punish the world, convert parents, express fear of difficult situations, and, in some, adapt to an unlivable world. When therapists no longer defend that world but share the patient's defeat by it, there may be less need to be psychotic.

Being and staying for its own sake! Nothing seems more remote from the usual therapeutics. Even the Sullivanian coun-terprojective method and certainly the analytic bringing-the-neurosis-to-consciousness have a more familiar ring. While consciousness, in which psychoanalysis puts such stock, may not seem the therapeutic power it once did, the power to know and the power to direct actions by knowledge still command wide respect.

Yet there are powers in being and staying familiar to all the schools. I do not mean now the companionship and normal-ization of experience, already touched on, that empathy ef-fects. I can introduce this difficult subject by staking out a claim for existential psychiatry. It would read: The existential method is the principal attempt to harness and bring into ther-apeutics the educational component of love.

The words that follow are from Freud, but they bear di-rectly on this mechanism of existential therapy. He is decrib-ing the resolution of the Oedipus complex. Note that, in ex-istential terms, the resolution evolves from a crisis and depends on entering the world of another and taking away from it some characteristics of the other, the latter being what Freud called an identification.

In its simplified form the case of a male child may be described as follows. At a very early age the little boy develops an object-cathexis for his mother, which originally related to the mother's breast and is the prototype of an object-choice on the anaclitic model; the boy deals with his father by identifying himself with him. For a time these two relationships proceed side by side, until the boy's sexual wishes in regard to his mother become more in-tense and his father is perceived as an obstacle to them; from this the Oedipus complex originates. His identification with his father then takes on a hostile colouring and changes into a wish to get rid of his father in order to take his place with his mother. Hencefor-ward his relation to his father is ambivalent; it seems as if the am-bivalence inherent in the identification from the beginning had become manifest. An ambivalent attitude to his father and an object-relation of a solely affectionate kind to his mother make up the content of the simple positive Oedipus complex in a boy.

Along with the demolition of the Oedipus complex, the boy's object-cathexis of his mother must be given up. Its place may be filled by one of two things: either an identification with his mother or an intensification of his identification with his father. We are accustomed to regard the latter outcome as the more normal; it permits the affectionate relation to the mother to be in a measure retained. In this way the dissolution of the Oedipus complex would consolidate the masculinity in a boy's character. In a precisely analogous way, the outcome of the Oedipus attitude in a little girl may be an intensification of her identification with her mother (or the setting up of such an identification for the first time)—a result which will fix the child's feminine character [9].

The crisis of the oedipal situation is precipitated by the child's possessive love. The crisis is resolved, Freud suggests, by giving up the loved object and taking into the self what the beloved himself or herself loved, the parent of the same sex as the child. Fear is one motive for this identification; love is another. Failures of identification abound in which the child either does not have a loved parent or cannot also love the feared parent or has no reason to fear either parent: That is, absence of love, on the one hand, or absence of fear, on the other, makes impossible both the oedipal crisis and its resolution through identification.

Love and fear are here, as perhaps everywhere, the great educators. Education, in turn, is marked by a taking in—in this case of features of a parent, in others of information, habits, learning of any kind. We test the occurrence of learning by memory: Can the subject reproduce what has been taken in?

The oedipal crisis is a maturational crisis. It is one of the graduation points from childhood into adulthood. Because the maturation is a kind of joining up with features of the parent, the maturation can be only as complete as the figures one identifies with are mature, as well as appropriate to the particular developing young person. Later there will need to be as many other maturational crises as there are occasions to replace or add to one's internal objects.

I present the oedipal crisis as a model for the existential crisis and encounter because nowhere else is the educational component of love more prominent. There is not a great understanding of the conditions which make successful oedipal resolution likely. There are, however, many contributions to our understanding of oedipal *failure*. As I noted, if one parent is absent, if the relationship between parents is so distant as to permit the child to keep its dependent love relationship with one or both parents—that is, so distant as not to exclude the child—there need be no crisis, and as a result no need for the encounter, and no one with whom it can be experienced. On the other hand, where there is a sufficiently loving relationship between parents to exclude the child's possessive love, and where there is a parent it is possible to get close to, the conditions for crisis and coming together are present. The result is the identification.

The educational component of love is therefore love's capacity to engender identifications. One of the technical requirements for this capacity to emerge is closeness, the being and staying. Another is the crisis which precipitated the need for the encounter, and then come the successive emotional crises which being and staying necessitates. Identifications occur in a needful, emotional field; the personality must be in solution, as it were, in transit. Then the therapist leaves pieces of himself behind in the patient.

I suggest that leaving pieces of ourselves behind in the patient is the chief mechanism of existential treatment. The method of existential psychiatry sets up the conditions necessary for the leaving behind.

It would be easy enough to put the goal of the method, and

even the method itself, in the language of the other schools. Some behaviorists, for example, have argued that learning proceeds best under conditions of "positive reinforcement," which has several features in common with the process just described. I think, however, that the distinct features of the existential method will come clearer if I contrast it to the methods of other schools.

Existential "being with the patient" may seem like the therapeutic alliance of psychoanalysis, but in fact the two are far apart. The therapeutic alliance is a rapport between the working egos of doctor and patient; the *neurotic* formations of either doctor or patient do not participate. Existential "being with the patient," on the other hand, means being with whatever one can find of the patient; one does not decide what is well or sick before one has arrived there. Existential psychiatry, like interpersonal psychiatry, warns analysis that its therapeutic alliance too often means an alliance with the characterological, highly organized part of the personality, which may prove more rigid and difficult than even the psychotic elements. Psychoanalysis, for its part, warns existential psychiatry that "being with the patient" easily becomes sentimentality, gives way to a mystic communing from which nothing but vague feelings emerge.

Secondly, psychoanalytic descriptions of the "narcissistic transference" may suggest the phenomenological reduction. The analyst is to interest himself in the interests of the patient, appear at least to be where the patient is. The idea is to encourage rapport and the therapeutic alliance. I wonder, however, whether those analysts bent on making a narcissistic transference seem persuasive; they are admittedly not sincere. The narcissistic transference is essentially role-playing or a manipulation. What, for example, will the patient feel when these interests that were once the basis of comradeship come under analytic scrutiny? Even more important, is the analytic search for "things back of it all" compatible with an existential relationship? The existential method is trusting; it means the therapist is to be "taken in." Nothing could be farther from the analytic method.

The existential method also asks the therapist to give up his partnership with the *establishments* of the world. He is not to think he knows what the patient's "reality" is, for instance; he therefore cannot help the patient reality-test, not knowing what his reality is. Thus, as I have remarked, he cannot ally himself with the "realistic" part of the patient because that civilized conservative part may be the worst enemy both doctor and patient have. Existential psychiatry wonders whether there is any neutralized or conflict-free part of the personality, at least any that is alive [10].

•

All the schools want to discover and correct what is wrong. The medical-descriptive method does it from outside, existentialists insist on going as far inside as possible, and analysis tries to draw the illness out, to be studied and affected once outside. We will see in the next pages that interpersonal psychiatrists attend to a still different area. The illness is *between* the patient and others and must be dealt with there.

INTERPERSONAL PSYCHIATRY

Sullivan sat beside his patients because he believed spoken sounds conveyed more than faces (here was an ear-to-ear, not a face-to-face technique) and because his sitting beside the patient expressed his alliance with the patient, literally being on his side. Besides, not being face to face avoided the forming of too intimate or soulful a relationship too quickly. Intimacy was not Sullivan's dish. He preferred expertise through observation and interaction; hence the method's name: participant observation. In addition, not looking directly at the patient avoided the suggestion that the sickness was in the patient; here was a way to prevent instant conflict with paranoid people. Also, because Sullivan believed that psychiatric troubles were usually in the patient's "situation," sitting beside the patient and looking with him out at the world directed the attention of both patient and doctor to where Sullivan thought the trouble was. Each of the great schools centers its observing somewhere, on the patient seen from outside, on the freely produced associative material, or on inner experience. Since Sullivan's was a social or interpersonal psychiatry, the focus of observation was on society.

The method is neither objective nor subjective, nor is it intent on reducing the subject-object distance, like the existential method. The operative term is *interview,* looking and talking back and forth, not an examination, hour, or encounter. Some distance between patient and doctor is accepted, and it is conceptualized as an active space across which are traveling communications that affect both parties. The effects begin at the onset of the interview, the first business of which is both to understand and to influence them.

For this method neither object nor examiner is static, as objective-descriptive psychiatry demands. Because patient and doctor are caught in an ongoing interactive flow, the efforts of the objective schools to step outside that flow only conceal and complicate the interactive process. There is no fixed position, Sullivan argued, from which human observations can be made.

The observer can also not listen and collect, as psychoanalysis claims is sometimes possible, again because no neutral, aloof position exists in the social field. Real neutrality and objectivity are goals to be achieved by understanding and managing the mutually distorting forces. Much of the analyst's neutral technique—the use of silence, for example—Sullivan claimed made even the eventual establishment of objectivity impossible.

Nor, from the standpoint of the interpersonal method, do the empathy and shared experience of existential psychiatry offer a realistic resting point. Being and staying where the patient is, expressing feelings insofar as is necessary to remain there, revealing oneself to the patient so that he will know where one is (and because self-revelation cannot be a one-way street), the radical *neutrality* of the existential technique (nothing will be presupposed as to who or whether anyone is sick)—all this makes *conceivable* a games-free interaction, the game beyond games, of spontaneity, intimacy, and receptiveness. The more completely phenomenological reduction is practiced, however, the more likely doctors and patients are to lose their heads and, in the communing of the existential method, concoct fresh games they cannot observe and remedy. Existential psychiatry approaches mindlessness. Existential psychiatry glorifies intimacy and disdains the roles and masks of everyday life. Interpersonal psychiatry deplores many games people play, too, and sets about actively to change them, but some degree of game-playing it finds a necessity. For all the sweet sound of the word, intimacy may not be the stuff of everyday life.

Intimacy not only opens the door to fresh games that observing the intimacy will expose. Concentration on intimacy also neglects the extraordinary obstacles to intimacy that most people carry. As we have noted, Sullivan believed that almost everyone is both more solipsistic and more projective than the other schools have assumed. In concrete terms, he believed people spend most of even their waking lives in their own heads, and that when they do look out on the world, what they see is heavily colored by what is already in their heads. Interestingly, Sullivan has been criticized for making these assumptions because he is thought to have illustrated them better than "normal" people do. Whatever their subjective roots, however, or the skewing of his judgment by particular clinical experiences, the interpersonal method is attention-seeking (to rouse patients out of their self-absorption) and counterprojective (to offset the projective distortions).

The need for both attention-seeking and counterprojective behavior is hard to demonstrate to people used to assuming high degrees of normalization or reality orientation in every-day life. Of course, salesmen have either to learn the Sulli-vanian method or to have it already in their bones if they want the doors opened and then not slammed in their faces. Pro-fessional people, however, tend to assume that they are attended to and understood; they do not maintain Sullivan's ex-quisite alertness to what the patients feel about their relation-ships with us. Even psychoanalysis, despite the credit it merits for discovering the closely related transference phenomena, keeps its attention on the meaning of the present relationship in terms of past relationships. In practice, this is a far cry from noting moment to moment how the patient is feeling about the attitudes we impart to him. For one thing, analytic trans-ference observations rather neglect the contribution we and our professional situation are making to the misunderstanding, and tend to set the therapist's mind on the line of a few possi-ble misunderstandings (the patient is becoming dependent on me as he was on his mother, for example) rather than requir-ing him to form a precise idea of how the patient is misunder-standing and then look for prototypes in the past. Because interpersonal psychiatry is focused on the present and on the social realities of the patient's experiences, including the fact that he is now talking to someone supposed to be helpful, the relationship of interpersonal psychiatry to transference or para-taxic phenomena is the reverse of that in psychoanalysis: pres-ent, not past; reality first, fantasy later.

I do not know how much projection does occur in everyday

life, or even how to measure it. Yet the more experience I have, the more prevalent projection seems to me, more common perhaps than denial or repression, once the kings of defense mechanisms. This presumption, in turn, may be the result of *my* distortions or due to the skewing of my experience. I have seldom, however, been mistaken in *assuming* extraordinary amounts of projection in both clinic and neighborhood.

Sullivan eschewed intimacy not only because it was difficult for him but because there was literally no time, at least early in a relationship, to do anything but attend to the projections. Here is the clearest possible contrast to analytic method. The latter uses neutrality as a tool—or a screen on which to throw the projections—to encourage them. For Sullivan neutrality was a *goal,* to be achieved through recognizing and correcting the projections. In order to achieve rationality, in order to establish a clinical field free of projections and therefore possible to judge coolly and objectively, all kinds of unneutral behaviors were necessary.

Of course, analysts analyze the resistances in order to reduce them. This use of reason, insight, and consciousness is the hallmark of psychoanalysis. Sullivan found such an approach to the resistances inadequate, perhaps because the strength of the resistances he encountered in his psychotic and near-psychotic patients made an intellectual approach fruitless. Sullivan therefore made remarks to patients sharply critical of their parental figures, or, if the parents were still being protected by the patient, remarks systematically ambiguous. He used sarcasm and irony; he even role-played—all with the intention of removing himself from the patient's projections, of making it more difficult to respond to Sullivan as if he were the patient's excessively loved and hated figures. Such behaviors are included under the term *action against the resistances.* Many psychoanalysts would respond: In the case of psychotic people, yes; with the neuroses, never. However, too many analysts have been defeated by the resistances of supposedly neurotic patients for us to rest easy with such a rebuttal.

At this point the reader may protest that I have neglected *ego psychology.* Actually I have not neglected it but avoided using the term because ego psychology is a *hybrid,* springing from psychoanalysis on the one hand and social psychiatry on the other. To have used the term would have suggested an easy mating of these two roots of ego psychology, which in fact does not exist. The reason is now clear. In practice ego psychology means for both psychoanalysis and Sullivanian psychiatry *recognizing* the defenses or resistances. But the types of *action* each takes against the defenses are at sharp variance: in one case, analysis of the resistances and bringing to consciousness the defenses; in the other, action against the resistances, even role-playing, and attempting to diminish the defenses, without prime concern for the patient's insight.

Finally, in contrast to *existential* psychiatry, Sullivan warned against falling into a comfortable, easy, loving relationship with the patient, and against enjoying the work. Either invites a coming together in projection which promises trouble for tomorrow. It is not too much to say that Sullivan saw most therapeutic efforts in psychiatry as little short of folie à deux between doctor and patient, or, at best, writing on water.

·

The methods of social psychiatry developed from direct observation of homes and industry and proceeded to the study of social processes in institutions (family and industries, too, but now also hospitals and the relationship of doctor and patient). The most powerful and subtle tool developed for the study of social processes was the interpersonal or Sullivanian method, the psychiatric *interview,* by which the actual social experience of the patient could be determined and sometimes improved. This method studies social processes by participating in them (just as psychoanalysis studies fantasies by participating in them—the transference neurosis), and then applying tests and correctives to determine and alter the *social unconscious*. Here was a fresh region of unconsciousness. Social processes were no more open and obvious than intrapsychic ones. They had to be discovered just as elements and atoms did. The commonest unconscious social process appeared to be projection (parataxis). One tested for it either by playing into the projections (and watching anxiety rise) or by doing something counterprojective (and watching anxiety fall). Anxiety was the central indicator of parataxic processes (like fever in bodily disease processes), and testing the patient's anxiety level was continually necessary if the participant observer hoped to retain any grasp of the actual social forces at work. This was a method for dealing with the "other people in the room": those figures in the patient's life whom he brings into any social situation, however much he appears alone.

The goals of the method were at first investigative, like those of the other schools. Sullivan was able to describe the behavior of schizophrenic patients with their parents and something of the latter's behavior with their children, a current of investigative work running strong and full since [11]. The investigative interest was soon therapeutic, and, because Sullivanian psychiatry owed so much to psychoanalysis, it was easy to confuse the treatment devices of the one with those of the other. As a result, the sharp differences between transference interpretation and what we can call transference correction, or action against the resistances, have been blurred.

Sullivan argued that all psychiatric illness was social illness. (His method of work made discovering anything else impossible, just as Freud's method restricted him!) It was therefore vital for Sullivan to correct pathological social processes such as "self-fulfilling prophecies," not the intrapsychic ones. If the neurotic and psychotic games could be broken up by having the parataxes cut down or eliminated, the ongoing sociopathic processes would stop. No effort was made to correct intrapsychic processes; these were assumed to take care of themselves when the social processes were changed. Nor was it central for the patient to understand the social processes at work (that was intrapsychic insight). The important thing was that *social consciousness* be raised; the people involved were no longer to see each other the old projective way. What was being sought was true awareness of the *other*, not of oneself. Or similarly, one sought to be seen by others for what one was. Self-knowledge was therefore secondary or peripheral.

11

DILEMMAS AND SOLUTIONS

From cases like this I learned to adapt my methods to the needs of the individual patient, rather than to commit myself to general theoretical considerations that might be inapplicable in any particular case. The knowledge of human nature that I have accumulated in the course of 60 years of practical experience has taught me to consider each case as a new one in which, first of all, I have had to seek the individual approach. Sometimes I have not hesitated to plunge into a careful study of infantile events and fantasies; at other times I have begun at the top, even if this has meant soaring straight into the most remote metaphysical speculations. It all depends on learning the language of the individual patient and following the gropings of his unconscious toward the light. Some cases demand one method and some another.

Carl Jung

T HE DILEMMAS presented by the schools are innumerable, but I will list, illustrate, and then discuss some of the principal ones. As long as one school or another is blindly followed, these dilemmas are obscure. However, once one is outside the method of any individual school, alternatives emerge that are not easily united even by what Glover has called "terminological sutures."

The therapist must decide whether to sit close to the patient or at a distance, in sight or out of sight, beside or in front so as to hear or see best, with or without some objective instrument between. He can equip himself with as much knowledge of the patient as possible before seeing him and remember all he can of what transpires between visits, or each time the approach may be new and fresh. Then he must consider whether to ask questions or to wait, engage himself or remain aloof. He might permit the development of misunderstandings in the clinical situation or he could attempt to keep abreast of these misunderstandings and reduce them whenever possible. What the patient says can be accepted at face value and only his point of view enlarged, or the therapist could search out hidden meanings from the start. Would it be wiser to apply this method in the group setting or to one patient at a time? Does the therapist remain neutral with his patient, or ally himself with him against the world, or ally himself with the world and against the patient perhaps? Shall attention be directed to the associative material, or to the interaction between patient and therapist, or to the patient's felt conscious inner experience, or to the details of his appearance, or even to the symptoms he brings? The therapist must decide what to give priority to next—the past, present, or future—and whether to allow himself expression of feelings in some clinical situations or to assume that he must operate rationally and verbally, but seldom affectively. The focus can be on the individual (or the individual disease entity), or on the interaction between individuals, or on the "transactional field," in which there are no individuals but only "systems" influencing each other to produce phenomena previously thought of as entities.

No school, of course, sees these as dilemmas [1] because, by definition, the schools have internally consistent methods that resolve each issue. Once set to develop a transference neurosis, or to be where the patient is, or to diagnose and treat the symptoms, or to determine and reduce the parataxes, therapists can act promptly and consistently.

AN ILLUSTRATION: DEALING WITH ANGER

Almost any clinical situation will illustrate the schools in action:

The patient is angry; he verbally attacks a family member as unfeeling or obstructive, and more indirectly, the doctor, too, for the same reasons. All this has taken place in the first minute or two of contact. What are the possible responses?

Some are tempted to call attention to the patient's anger, naming the mood and asking the reason. This directness, plus use of a question, alerts us to an objective-descriptive approach. Other questions may follow, to uncover, perhaps, paranoid delusions, similar past convictions, persecutory voices, etc. The focus is on the patient as a carrier of psychopathology. The technique is effective because, even if the patient resents the implications of the questions, his resentment may make him appear still more paranoid, confirming the diagnosis. In short, the questions are not only information-gathering but testing, as in Kraepelin's catatonia tests. What may be lost, however, is rapport. When the doctor is tired or the patient particularly difficult or brought to the doctor against his wishes, the loss of rapport need not be experienced as a loss. Further, what distinguishes protagonists of the objective-descriptive approach is their conviction that precise diagnostic information is worth possible losses of rapport because precise diagnosis makes possible appropriate treatment. This relationship of early diagnosis to treatment is at the heart of the objective-descriptive method.

In psychoanalysis, by way of contrast, accurate diagnosis does not precede treatment; the two go hand in hand. Diagnosis may even be the result of treatment, reversing the familiar order.

In response to the angry patient an analyst might remain

silent, listening expectantly, or repeat words or phrases the patient used. This process might continue until the patient fell silent. The analyst would then attempt to remove whatever resistances to the patient's continual flow he could reach. "Perhaps you thought I would react to your observations in the same way you felt your parents did." (Contrast this with the Sullivanian "Well, it must be hard, on this short acquaintance, to know whether I am not as supersensitive or closed-minded as, from what you tell me, your parents seem to be.") Note the analyst's statement is relatively neutral in its judgment of the parents; also there is no attempt to deal wih the patient's feelings about the interview situation, specifically the difficulties the patient must have knowing the doctor's personality. Analysis, of course, wants to keep the doctor's personality a secret, so that the patient's projections can be drawn out. The more hostile the patient is or the more aloof the doctor seems, the more tension will occur in the hour, with increasing pressure on the patient to surface the doctor's real attitudes and on the doctor to modify his neutrality in order to reduce possible misunderstandings. If the doctor refuses to modify his neutrality and the patient explodes or becomes psychotic, the doctor will probably conclude that this is not a suitable patient for the classical technique. Hence the objective methods of both medical-descriptive psychiatry and psychoanalysis are also testing methods. And, as in most testing methods, one has to jump nimbly if the weights bring down the bridge.

This description will put off a great many contemporary analysts because today the literature on analytic technique is more existential and Sullivanian than even Ferenczi's writings, or Franz Alexander's [2]. Some psychoanalysts, in other words, believe the goal of a transference neurosis permits a greater range of emotional responsiveness and freedom of intervention on the analyst's part than was once considered desirable. The clinical evidence for this position seems weak to me, and certainly its theoretical defense is still weaker, even in structural and object relations terms. It is difficult, moreover, to get enough precision into the terms and discussions for a clear decision. The activistic mood of contemporary psychotherapy, furthermore, pits itself more and more strongly against the technique of listening and waiting described.

Both the objective methods screen out patients who will not accept being targets of pathological investigation. The result is that comparisons of objective with existential and Sullivanian methods are comparisons of different methods on different patients and on different problem areas of the same patient. Undoubtedly there is as much selection of what the patients bring different doctors as there is of which patients arrive in the first place.

Existential therapists, on the other hand, *welcome* the patient's anger because any strong, emotional presentation of the self shows where the presenter is and also integrates the presenter, if only temporarily! Therapists are that much closer to that much more of their patients. Welcoming anger, however, demands at least a nonjudgmental attitude toward an emotion usually condemned. More than that, a positive rather than a neutral attitude is favored, and before anything can be known of the anger's justice or appropriateness. Such an indiscriminate acceptance of the patient's feelings instantly condemns existential work in the eyes of many because it seems to encourage what may be irrational actions and ideas; the psychiatrist is taken from one of his traditional posts as the spokesman and guardian of society's values against the mad. When this traditional position is strongly held, even the *scientific rationale* for existential method may be overlooked: that we really cannot decide much about a person (if we see that as our job) until we get where the person is; and we are not likely to be permitted there if he is judged sick until proved well. (In medicine, presumably for safety's sake, the traditional assumptions of Anglo-Saxon criminal law are reversed.)

How does one take an existential position toward the angry patient? [3]. "You have really felt taken advantage of. No wonder you feel furious." Or, "It's astonishing you don't feel even angrier than you do in the light of what you've been experiencing." Surprisingly, this sort of thing quiets more angry people than it excites, perhaps because it translates feelings into words or because confronting the patient with his feelings may temper them. In any case, if it is successful (and no technique is always successful) the patient should feel understood, closer to the therapist, which association itself may reduce fear and any anger secondary to fear. Of course, particularly if the therapist is insincere, patients may become *more* suspicious.

Once closer to where the patient is, the therapist learns quickly whatever "justice" there is to the patient's furies. And once this has been acknowledged, the chances of getting the patient to acknowledge any "injustices" of his own behavior increase commensurately. The existential method involves a quid pro quo, or, again to use Binswanger's language, in a true relationship both parties change.

Of course the existential therapist may *not* be able to welcome the patient's anger. He may, in other words, have to demand some change in the patient before rather than after the two get closer (as occurred in the Minkowski case discussed). In accomplishing this, unless therapists are prepared for shouting matches right off, they had best listen and bear awhile, as empathically as possible. (Again, like Minkowski.) At least the appearance of receptivity may make the patient more receptive when the encounter occurs.

An emphasis on felt experience and its sharing is, of course, the hallmark of the existential method. It is therefore likely that *affective* disorders will yield most to this method. Sullivanian technique, in contrast, seems particularly appropriate for *paranoid* patients.

I mentioned earlier a Sullivanian response to the angry patient. It was marked by more attention to the doctor-patient situation than are typically analytic comments, and also by a less neutral position on family members. These emphases on the present and the actual are, of course, characteristic of the method. Like analysts, however, interpersonalists *comment* on experience; they do not share it, existentially.

The emphasis on social experience, present and past, diffuses the patient's responsibility for illness. The parataxes are assumed to spring from parental interactions and can be "blamed" on the parents. Something similar is achieved by the existential partisanship with the patient. With both methods, facile scapegoating is a danger.

Since actual experience rather than fantasies and wishes are being searched for, we can speak of social psychiatry as more historical in the traditional sense than psychoanalysis. The latter makes light of the difference between fact and fancy which is at the heart of traditional historiography. The Sullivanian psychiatrist, like the historian, wants to know what really happened.

"God forbid," Sullivan might have muttered, "you should ever confuse me with your blessed parents!" well aware that the patient was already hopelessly confused between the two. "Well, sooner or later I'm bound to receive that happy inheritance of good will she has stored up in you"—all this dripping with sarcasm.

Objective psychiatrists cannot tolerate the subjectivity and emotionality of such utterances. Paradoxically, however, interpersonalists are using this apparently wild technique in part to establish the actualities. They question any statement about what is fantasy before one knows what is fact. Granted that our fantasies about one another constitute perhaps the greatest social reality, there is still a remarkably important difference between fact and fancy; of course the concept of transference interpretation implies that, too. Similarly, ideas about the past were not to be treated as if they were fantasies alone or as if it did not matter whether they were facts or fantasies. One had to attempt the fullest possible historical reconstruction (another reason for seeing the whole family) because the patient could otherwise never establish a firm reality sense, and without that he was crippled socially; there would be no separating false from true expectations of others. The issue—What did I contribute and what did you contribute?—is central to social psychiatry, both in its historical reconstructive phase and in its efforts to help people make sense of their ongoing social experiences.

The patient is operated on by Sullivan, manipulated, as in objective-descriptive psychiatry, but by means of affect-laden strokes and parries. Sullivan was almost as "emotional" as existential psychiatrists. The social masks, however, were being flicked on and off, not put aside.

Watch how he would try to bring both sides of an ambivalent relationship forward almost at once, so that the whole, complex social picture could be exposed: "I do not suppose your parents could have been better intentioned," still dealing with the angry patient.

The goals are to separate himself from the parents and at the same time help forward both sides of the patient's feelings about the parent: The remark defends parents at the very moment it suggests blundering. How else, Sullivan would have argued, can we learn what is actually going on between the people involved, for if the patient confuses me with his parents, he must hide from me too? And unless I surface both sides of his ambivalence toward the parents, I cannot fully know what he has experienced with them.

Pros and cons are played off against one another by this

manipulative technique. Having acknowledged the devoted protectiveness of the parents, and secured extensive evidence of it, Sullivan is in a position to explore the limitations of this method of child-rearing, and therefore to understand the basis of the patient's negative feelings toward the parents. The patient is afraid of and even grateful toward his parents; he is therefore hesitant to criticize them or to expose what in fact went on. Sullivan first placates the "hostile introjects," then allies himself with the patient. The two get the parents, real and introjected, into perspective. Note that an awareness of *conflict* is central to this method, as in analysis, but the interest of dealing with the conflict is in exposing actual social experience, not fantasy.

Thus, *interviewing*, with all its sense of interacting, participating, adapting to each other, even manipulating each other, is no *examination* in which detached observers look over static objects. Neither is it an *encounter*, for interviewer and interviewee stand apart, not sharing feelings but reacting. Nor is it an *hour*, that temporal receptacle for associations and interpretations in which analyst and analysand move through time.

Again, by way of contrast, medical-descriptive psychiatry is increasing the clinician's power of recognition; Sullivanian psychiatry, his power to act. Psychoanalysis has brought psychiatry a great power of explanation [4]; phenomena hitherto separate now seen related, some even identical. Existential method, in turn, has brought to clinical work new power to feel.

THERAPISTS' DECISIONS

The psychiatrist must choose his method as a surgeon or an internist chooses his tests or medicines or operations, depending on the goals sought, information needed, stage of the work, or type of person and illness. But because psychiatric development is at a more uncertain stage than that of medicine or surgery, psychiatrists experience these decisions as dilemmas among which our incomplete understanding hesitates.

Many influences play over therapists' decisions. We can recognize national styles, however problematic such mass judgments are. Personal, temperamental factors enter everywhere, especially today when much is said about the importance of therapists' feeling comfortable in what they do. The example of charismatic teachers has great influence not only in teaching but whenever there is need for confidence and authority. Styles in thought change, too, so that now people believe in existentialism, social psychiatry, or behaviorism, where once psychoanalysis was believed in. Finally, among these extraclinical influences, the patients affect us through unconscious social mechanisms. Processes of emotional contagion, for example, are set going between doctor and patient that may escape conscious clinical control.

Happily, in addition, clinical considerations enter. Because psychiatry is a practical art with scientific aspirations, clinical considerations have to make their way against heavy stylistic, temperamental currents, but psychiatry's goal is to increase the power and accuracy of clinical considerations, and significant gains have been made.

When we read a psychiatric account by Charcot or Janet, we are immediately struck by its *dramatic* values. The patients wail, cling together, or fall down in faints. Even allowing that hysteria was the condition most often described, we recognize a French style, evident in Pinel from an earlier time. These writers can make even obsessions exciting. Certainly nothing similar occurs in Kraepelin or Jaspers. Theirs are objective accounts. Items of description and sequences of clinical events march along inexorably with the writers' ideas to their conclusions, often as sharp and definite as a pistol shot. Or the German word forms pile up, gathering conviction by sheer weight. From a different origin, the descriptions of Weir-Mitchell and Sullivan have a piquancy, a sympathetic irony, that barely conceals these psychiatrists' eagerness to take the patients' side against the world. There is an anti-institutional air, an unmistakable nose-thumbing which reminds us of the Boston Tea Party and the continuing resentment of the old, perhaps especially of the Old World.

These differences are not merely stylistic. Each account gains some of its individuality from what the author selects as starting points or causes. The French highlight events or relationships, as in the theater. For all Janet's talk of falls in the level of energy or synthetic weakness, in case after case he puts emphasis on a fright 20 years before or on some catastrophe. With many of the Germans there is an internal independent process at work, a subtle monkey-wrench in the machinery. This is evident in Kraepelin's or Jasper's accounts of psychoses, a little less so in Bleuler's and in Freud's. The latter's epigenesis of desires is touched and sometimes even shaped by events, but it has its own fate. To give a third example, the Americans condemn parents, the old people. If only mother had been wiser or more understanding!

We can also recognize fashions that change with the psychiatric times. Adolf Meyer praised Kraepelin for rescuing psychiatry from the "paranoiification" of its nomenclature introduced by Ziehen. Nearly every patient had become an example of paranoia this or paranoiissima that. In its turn, the diagnosis of dementia praecox was overused. The patient totals in the Heidelberg Clinic for that entity had to be steadily reduced. With the psychoanalytic discovery of homosexual fantasies and fixations in many cases of alcoholism and obsessional neurosis, as well as in paranoia, homosexuality became widely used as an explanation. Later, everything pathological

seemed due to "ego defects." As in times of colonial exploration, we do not know whether the phenomena freshly discovered are representative of the best achieved by newly-come-
upon people, are occasional aberrations, or are signs of a
malignant process. We *do* know that each new discovery is
likely to be overrated (telegraphed frantically home) and
given *causal* importance.

Recently, the word *depression* has been in fashion. "Underlying depression," "depressive equivalents," "depressive position" filled the talk of clinic and conference. Everyone
searched for "lost objects" as they once did for lost fantasies.
The great thing was to mourn. Now the magic word is "bor-
derline!" Certainly it is true that not all fashions are merely
that; a permanent residue may remain; and other scientific
and humanistic studies bend to *their* fashions. Besides, styles
have value—through devotion to them, points of view can be
carried to their extremes and more fully understood. But only
art can afford a complete devotion to style. Science makes additional demands.

Temperament is also powerful. Keen decisive types take
naturally to objective-descriptive work. They hope to recognize an entity and act against it. More passive types listen for
the processes "back of it all," in order to lure out something
for analysis. Then there are games-players, therapists who
grasp easily what others are "up to," who know right off
where they stand with people: embryonic Henry Jameses. Finally, many enter the helping professions for the felt, empathic, sharing experiences they provide. These students are
existential therapists often without knowing the name.

A stubborn drift occurs in training toward such teachers
and techniques as fit the learner's temperament. The result
at its worst is a practitioner skilled in one method alone and
eager to apply it to all patients. Or, hardly better, the student
may learn a little about everything and do nothing well, so

that he works at the level of first aid. Of course, therapists must develop in accord with their temperaments, but the main purposes of training are surely both to refine natural gifts and to supply some absent ones. At the very least, practitioners should learn their limitations. Where they seem unlikely to do so, the community's only recourse is to wise referring sources, able to judge quickly what patients need and who has it.

Training is not nearly so important as temperament in the determination of what a therapist does. For this reason even graduates of psychoanalytic institutes, despite all the learning, treatment, and supervision they undergo, may be more existential in their methods than analytic. I have also known therapists trained in objective-descriptive work who did participant observation naturally and did not know it until they read Berne or Perls. Nor is it possible to determine a therapist's actual allegiance by what he says. I recall one debate over technique in which the very objective therapist made the case for existential confrontation and the empathic physician advocated objectivity; each was defending what he needed. "Psychotherapeutic technique" meant what each had had to learn, not what he did without thinking.

The example of charismatic teachers is also more decisive than any training program or syllabus. Amid the uncertainties of psychiatry, with its fragmentation and often open conflict, students fall easy victims to identity diffusion. Confident, attractive, answer-giving teachers therefore attract enormous followings and may turn out versions of themselves like Fords. If, in addition, the style of the teacher fits the temperament of the student, development may stop right there.

In my own training, I had two teachers who were charismatic as well as technically consistent, and each offered a strikingly different example. Many who came within their orbits wanted to do what they did; anyone who came within both their orbits did not know what to do. But the reward of early indecision was eventual clarity because, by very reason of the contrast they offered, the definition and selection of method was made easier in the end.

Interviews by the first teacher were marvels of subterranean passage. The patient hardly knew what he was revealing. A phrase here, a gesture there, listened to by our teacher with a suddenly quickened interest, eliciting perhaps an exclamatory grunt, started trains of associations that laid bare deep-running conflicts, often totally unexpected revelations of the past. There was no alliance with the patient, in the sense of any conscious contract; the alliance was between the *un*conscious of both instructor and patient. When this man was through, it was as if the patient was waking from a trance or operative anesthesia, to depart unknowing what had been revealed.

The second teacher worked in a quite different way. Everything he did had the patient's warmhearted conscious acceptance. First, listening to the presenting therapist's history, he nodded sleepily, caught a point here and there, but did not want to know too much. He did not want to approach the patient with too heavy a burden of facts and ideas. Above all, he did not want to have decided the patient *was* something, to let material come between the patient and himself. He found one key or a little lever, then gently applied it: "Oh, you are still in love," he said to the patient of her long-dead fiancé, "after all these years." He said it so kindly, so sympathetically, with so much conveyance of what pain this must mean, that the patient gave up all her denials and projections at a stroke. Quickly, almost imperceptibly, the doctor was where the patient was. There was this "being there together" and the relief it brought to discuss afterward.

The lessons for pedagogy seem clear. It is necessary to select teachers who represent all the schools and to warn the students that psychiatry's methods are multiple and conflicting.

Perhaps most important of all, we must be prepared to say, "Often we do not know which to use! You students are the future. It is you who must discover new methods and learn when to use them!"

The patients, too, shape us in ways apart from conscious clinical deciding. Who has not been richly existential with young hysterics whose problems were seemingly understood, or proudly objective with annoying depressed or paranoid people? How often the patient's revelation of something primitive or shocking in his behavior puts us in a classificatory mood or sets us to fencing interpersonally. The physician who has been depressed by a depressed patient or excited by a manic one finds his behavior shaped toward less or more activity.

These *observer effects*—that is, the effects of the patient on the observer—have not yet taken their full place in clinical calculation. Awareness of praecox gefühl, the eerie feeling schizophrenic people convey, is old. There has been backstairs talk for years of what we call in Boston Hendrick's signs: what young female hysterics convey to the doctor's penis. But the number of distinct observer effects are few. Obsessional patients make us yawn. I named another Sullivan's sign from the following anecdote: Sullivan is rumored to have said, "I can detect when I am in the presence of a strongly homosexual person by a tightening of the anal sphincter." A clever but foolish colleague asked, "Whose?"—clever because that brings a laugh, foolish because none but a proctologist learns much about the patient's anal sphincter in the course of the average examination. Finally, I like to call Havens' sign what the praecox gefühl does to many: Like a horror movie the young schizophrenic's account of derealization or of déjà vu or of strange bodily feelings produces pilo-erection; one can feel the small hairs on one's neck go up.

Such phenomena have diagnostic importance. They also

signal that a battery of influences is streaming across to us from the patient, of most of which we are unaware. The interviewer is "at sea." He swims in a turbulent medium whose temperature and buffetings the patient affects as much as the therapist ever does.

PLURALISM IN PSYCHIATRY

Medical-descriptive psychiatry allows the first glimpse of patient types and diseases. As Jaspers wrote, we discover something in the first moment with a patient that may take years to reappear. Psychoanalysis, in contrast, deepens our understanding of mechanisms, so that events, feelings, fantasies, and symptoms can be for the first time ordered into sequences and processes. The biological understanding of mental processes, still embryonic, will cast a similar light on physical processes. Interpersonal psychiatry indicates what to do in order to expose and control the situations before us, while phenomenology and existential psychiatry, asking us to be in the patient's world, create the feelings and awareness that allow empathic contact and knowledge. In short, the schools comprise a rich psychiatry, perhaps already ordered into a rough succession of tasks.

If we do not know where to sit or how friendly to be at the start, at least we see the value of Jaspers' first moment of observation, and we can catch other objective glimpses between our listening, interacting, and encountering. Nor will the most phenomenologically reduced existential psychiatrist want to surrender the analytic grasp of processes. He may not want to insist on it; he will want to abandon it when a fuller inward understanding is achieved. But surely the hard-won psychoanalytic knowledge can be carried, if lightly, however much the existential method will compromise the conditions necessary for developing the transference neurosis!

Moreover, when an understanding of pathological processes has been achieved, both interpersonal and existential methods come forward quickly in the "working through." In fact much of the contemporary psychoanalytic description of the working-through process sounds very Sullivanian and existential: If the transference neurosis is not to be bored to death, it must be acted against, à la Sullivan, or encountered existentially. So already we imagine a crude sequential outline of the place of the schools, each taking up a spot in the course of treatment, as recognition, understanding, control, and empathic identification succeed one another.

Similarly, we can spot patients seemingly designed for each method [5], although it is more likely that the methods developed from the patients. Affective disorders often need the battering encounter of existential work to surrender their denial. Paranoid patients, almost by definition, need the counterprojective techniques of interpersonal work. How readily some hysterical patients develop their transference neuroses and almost work them through by themselves, on couch or chair; perhaps these are the relatively adult hysterics Elizabeth Zetzel described [6], whose experience of family life has taken them far enough into the oedipal situation to complete its resolution with little help. Finally, many patients need, despite our most sophisticated intentions, the observation, manipulation, and medical control of the oldest school. It is not possible to deal existentially with some. They just do not call up in us the feelings necessary for the encounter. With others, often free association proves impossible!

Or we may use the existential scheme: The objective schools, psychoanalysis, and objective-descriptive psychiatry deal with the *umwelt*, the world of the body and its demands; interpersonal psychiatry explores the *mitwelt*, the world of those around us; and existentialism discovers the *eigenwelt*, the inner world of purposes and feelings. If only we can *locate* the patient's disorder, perhaps a method of the schools speaks to it.

Such schemes suggest, however, a degree of psychiatric completeness nothing else supports. Indeed, knowledge of what place present methods should have probably awaits knowledge of the methods still undiscovered! [7].

•

Of course every period produces manuals of practice in which the clinical lore of the time is collected. These books offer solutions rather than dilemmas and slide over the systematic difficulties of mixing methods. Janet's was perhaps the best in the first half of the century; Wolberg's is certainly impressive in the second half [8]. Each offers superb advice: specific prescriptions for specific problems. Reading them, we feel that nothing is beyond us.

Eclecticism is the name for these efforts at synthesis. Usually it has meant grasping the ideas of all the schools and taking from them those most appealing to us. It has usually not involved the much more taxing matter of mastering all the methods of the schools and discerning when to use them. Eclecticism has tended to underplay differences, to homogenize complexities, so that the powerful school methods and ideas lose their edge.

I believe that the future lies with refining methods, not mixing them, just as physical treatments have moved toward more and more precise methods and medicines. Such a refinement would mean *pluralism* in psychiatry, the goal that Adolf Meyer more than anyone represented. Having achieved that pluralism, we could look back on psychiatry's *school* days with both nostalgia and relief.

NOTES

Chapter 1

1. I make no apology for the term *objective* in characterizing this school, but *descriptive* is not quite right. Kraepelin took pride in his conviction that he was moving *beyond* the descriptive attempts characteristic of the psychological formalists who had preceded him and carrying psychiatry to a disease orientation. A more accurate name for the school would therefore be objective-syndromic or objective-pathological. I have, however, followed common usage.

2. Kraepelin's relationship to Wundt would be a fine subject for investigation. Wundt and Kraepelin went in opposite directions professionally, reversing their respective starting concerns. It is also interesting to note the number of distinguished psychologists who, like Wundt, had been medical men: Locke, Fechner, Lotze, James. (Of course some people would put Freud in that list!) I suppose the reason is at least partly that physiology is one of the bases of psychology. It would not be so popular to put it the other way round.

3. There is no complete English translation of any edition of Kraepelin's textbook. To my knowledge the closest is A. Ross Diefendorf's abstraction and "adaptation" from the seventh German edition: *Clinical Psychiatry: A Textbook for Students and Physicians* (New York: Macmillan, 1915). In this reader's opinion the best English introduction to Kraepelin's work is his *Lectures on Clinical Psychiatry*, revised and edited by Thomas Johnstone (London: Baillière, Tindall, and Cox, 1904) and reissued by Hafner (New York) in 1968. This is the source of the case material in the chapter. Unlike Kraepelin's *Textbook*, the *Lectures* present individual cases and give full play to his remarkable capacity for psychiatric portraiture (a capacity perhaps rivaled only by Wilhelm Reich).

4. Kraepelin, E., *Lectures on Clinical Psychiatry* (see note 3).

5. For an excellent review of this syndrome see Lewis, A. J., Melancholia: A historical review, *J. Ment. Sci.* 80:277, 1934.

6. Kraepelin provided a fascinating review of his psychiatric experience and views, as of 1917, in *One Hundred Years of Psychiatry* (New York: Citadel, 1962). (Translation from *Hundert Jahre Psychiatrie*, 1917; available in paperback.)

7. The statement about delirium tremens is taken from Hunter and Macalpine's superb *Three Hundred Years of Psychiatry*, *1535–1860* (Hunter, R., and Macalpine, I. [Eds.], *Three Hundred Years of Psychiatry, 1535–1860* [New York, London: Oxford University Press, 1963]). (This makes a wonderful birthday or holiday present for anyone interested in psychology or psychiatry.) Hunter and Macalpine have brought a degree of sophistication and love of detail to psychiatric historiography reached previously only by Gregory Zilboorg (*History of Medical Psychology* [New York: Norton, 1941]).

8. The claim about Kraepelin's statistics comes from vol. IV of Adolf Meyer's *Collected Papers* (Meyer, A., *The Collected Papers of Adolf Meyer*, vol. IV [Baltimore: Johns Hopkins Press, 1950]). (See Chapter 5.) I do not know where Meyer found his information—perhaps on a visit to the clinic.

9. Kraepelin, E., *Dementia Praecox and Paraphrenia*, trans. from the Eighth Edition of the *Textbook* (Edinburgh: Livingstone, 1919).

10. The complexity that any adequate description of the outcome of schizophrenia requires is evidenced by Kraepelin's need

to distinguish eight types of residual states. Moreover, when it becomes clear that some patients not only recover from their acute psychoses but improve over their premorbid states (for example, see Sullivan, H. S., *Schizophrenia as a Human Process* [New York: Norton, 1962]), perhaps every possibility has been realized. This last outcome is sometimes dealt with in the Kraepelinian system by claiming that the patient could not have been schizophrenic in the first place. (Kraepelin himself, however, claimed only a *tendency* to deterioration.) Other workers draw out a group of "good prognosis" cases which may or may not be called schizophrenic (see Vaillant, G. E., An historical review of the remitting schizophrenias, *J. Nerv. Ment. Dis.* 138:48, 1964). Sometimes these are called reactive cases (as opposed to process or endogenous) or schizophreniform; Sullivan called the more promising patients schizophrenic and the others examples of dementia praecox.

In any case there is excellent agreement on the criteria governing admission to one group or the other (see also Vaillant). So strong is this agreement that one is tempted to abandon the disease-naming business altogether and speak of bad- and good-outcome cases. On that basis there would still be two major functional psychoses, and the two would heavily overlap respectively Kraepelin's dementia praecox and maniacal-depressive insanity! Finally, the most economical names for the two groups would be chronic and acute psychoses, since the outcome criteria seem mostly functions of chronicity or acuteness.

I suspect few had noticed that the schizophrenic patients sometimes were better after the attacks than before because little was known about how they had been before. And perhaps because schizophrenia has been thought to be a "disease," it was difficult to imagine improving as a result of it! Further, as one could perhaps conclude from William James's *Varieties of Religious Experience* (New York: New American Library Mentor, 1958), those individuals whose hallucinatory and delusional episodes turn out happily may be saints!

Nevertheless, these considerations do not settle the argument. Kraepelin believed there *were* differences *among the acute forms* that distinguished those going on to dementia or paranoia from those not doing so. (Bleuler credits Kahlbaum with first suggesting this possibility.) However, the claim is still argued.

11. For those who feel I overcredit Kraepelin, Bleuler's words

are to the point: "After paresis was excluded from among the functional psychoses and the other organic forms followed of themselves, for over seventy years theoretical psychiatry stood entirely helpless before the chaos of the most frequent mental diseases" (Bleuler, E., *Textbook of Psychiatry* [New York: Macmillan, 1924]). Kraepelin ended this chaos.

True, Kraepelin had to retreat from his extreme emphasis on etiology. The hope that his disease pictures were so distinct that they must have distinct causes was shattered for many entities (for example, the infectious psychoses; see Bonhoeffer, K., in Aschaffenburg's *Handbuch der Psychiatrie* [Leipzig: Deuticke, 1911]). Today it would be more popular to speak of workable units for clinical intervention than of diseases. Yet even the much-attacked schizophrenia diagnosis remains in worldwide use and has recently received support on the basis of fresh evidence (Kris, A. O., Developmental arrest and regression, *Arch. Gen. Psychiat.* [Chicago] 26:321, 1972; Case studies in chronic hospitalization for functional psychosis, *Arch. Gen. Psychiat.* [Chicago] 26:326, 1972). It is important, too, that Kris's definition of schizophrenia is closer to that of Kraepelin than the present-day, wider-limits definition that owes so much to Bleuler. In fact, Kris faults Bleuler for his lack of a clear developmental framework and excessive dependence on formalistic categories—for example "thinking disorder." In this formulation Bleuler is seen as partly a pre-Kraepelinian! (A somewhat similar criticism is made by Stierlin, H., Bleuler's concept of schizophrenia: A confusing heritage, *Amer. J. Psychiat.* 123:996, 1967.)

12. It would have been as appropriate to write this second half of the objective-descriptive chapter about Eugene Bleuler as about Janet. Bleuler played a role in regard to psychotic symptoms and signs very like Janet's role in regard to neurotic phenomena. Both categorized (for example, into fundamental and secondary) the lists of phenomena Kraepelin had collected; both rested heavily on the concept of dissociation. It is also true that both Janet and Bleuler were "conservatives," for some time inclined to fence-sitting and then ending up squarely in the objective-descriptive camp.

Both are also first-rate expository writers. Bleuler is usually presented to English-reading audiences through his monograph on dementia praecox (*Dementia Praecox, or The Group of Schizo-*

phrenias [New York: International Universities Press, 1950]). To me, however, his *Textbook* (cited in Note 11) is a better introduction, gives a clearer idea of his ways of work, and is still clinically useful.

13. The interesting question of whether somnambulism occurs during dreaming has been approached with the new techniques for identifying dream occurrences (Jacobson, A., Kales, A., Lehmann, D., and Zweizig, J. R., Somnambulism: All-night electroencephalographic studies, *Science* 148:975, 1965). "The somnambulistic incidents occurred predominantly during the first few hours of the night and were not temporally related to REM periods," during which dreaming is most often recalled. "The time spent dreaming did not differ when nights in which several somnambulistic incidents occurred were compared with nights without such incidents."

14. Janet, P., *The Major Symptoms of Hysteria* (1st ed.) (New York: Macmillan, 1907).

15. Binet, A., *La Suggestibilité* (Paris: Schleicher Frères, 1900).

16. Janet, P., *Psychological Healing* (New York: Macmillan, 1925).

17. Lasègue, E. C., De l'anorexie hystérique, *Arch. Gen. Med.* 21:385, 1873. Also in Kaufman, M. R. (Ed.), *Evolution of Psychosomatic Concepts; Anorexia Nervosa: A Paradigm* (New York: International Universities Press, 1964).

18. Among these, I have not discussed the "disposition to equivalences." This refers to an old observation on hysterics: Cure one symptom and another appeared to take its place. The old magnetists literally chased hysterical manifestations around the patients' bodies. A sign gone from the left side appeared on the right; hysterical coughing alternated with fits of sleep; vomiting gave way to confusion and delirium (a common exchange important to the later concept of "oral" hysteria). The best teaching is still that hysterical symptoms and signs are easy to cure, but the disposition to form them is not. Recently behavior therapists have been claiming that, at least when their methods are used, the "disposition to equivalences" disappears. It is not clear, however, how often their patients are truly hysterical or whether the illnesses are not occurring in unnoticed forms.

19. This acceptance is characteristic of objective-descriptive psychiatry. Psychoanalysis is less ingenuous.

20. Janet, P., *Les Névroses* (Paris: Flammarion, 1910; my own translation). This last very readable book gives a broader spectrum of neurotic phenomena than *The Major Symptoms* and should be in English.

21. For example, Janet is often given credit for discovering the cathartic method, and certainly he helped bring the technique into medicine. Recently, however, Henri Ellenberger (*Discovery of the Unconscious: The History and Evolution of Dynamic Psychiatry* [New York: Basic Books, 1970]) has pushed this discovery back to Benedikt; also one can find evidence of cathartic techniques surely in Mesmer's work and probably much earlier. Priority in psychiatric discovery is a vexing matter. At times one wonders whether Shakespeare didn't discover everything! And is one to put the discoverer of the following beside Pavlov and Skinner?

And this fanciful humour has just come into my mind through the recollection of a story told me by a domestic apothecary of my departed father, a simple fellow and a Swiss, a nation little given to vanity and lying, of a tradesman he had long known at Toulouse, a valetudinarian afflicted with the stone, who often had need of enemas, of which he had several sorts prescribed by the physicians according to the incidence of his infirmity. When they were brought, none of the usual forms were omitted, and sometimes he would feel if they were too hot. Behold him then lying prone on his bed, the usual operation performed, except that no injection was made! The apothecary having retired after this mummery, and the patient made comfortable, he felt the same effect as if he had really taken a clyster.

(Montaigne, M. E. de, *The Essays of Montaigne*, vol. 1, trans. E. J. Trechmann [New York and London: Oxford University Press, 1946, pp. 98–99].) And for an example of cathartic cure, see p. 94 of the same chapter. (Much of that chapter, incidentally, is good early Masters and Johnson!)

22. Janet, P., *Les Obsessions et la Psychasthénie*, vol. 1 (Paris: Alcan, 1903, p. xiii).

23. Mayo, E., *Some Notes on the Psychology of Pierre Janet* (Cambridge, Mass.: Harvard University Press, 1948).

24. Janet, P., *L'Amour et la Haine* (Paris: Maloine, 1932).

25. I could have discussed here Bleuler's closely related "autism concept" (or the psychoanalytic idea of "reality-testing"). Perhaps, however, if Bleuler is right, credit should go to the French. "Of

old, autism attracted attention, particularly among the French. The latter have described and stressed one aspect of it under such terms as autophilia, egocentricity, ego-hypertrophy, or *augmentation du sens de la personalité*, whereas the negative side was diagnosed as *perte du sens de la réalité*, or *perte de la fonction du réel*. Pelletier says that, above all, the patient does not differentiate anymore between reality and fantasy" (Bleuler, E., *Dementia Praecox* [New York: International Universities Press, 1950, p. 373]). Again note my p. 60, how close these "functional" concepts are to psychoanalytic ego concepts (for example, of reality-testing).

26. Janet, P., *La Force et la Faiblesse Psychologiques* (Paris: Maloine, 1932, pp. 24–25).

27. This phrase is from the second edition of *The Major Symptoms of Hysteria* (New York: Macmillan, 1929). Here there are many antecedents, as well as modern versions. The nineteenth-century *vesania* concept is perhaps the most important. This is the concept of a unitary psychosis (*Einheitspsychose*) of one or more phases of which numerous other illnesses are only an expression. Thus the patient first becomes anxious or sad (or sometimes hypochondriacal), later angry or manic, then delusional, and finally demented. We can compare this way of thinking to psychoanalytic regression theory and to Karl Menninger's adaptational or ego psychological version of regression theory (*The Vital Balance: The Life Process in Mental Health and Illness* [New York: Viking, 1963]). Kraepelin's disease theory was, of course, sharply at variance with these. "Snell and Westphal demonstrated that the Zeller-Griesinger Theory (Vesania Theory) was untenable by showing that lunacy was not always the terminal point of a mental disorder associated with emotional agitation but that it could develop independently and as a 'primary' condition" (Kraepelin, E., *One Hundred Years of Psychiatry* [New York: Citadel, 1962, pp. 114–115]). Simple schizophrenia offered perhaps the most convincing support for Kraepelin's claim, of a distinct clinical picture emerging de novo. I do not know of a single simple schizophrenic patient studied closely enough to rebut the claim.

28. "Consciousness" is once again a major topic of research, whether by means of "consciousness-expanding" drugs or neurophysiologically (Hernandez-Peon, R., Scherrer, H., and Jouvet, M., Modifications of electrical activity in cochlear nucleus during "attention" in unanaesthetized cats, *Science* 123:331, 1956; and Kuf-

fler, S. W., Discharge patterns and functional organization of mammalian retina, *J. Neurophysiol.* 16:37, 1953). Not long ago, the great interest was in *un*consciousness.

29. Ey, H., La Psychopathologie de Pierre Janet et la Conception Dynamique de la Psychiatrie, in *Mélanges Offerts à Monsieur Pierre Janet* (Paris: Editions d'Artrey, 1939).

30. Janet, P., *The Mental State of Hystericals* (New York: Putnam, 1901).

31. Sometimes it is heartbreaking to see how close Janet comes to Freud's discoveries. "Pby, (male, 29) is walking arm-in-arm with a woman whom he loves, and they are watching the sunset at the seaside. 'My heart is flooded with a joy that is purer and more beautiful than I have ever known before. Life is suffused with splendor. Then something seems to go crack in my head, and all turns black and gloomy. I am seized once more by the obsession that I have to fight a man, whom I used to know at college, a man I detested, but whom I have not seen for ten years'" (*Psychological Healing* [New York: Macmillan, 1925]). Janet's account is of an action, or function, checked, not of specific patterns of fantasies or of social facts.

32. Janet, like Kraepelin (1856–1926) and Freud (1856–1939), lived a long life, and at much the same time (1859–1947). (Indeed, longevity—and at that specific period—may be the attribute most highly correlated with psychiatric fame: Bleuler, 1857–1939; Meyer, 1866–1950). Like Kraepelin and Freud, Janet kept developing his thoughts. What I have written must be seen in that perspective and with the understanding that my focus is on illustrating objective-descriptive psychiatry and its methods. For material on almost the whole range of Janet's development, see Henri Ellenberger's fascinating *Discovery of the Unconscious: The History and Evolution of Dynamic Psychiatry* (New York: Basic Books, 1970).

Chapter 2

1. The uterine hypothesis not only was a clever idea to connect some symptoms and signs of hysteria but also served to specify those symptoms and signs most dependable clinically, that is, to specify a syndrome. Later-discovered aspects of hysteria add to the full disease picture, but the use of them alone—for example, use of

the conversion phenomenon to diagnose hysteria—gives many false-positives. (One could pursue this line of thought further, remembering Freud's remark that psychoanalysis was to psychiatry as histology is to anatomy.) Once again, objective-descriptive psychiatry provides *power of recognition*. (Guze, S. B., The diagnosis of hysteria: What are we trying to do? *Amer. J. Psychiat.* 124:491, 1967.)

2. The Dialogues of Plato, vol. II. *Timaeus*, trans. B. Jowett (New York: Scribner, 1889).

3. Charcot, J. -M., *Clinical Lectures on Certain Diseases of the Nervous System*, Lecture VII, trans. E. P. Hurd (Detroit: Davis, 1888).

4. Hunter, R., and Macalpine, I. (Eds.), *Three Hundred Years of Psychiatry*, 1535–1860 (London: Oxford University Press, 1963).

5. Bernheim, H., *Hypnotisme et Suggestion* (Paris: Doin, 1910, pp. 215–216), and Janet, P., *The Major Symptoms of Hysteria* (New York: Macmillan, 1907, p. 275).

6. Guillain, G., *Jean-Marie Charcot, 1825–1893, His Life and Work*, trans. P. Bailey (New York: Hoeber Med. Div., Harper & Row, 1959).

7. Charcot, J. -M., *Clinical Lectures on Diseases of the Nervous System*, Lecture XXI, trans. T. Savill (London: New Sydenham Society, 1889).

8. The statements about the reproducibility of hypnotic phenomena without hypnotic preparation and the comparison of hypnotized subjects with simulators, pp. 75, 76, are based on the work of Martin Orne and his associates (for example, Orne, M. T., *Hypnosis, Motivation, and the Ecological Validity of the Psychological Experiment*, Nebraska Symposium on Motivation, Arnold, W. J., and Page, M. D. [Eds.] [Lincoln: University of Nebraska Press, 1970]). More and more the concept of hypnosis is coming to seem an explanatory carbuncle, like the ether of phlogiston, able to disappear and leave the whole structure of observation and explanation intact. Nevertheless, Orne and others continue the search for objective correlates of the subjective state.

9. Charcot, J. -M., *Clinical Lectures on Diseases of the Nervous System*, Lecture I, trans. T. Savill (London: New Sydenham Society, 1889).

10. Charcot, J. -M., *Clinical Lectures on Diseases of the Nervous System*, Appendix I, trans. T. Savill (London: New Sydenham Society, 1889).

11. The importance of Charcot's contribution can hardly be exaggerated. By the end of the nineteenth century psychological causes were under great attack: There were too many; they bore little relationship to one another (see Chapter 7); they could not be measured. By taking the psychological and social events noted to precede hysteria and ordering them into a sequence, with a hypothetical underlying process, Charcot had made not so much a discovery as a change in our whole way of thinking. A structure was provided for understanding psychopathological events.

12. Wölfflin, H., *Principles of Art History*, trans. M. D. Hottinger (New York: Holt, 1932).

13. Breuer, J., and Freud, S., *Studies on Hysteria* (1893–1895). (Standard Ed., vol. II [London: Hogarth, 1955].) See text footnote for full data.

14. Henri Ellenberger has written two invaluable accounts of the Anna O. case. In *Discovery of the Unconscious* (New York: Basic Books, 1970) he suggested an understanding of the material along Jungian lines; this must be read carefully and with an appreciation of existential ideas. More recently (The story of "Anna O.": A critical review with new data, *J. Hist. Behav. Sci.* 8:267, 1972) he has presented fresh information about the case, some of it correcting the account in Ernest Jones's biography of Freud (*The Life and Work of Sigmund Freud* [New York: Basic Books, 1953]). There is more evidence of Anna's intense attachment to her father, and a revealing explanation of why the father's death was so traumatic—she had been kept from him and deceived about the seriousness of his condition. Ellenberger also discovered that the physician who blew smoke in her face, from a burning piece of paper (compare Kraepelin's catatonia tests), was none other than the great objective-descriptive psychiatrist Krafft-Ebing.

Chapter 3

1. Breuer, J., and Freud, S., *Studies on Hysteria* (1893–1895). (Standard Ed., vol. II [London: Hogarth, 1955].) See text footnote for full data.

2. Freud, S., Fragment of an Analysis of a Case of Hysteria (1905 [1901]). (*Collected Papers*, vol. III [New York: Basic Books, 1959].) See text footnote for full data.

3. Freud laid his "failure" in the Dora case to various causes. At

a different point he gave responsibility to his failure to analyze the transference.

4. The study of fantasy also led to schemata of development and of modes of relationship which made possible investigations extraordinarily more subtle than any before. Concepts were provided that made possible the perception of phenomena of remarkable variety and importance. It was a child psychoanalyst, Bowlby, for example, who suggested to an animal psychologist, Harlow, that he determine whether oral or tactile needs were the more fundamental in the monkey. The result was an experimental demonstration of what forms of deprivation can drive monkeys mad! (For example, see Harlow, H., The heterosexual affectional systems in monkeys, *Amer. Psychol.* 17:1, 1962.) It is true that tactile, not oral, interests proved predominant in Harlow's monkey experiments—not the result anticipated. Similarly, the early theory of gene distribution in mitosis proved wrong, but it led to knowledge that was fundamental to many present-day genetic conceptions. In short, although fantasy was removed from reality, it was also in touch with parts of reality difficult, perhaps impossible, to perceive without it. This is perhaps answer enough to those for whom psychoanalytic concepts have no apparent scientific usefulness.

The very richness of psychoanalytic ideas often led to the provision of alternatives rather than conclusions in clinical discussions. The result has been a *topography* for locating problems that greatly enlarges the data of psychiatric relevance. The conceptions, in turn, have proved flexible enough to contain the data of many other schools. Thus psychiatry was finally given a vocabulary of terms and concepts rich enough to deal with the phenomena of individual human life.

5. It is also true that the analytic method can throw a very bright light on actuality. As one listens to analytic associations, the picture that emerges of other people in the patient's life is often remarkably faithful. It is as if the unconscious had its own method of recording actuality. The result is that one can sometimes recognize instantly a person described in analysis only briefly.

6. The widening out of the material of accumulating relevance to psychiatry is dramatically illustrated by the successive phases of Freud's work: from neurocellular speculation, to traumatic psychopathology, to the farthest reaches of individual experience, to the social and cultural setting, and finally to the historical background

of certain world figures. Roughly the same sequence is recapitulated in the successive chapters of Jaspers' *General Psychopathology* (see Chapter 4).

7. I do not make any attempt to discuss the various schools of psychoanalysis, such as those of Adler and Jung, largely because none is methodologically original. Jung, for example, did not make methodological contributions, to my knowledge, beyond his free association test and the technique of active imagination. In practice he was a versatile, pluralistic therapist.

Chapter 4

1. Griesinger's solution is of particular interest and quite different from either Kraepelin's or Jaspers'. Griesinger put the paranoid cases, his monomaniacs, with the maniacs and melancholics, on the basis that the three shared disordered affect—in the case of paranoia a disorder of anger (*Mental Pathology and Therapeutics* [New York: William Wood, 1882]). There certainly is a prominent fixed affect in the paranoid cases, as with maniacs and melancholics, and no predictable thought disorder in the dissociative sense.

2. Jaspers, K., Eifersuchtswahn. Ein Beitrag zur Frage: "Entwichlung einer Personlichkeit" oder "Prozess"? Z. Ges. Neurol. Psychiat. 1:567, 1910. I am indebted to Erika Davis for help with the translation.

3. For a similar patient with quite a different outcome (and a different wife!), see the following from Bleuler (*Textbook of Psychiatry* [New York: Macmillan, 1930]): "A skillfully dissimulating paranoiac used to confide his delusions only on toilet paper; and as his wife, who suffered severely in consequence of his disease, collected these documents, she obtained the necessary material for divorce and guardianship." Note the typical paranoiac need to comment in writing, plus the typical hostility and relationship to feces.

4. Jaspers, K., *General Psychopathology*, trans. from the German by J. Hoenig and M. Hamilton (Chicago: University of Chicago Press, 1963). Although in Jasper's book there are no references from the literature of the last 20 years, and almost nothing from the American literature of any time, it is a work of extraordinary interest, standing as the still unsurpassed high-water mark of psychiatric erudition and sophistication.

Jaspers' account of existential method is, however, particularly dated. He makes the popular mistake of equating existential method with friendship ("professional friendship"). It is more correct to state that existential method forbids *any* a priori account of what the relationship will be like. To suppose it will be friendly is to impose a meaning on the relationship in advance.

5. Minkowski, E., *Lived Time: Phenomenological and Psychopathological Studies*, trans. Nancy Metzel (Evanston, Ill.: Northwestern University Press, 1970). In a personal communication Henri Ellenberger remarks that Minkowski's main inspiration came from Bleuler and the latter's concept of the "affective rapport" and the idea that the psychiatrist's immediate feeling toward the schizophrenic patient was one of the main signs of schizophrenia.

6. May, R., Angel, E., and Ellenberger, H. (Eds.), *Existence: A New Dimension in Psychiatry and Psychology* (New York: Basic Books, 1958). This splendid volume repays reading and re-reading. The only summary material of comparable value on existential psychiatry in English is in Dieter Wyss's *Depth Psychology* (New York: Norton, 1966). As a starting point to read Binswanger's own writing I recommend *Being-in-the-World* (New York: Basic Books, 1963). His remarkable essay on psychoanalysis in that volume is especially rewarding.

7. Laing, R., *The Divided Self; A Study of Sanity and Madness* (Baltimore: Penguin Books, 1965); *Politics of Experience* (New York: Pantheon, 1967).

8. I have lumped together Szasz and Laing, which is rich company but does not do full justice to either. The two writers are very different in many respects; they perhaps come together only at the intersection I mention: Both divert pathological emphasis from the patient, or, put the other way round, both are trenchant critics of institutions. They see the individual's state of mind from the viewpoint of the failure of the world. This is the equivalent of stating that both share some elements of existential *and* social psychiatry. Such a union of the two newest developments in psychiatry may explain the extraordinary popularity of these writers with the young. It is true, however, that Szasz is closer to the concerns of social psychiatry, especially adaptational notions, than to existential thought. See Szasz, T., *The Myth of Mental Illness: Foundations of a Theory of Personal Conduct* (New York: Hoeber Med. Div., Harper & Row, 1961).

9. I have not, of course, attempted to cite all the existential psychiatrists; that would have required another book. Some workers, in many critical respects existential, are often not identified as such—for example, Carl Jung (*Collected Works* [New York: Pantheon, 1961, vol. IV, pp. 83–226]) and Carl Rogers (*On Becoming a Person* [Boston: Houghton Mifflin, 1961]). A number of psychoanalytic writers also reflect elements of existential methods and ideas, as, for example, in Winnicott's discussions of the value of feeling hate for the patient (Hate in the counter-transference, *Int. J. Psychoanal.* 30:69, 1949).

Chapter 5

1. Main currents of psychiatric development, *Int. J. Psychiat.* 5:288, 1960. Donald Schon's discussion of that article in the same issue is one source of the further development of the present writer's ideas.

2. Throughout this chapter I have slighted Adelaide Johnson, who may be the most inspired student of sociopathological facts. Happily her splendid work has been collected (*Experience, Affect and Behavior* [Chicago: University of Chicago Press, 1969]). She too developed a fresh method of getting at social events, her "collaborative psychotherapy." I do not give it the attention I give Sullivan's method because Johnson's method is considerably more difficult to use on a clinical basis. Nevertheless, I would put Johnson among the half-dozen principal American contributors to psychiatry.

Karen Horney (for example, *New Ways in Psychoanalysis* [New York: Norton, 1939]) has also been neglected here. She shares much with Sullivan: his emphasis on society and the present, his de-emphasis on sexuality and the instincts, his emphasis on the importance of narcissism, and above all his conception of neuroses as disturbances of human relationships. (Later she took the position that neuroses were also disturbances in the relationship to the self.) I have not called attention to her work for the same reason I have neglected Jung; I am not aware of her having made systematic innovations in method.

Such a principle of exclusion does not justify my ignoring the group therapy writers, many springing out of Sullivan's work or running in parallel to it. Here my neglect springs from ignorance (I do not like to write about methods I have not used extensively) and from the perhaps mistaken belief that the group and family therapy movements reflect the main methods herein described. Some group workers seem clearly psychoanalytic, others interpersonal or existential, still others even behavioristic and objective-descriptive.

3. Other prominent Sullivanians include Lewis Hill (*Psychotherapeutic Intervention in Schizophrenia* [Chicago: University of Chicago Press, 1955]), Frieda Fromm-Reichmann (*Psychoanalysis and Psychotherapy* [Chicago: University of Chicago Press, 1959]), Patrick Mullahy (*Psychoanalysis and Interpersonal Psychiatry; the Contributions of Harry Stack Sullivan* [New York: Science House, 1970]), and Eric Berne (*Games People Play* [New York: Grove Press, 1969]). The Gestalt therapy movement of Fritz Perls shares a good deal with Sullivanian psychotherapy (see Fagan, J., and Shepherd, I. [Eds.], *Gestalt Therapy Now* [Palo Alto: Science and Behavior Books, 1970]), the old cathartic techniques being wedded to an interest in social gestalts.

Finally, Robert Coles has made himself the leader of those who look for facts in a fresh social psychiatric area, the lives of children, especially poor children (see Children of Crisis: vol. II, *Migrants, Share-Croppers, Mountaineers*; vol. III, *The South Goes North* [Boston: Atlantic–Little, Brown, 1972]). This late interest in children and the poor suggests Auerbach's material on the order in which reality reaches the Western mind (*Mimesis* [Princeton, N.J.: Princeton University Press, 1953; Princeton Paperback, 1968]).

4. *The Collected Papers of Adolf Meyer*, vols. II and III (Baltimore: Johns Hopkins University Press, 1950).

5. Alfred Leif, *The Common-Sense Psychiatry of Adolf Meyer* (New York: McGraw-Hill, 1948).

6. The sources of Meyer's practical and environmental orientation, particularly his concept of a therapeutic community, have been illuminated by Manfred Bleuler; see Early Swiss sources of Adolf Meyer's concepts, *Amer J. Psychiat.* 119:193, 1962.

7. Breuer, J., and Freud, S., *Studies on Hysteria* (1893–1895). (Standard Ed., vol. II [London: Hogarth, 1955].) See text footnote for full data.

8. Meyer's interest in the life course, which he exemplified in his life charts, has been continued by a number of workers, for example, Jack Block (*Lives Through Time* [Berkeley, Calif.: Ban-

croft, 1971]), and George Vaillant on the Grant Study, this last still largely unpublished.

9. Auerbach, E., *Mimesis: The Representation of Reality in Western Literature*, trans. W. R. Trask (Princeton, N.J.: Princeton University Press, 1953; Princeton Paperback, 1968, pp. 319–320). Is there a more interesting book?

10. The interest both Meyer and Sullivan had in the facts, at the expense of the fantasies, is of course one hallmark of interpersonal psychiatry. It is of great value to follow a psychoanalyst who is also interested in facts, W. Niederland, integrating them into analytic thinking (for example, Schreber's father, *J. Amer. Psychoanal. Ass.* 8:492, 1960). Niederland's work is of further interest because it offers direct support to the Sullivanian school. The probable facts of Schreber's upbringing are as "mad" as any madness of Schreber's psychosis.

11. Sullivan, H. S., *The Psychiatric Interview* (New York: Norton, 1954).

12. In respect to Sullivan's style, a book of clinical maxims should be put together from his writings. Perhaps Helen Perry or Patrick Mullahy already has the job in hand. Here are two fine ones for a start. "The therapeutic 'test' is no test at all; witness chiropractic and Eddyism." "That certain of the most important investigators in psychoanalysis reached divergent results from contact with supposedly identical or homologous facts in one manifestation. That certain individuals among them move the accent of importance to this or that 'mechanism,' as for example Ernest Jones with Anal Erotism, Coriat with Urethral Erotism, or Rank with the Birth Trauma, Adler with the Masculine Protest—seems to reflect more than a little of personal warp." Both are from *Schizophrenia as a Human Process* (New York: Norton, 1962).

13. See, for example, Rennie, T. A. C., Srole, L., Michael, S. T., Langner, T. S., and Opler, M. K., *Mental Health in the Metropolis: The Mid-Town Manhattan Study* (New York: Blakiston Div., McGraw-Hill, 1962). The work of Leighton and his collaborators is also of great interest: Stirling County Study of Psychiatric Disorder and Sociocultural Environment—vol. I, Leighton, A. H., *My Name Is Legion: Foundations for a Theory of Man in Relation to Culture* (New York: Basic Books, 1959); vol. II, Hughes, C. C., Tremblay, M. A., Rapoport, R. N., and Leighton, A. H., *People of Cove and Woodlot: Communities from the Viewpoint of Social*

Psychiatry (New York: Basic Books, 1960); vol. III, Leighton, D. C., Harding, J. S., Macklin, D. B., Macmillan, N. M., and Leighton, A. H., *The Character of Danger: Psychiatric Symptoms in Selected Communities* (New York: Basic Books, 1963).

14. Here there is need for a longer discussion of "ego psychology." As psychoanalysis turned its attention to the resistances to analysis, there grew up a knowledge of the forms and deformities of the ego, which was then being used as an equivalent term for defensive processes. The classic work was Anna Freud's *The Ego and the Mechanisms of Defense* (London: Hogarth, 1942). As I have indicated, part of this development took place in the area of intrapsychic processes, part in relation to social processes. The result has been that interpersonal psychiatry, object-relations theory, and ego psychology all have overlapping meanings, with resulting confusion.

A number of workers, including Sullivan, took a social rather than somatic or sexual view of fundamental human interests. We might say they chose to define human interests from the outside rather than from the inside; emphasis fell on the objects of instincts rather than the instincts themselves. For an example of this adaptational approach, see *Homosexuality and Pseudo-Homosexuality* by Lionel Ovesey (New York: Science House, 1969). Such an approach does not solve the problem of data difficult to interpret without the concepts of drive, wish, or instinct, but it does get the personality out into the world of observable experience.

In discussing object-relations theory I chose Sullivan rather than Fairbairn, as another possibility, again because of Sullivan's methodological contributions. When the term *ego psychology* is used interchangeably with *object-relations theory*, it is plain that only one function of the ego is being considered, its management of and relations with the outside world. Fairbairn's and Sullivan's assumption is that the ego has no other relationships—for example, it has no relationships with the body per se or with somatic drives, but only with their object representations or introjects. This seems to me nonsense. (See Fairbairn, R., Synopsis of an object-relations theory of the personality, *Int. J. Psychoanal.* 44:224, 1963, as an introduction to his work.)

15. Sullivan, H. S., *Conceptions of Modern Psychiatry* (New York: Norton, 1953).

16. Sullivan, H. S., *Clinical Studies in Psychiatry* (New York: Norton, 1956).

17. Sullivan, H. S., *The Fusion of Psychiatry and Social Science*. The Collected Works of Harry Stack Sullivan, vol. II (New York: Norton, 1964). The sentence just beyond "For all I know . . ." makes the same point. It is also an example of the "psychology of School-Founders." We see for a moment into the temperament of those able to push against the tide. But lose our fear of this single-mindedness (as we must with Freud), and Sullivan teaches us at once about the ego and about society.

18. Personal communication from Herbert Spiegel, M.D., of New York.

19. Pinel, P., *A Treatise on Insanity* (New York: Hafner, 1962).

20. Rush, B., *Medical Inquiries and Observations upon the Diseases of the Mind* (New York: Hafner, 1962).

21. Sullivan, H. S., *Schizophrenia as a Human Process* (New York: Norton, 1962).

22. Jones, M., *The Therapeutic Community; A New Treatment Method in Psychiatry* (New York: Basic Books, 1953).

23. "Presumably" unaware: See the work of Martin Orne (*Hypnosis, Motivation, and the Ecological Validity of the Psychological Experiment*, Nebraska Symposium on Motivation, Arnold, W. J., and Page, M. D. [Eds.] [Lincoln: University of Nebraska Press, 1970]). He has demonstrated how much easier it is to fool doctors than it is to fool scientific subjects and perhaps patients!

24. Bleuler, E., *Textbook of Psychiatry* (New York: Macmillan, 1924).

25. I mention Muncie because he wrote the most systematic exposition of Meyer's psychiatry (*Psychobiology and Psychiatry: A Textbook on Normal and Abnormal Human Behavior* [St. Louis: Mosby, 1939]) and Campbell because he gave the most eloquent exposition (see *Destiny and Disease in Mental Disorders* [New York: Norton, 1935]). There are many others—for example, Henderson and Gillespie in England. One of Meyer's last residents, Theodore Lidz, has demonstrated how smoothly psychoanalytic ideas can find a home in Meyerian foundations (*Person: His Development Throughout the Life Cycle* [New York: Basic Books,

1968]). Lidz has also written a wonderful tribute to Meyer (*Amer. J. Psychiat.* 123:320, 1966).

26. The Hawthorne effect is another example. (Roethlisberger, F. J., and Dickson, W. J., *Management and the Worker* [Cambridge, Mass.: Harvard University Press, 1966]).

27. The "Stanton-Schwartz Phenomenon" is described in *The Mental Hospital: A Study of Institutional Participation in Psychiatric Illness and Treatment* (New York: Basic Books, 1954).

28. Meyer, A., The approach to the investigation of dementia praecox, *Chicago Med. Recorder* 39:441, 1917.

29. Perhaps the best test of where interpersonal psychiatry has taken us is provided by reading the following clinical account from one of Kraepelin's chapters on dementia praecox. This is a "specimen of writing," a patient's letter, and Kraepelin calls attention to "the shallowness of the contents, the incomprehensibility, the laboured style, the incoherence of the train of thought, as well as the slovenly external form, which is scarcely decipherable on account of the many crossings-out and alterations."

When you on the 19th May of this year, namely on a beautiful Sunday afternoon, constructed the plan for yourself to do me the honour to visit me by the railway in the Hospital for the Insane at H., care of Professor K., Littera Voss-strasse Nr 4, you thought then perhaps to give your dear and good son a special pleasure, visiting him in the institution!—Or was it not so?!—When I further recapitulate again the many unjust things and abusive epithets which I threw at the head of my dear mama, I think that I really cannot avoid being obliged to confess that I should have rather [never?] expected a visit first from the maternal side. [Had the mother been late in visiting or does he mean paternal?] Supposing namely the case that the above mentioned should not only have been ill, but had actually been so, so would my humble self have first strongly advised in her case a visit to her firstborn! Now as *happily* my 22nd birthday coincided with Ascension day, as God and fate would have it, but in the Asylum, the visit of my mother in person certainly caused me a great momentary joy, especially as she from motherly love showed me the honour and kindness to promise to bring me another cake and a silver chain, but in any case her visit would not and could not be a visible comfort for me for the old reason, namely my father's dissatisfaction with my diligence at home, regarding conscientiousness! Further I thank you also most heartily for the beautiful artistic card with the special signature Fam-

ily G. But wait! Who should the Family G. be then in this case, if its principal member is crouching in a madhouse? [and so on].
(*Dementia Praecox and Paraphrenia*, trans. from the Eighth Edition of the *Textbook* [Edinburgh: Livingstone, 1919].) Of course, Kraepelin's interest is in the *formal* characteristics, but once grasp Sullivan's perspective on family life and this specimen suggests Marcel Proust.

The social data also fits nicely with the dissociation concept. It surely must be impossible or nearly impossible to integrate experience with some parents. This is the message of Bateson's double-bind conception (see Jackson, D. D. A. [Ed.] *Etiology of Schizophrenia* [New York: Basic Books, 1960]) and of Laing's *Divided Self* (Baltimore: Penguin Books, 1965).

Chapter 6

1. Pinel, P., *A Treatise on Insanity* (New York: Hafner, 1962).

2. Esquirol, J. E. D., *Mental Maladies* (New York: Hafner, 1965).

3. Kraepelin, E., *Lectures on Clinical Psychiatry* (New York: Hafner, 1968).

4. Rush, B., *Medical Inquiries and Observations upon the Diseases of the Mind* (New York: Hafner, 1962).

5. Janet, P., *The Major Symptoms of Hysteria* (New York: Macmillan, 1929).

6. Erikson's work is so well known today that it hardly needs reference. For the matters most pertinent to this chapter the reader is referred to *Identity and the Life Cycle* (New York: International Universities Press, 1959). For a discussion of the few other contributions to our knowledge of adult phases, see Gould, R. L., The phases of adult life: A study in development psychology, *Amer. J. Psychiat.* 129:5, 1972.

7. The order in which different psychiatric tasks are taken up in successive life periods recapitulates the early development of much adult psychiatry. Originally there were only adults and children. The psychiatry of children is still not, however, as fully developed as that of adults. For example, there is relatively little agreement yet on diagnostic categories among children; also the social psychiatry of childhood is only now being developed; see particularly the work of Robert Coles (*Children of Crisis* [Boston: Atlantic–Little, Brown, 1972]). It would be fascinating to speculate on what the

existential psychiatry of childhood will prove to be (perhaps children treating children!). I predict that the various stages will be recapitulated, or at least approximated, with each new time period closely studied. Something like this can already be said about the psychiatry of adolescence.

For an engrossing treatment of the development of the concept of childhood, see Philippe Ariès' *Centuries of Childhood* (New York: Knopf, 1962). See also David Hunt's *Parents and Children in History, the Psychology of Family Life in Early Modern France* (New York: Basic Books, 1970).

8. Again, we could put the analysis in this chapter beside Auerbach's description of the changes in the representation of reality in Western literature. Perhaps Pinel's description of the restless man would correspond to the flat, brightly illuminated, everything-present, "unconceptual" quality of Homeric verse; and psychoanalytic descriptions, to the mixed-past-and-present, stream-of-consciousness, past-dominated writings of Virginia Woolf.

Chapter 7

1. Burton, R., *Anatomy of Melancholy* (London: William Kegg, 1876, pp. 78–79).

2. Rush, B., *Medical Inquires and Observations upon the Diseases of the Mind* (New York: Hafner, 1962).

3. List-making is still practiced. See Leff, M. J., Roatch, J. F., and Bunney, W. E., Jr., Environmental factors preceding onset of severe depression, *Psychiatry* 33:293, 1970.

4. Of course a great deal more than what I have described went on before this point *was* reached. For example, early in the nineteenth century the doctrine of monomania was widely subscribed to. This doctrine held that delusions were due to the peculiar attributes of the individual ideas; no personality-wide disturbance was noted. The concept of complexes was a later step in the same line of development. In the middle of the nineteenth century the doctrine of monomania came under increasing fire and was largely dismissed.

Another way of ordering the development of the understanding of causes would be through the idea of successive approximations. Thus, the frequency of mental illness was at one time thought related to immigration, then social class, and more recently community disintegration.

Still another way of ordering the development of causes would be through the idea of successive similes or metaphors. Rush saw mental illness as essentially a vascular disease. Charcot regarded hysteria as similar to epilepsy. Wernicke conceived of mental illness on the model of aphasia. Kraepelin's dementia praecox owed a great deal to syphilitic dementia, both in terms of its conception and because cases of syphilis were mixed in with the schizophrenic ones. Freud's metaphor was physical and hydraulic, a system of displaceable energies of fixed amounts. Today much social psychiatric thinking seems on a chemical model—elements relate to one another, react, form bonds, enter special relationships, and so on.

The development of treatment measures has followed a somewhat similar pattern. In this case advances in physical and organic sciences have regularly spawned therapies. The iatromechanical school applied Newtonian physics by means of various schemes of mass and energy and movement. The discovery of the circulation of the blood fostered great hopes from bloodletting. Electricity was put to use clinically. Discoveries in brain anatomy justified numerous procedures, perhaps the most widespread being lobotomy. Many of these measures seem in retrospect more lunatic than the patients they were meant to help, but their persuasiveness at the time was enormous. B. F. Skinner is one investigator who has been particularly assiduous in attacking such loose modes of thought, although it is not altogether clear that his own approaches do not suffer from more subtle metaphors. "Learned behavior was once commonly attributed to 'habit' but an analysis of contingencies of re-inforcement has made the term unnecessary. 'Instinct,' as a hypothetical cause of phylogenic behavior, has had a longer life." "Unable to show how the organism can behave effectively under complex circumstances, we endow it with a special cognitive ability which permits it to do so" (Skinner, B. F., The phylogeny and ontogeny of behavior, *Science* 153:1205, 1966). Special cognitive abilities include intelligence, attention, and, of course, ego.

5. On the theoretical side each school has had its particular dangers. The danger of the objective-descriptive school was that it repeatedly threatened to go over into premature theorizing on the basis of whatever was known at any particular time about brain anatomy. This was the failure of Wernicke and Meynert, and sometimes of Freud and Charcot. It was not the failure of Grie-

singer, Kraepelin, Janet, or Bleuler, all of whom let clinical observations speak for themselves without needing to translate them into brain anatomical concepts. Psychoanalysis is threatened both with premature brain theorizing and with metaphors from mythology and literature, those fertile parents of the possible. The existential school easily gives way to philosophizing. Social psychiatry is tempted to translate all its facts too facilely into the few established sociological concepts; Sullivan showed the way.

6. See Schildkraut, J. J., *Neuropsychopharmacology and the Affective Disorders* (Boston: Little, Brown, 1970).

7. Parsons, T., Illness and the Role of the Physician: A Sociological Perspective. In Kluckhohn, C., and Murray, H. A. (Eds.), *Personality in Nature, Society and Culture* (New York: Knopf, 1948).

8. One could prove that he often took a more inclusive view. Still he sometimes wrote as if he thought schizophrenia were "fundamentally" a "thought disorder." I have already suggested that this is part of the old psychological faculty thinking. Janet takes a further step, dividing illnesses by the functions affected. Thus we continue to speak of functional lesions.

The reader can judge for himself as to the success of attempts to show a specific thinking defect in schizophrenia (quite apart from the issue of whether such a defect is more "fundamental" than any affective or motor difficulty). A good starting point would be Trunnell's recent effort to set the whole problem up in terms of Piaget's theories; see Thought disturbance in schizophrenia, *Arch. Gen. Psychiat.* (Chicago) 13:9, 1965.

The most that comes clear to me is a general tendency of schizophrenic thinking to follow lines that seem immature, granted the vagueness or breadth of that term; granted, too, that such a term represents an advance over Bleuler's concept of primary splitting. (All these efforts remind me of efforts to characterize cancer cells as primitive or disorganized. Not only is such a description simplistic, but in fact cancer cells prove far *too* well organized, at least for our good!)

Freud's sweeping distinction between primary and secondary thought processes also seems simplistic in the light of at least several stages of thought development being described. (See, for example, Heinz Werner's *Comparative Psychology of Mental Development* [New York: International Universities Press, 1940].)

Piaget complicates the matter by showing how close, in some respects, "unconscious" or primary thinking is to mature thinking: Condensation can be seen as affective generalization, displacement as a form of abstraction, etc.

9. Scott, J. P., and Fuller, J. L., *Genetics and the Social Behavior of the Dog* (Chicago: University of Chicago Press, 1965).

10. I could have used a passage from Karl Abraham's account of the development of melancholia. The oral-narcissistic personality that, he argues, is the host condition of this development corresponds closely to the personal characteristics depicted by Binswanger (*Selected Papers of Karl Abraham* [New York: Basic Books, 1952]; see especially pp. 418–501).

11. May, R., Angel, E., and Ellenberger, H. (Eds.), *Existence: A New Dimension in Psychiatry and Psychology* (New York: Basic Books, 1958).

Chapter 8

1. Michel Foucault provides a remarkable account of how patients have been used in Western society in *Madness and Civilization: A History of Insanity in the Age of Reason* (New York: Random House, 1965).

2. Of course this was not a linear development, and it may have been a cyclic one. There is evidence, for example, from Foucault's account, that earlier times saw much more humane attitudes toward mental illness than were evident in the last 200 years. Some observers feel that the whole medical attack on mental illness is just that, an attack really directed at the patients!

3. The same attitude was a part of early dynamic efforts; see Marx, O. M., Morton Prince and the dissociation of a personality, *J. Hist. Behav. Sci.* 6:120, 1970.

4. Hollingshead, A. B., and Redlich, F. C., *Social Class and Mental Illness, A Community Study* (New York: Wiley, 1958). "Even Dr. Monro states in response to an investigative committee of the House of Commons that no one dared use chains on Noblemen, but that they were indispensable in dealing with the poor and with those in public institutions" (Kraepelin, E., *One Hundred Years of Psychiatry* [New York: Citadel, 1962]).

5. The following statement (from Leach, E., *Claude Lévi-Strauss* [Cambridge, Mass.: M.I.T. Press, 1970]) is a good summary of part of what Lévi-Strauss means by savage thinking. "The

distinction rather is between a logic that is constructed out of observed contrasts in the sensory qualities of concrete objects—for example, the difference between raw and cooked, wet and dry, male and female—and a logic that depends upon the formal contrasts of entirely abstract entities—for example, $+$ and $-$ or $\log^x$ and e^x."

Chapter 9

1. "But as soon as a *process* of illness defined the disease," vastly more people could be called sick. This concept extends to even commonplace descriptions. For example, people have probably always been noted to be secretive at times. Every one of us takes a hundred unnecessary precautions against having the most innocent things about us discovered. One goes to the doctor because of unhappiness and then cannot unburden his heart. Some measure of inhibition is in many contexts sensible, of course, and we should be suspicious of anyone who tells too much about himself. At one time the tendency to secretiveness was seen as quite natural, perhaps instinctive, or selected out for its obvious value in jungle situations. Such accepting ways of understanding secretiveness, and dozens of other human phenomena, were particularly customary in the nineteenth century. Since the coming of psychoanalysis, however, much of what was seemingly natural or inevitable or instinctive has grown suspect as possibly pathological. Secretiveness is left over not only from the jungle but from our upbringing, the result of unresolved conflicts, say, between holding and letting go. It has some relationship to toilet training and special attitudes toward this. One, and only one, result of modern lines of thought has been the evaluation of much behavior against a standard of ideal behavior, fully "appropriate" behavior, so that it can somehow or other be cleansed of all such atavistic elements. This is an important matter not only for psychology and psychopathology but for human life and especially human ideals. In essence modern psychopathology has radically challenged the casual air with which secular man regarded much of his behavior. (The Catholic church has, of course, long had as inclusive and frightening a catalogue of sins as modern psychopathology's catalogue of symptoms.)

2. See, for example, the work of Hunt, Alward, Bloomingfall, and Silverman of the New York State Psychiatric Institute.

3. Temme, H. S., Untitled, *The American Way*, March 22, 1972.

4. Coltrera, J. T., Psychoanalysis and existentialism, *J. Amer. Psychoanal. Ass.* 10:166, 1962.

5. Psychoanalysis is therefore attacked from both sides, as advocating too much permissiveness or tolerance of instinctual gratification and also as promoting resignation to social norms!

Chapter 10

1. In the *examination*, we study the patient piece by piece—perhaps first appearance, then mood or thinking, etc. There is an approach to the psychiatric *formalism* which was discussed a little in the chapter on Kraepelin. I have taken a generally negative attitude toward this when it was pursued for its own sake, but the values of such an approach should not be overlooked. Wernicke, for example, was able to describe "blunting of affect" in the course of surveying a large number of symptoms to determine whether they represented hyperfunctions or hypofunctions. See Wernicke, C., *Grundriss der Psychiatrie in Klinischen Vorlesungen* (Leipzig: Thieme, 1900); at least part of this was translated by W. Alfred McCorn, and appeared in *Alienist and Neurologist* 20:1, 1899. I have been unable to determine whether the whole volume was translated and reprinted.

2. Here is a common scene during the training of doctors. A teacher introduces the student to the patient: "Dr. So-and-so will be examining you." Young Dr. So-and-so: "How do you do? Tell me, in what way are you sick?"

3. Of course every school takes at least a little from the others, so that no one practices all one way. The great physician Osler advises students of medicine, "The motto of each of you as you undertake the examination and treatment of a case should be: put yourself in his place. Realize so far as you can the mental state of the patient, enter into his feelings—scan gently his faults. The kindly word, the cheerful greeting, the sympathetic look—these the patient understands" (Osler, W., *Aequanimitas, With Other Addresses to Medical Students, Nurses and Practitioners of Medicine* [New York: Blakiston, 1952]). My point is that the objective-descriptive school gives only the most rudimentary counsel as to how one puts himself in another's place and what he can anticipate.

4. See Jaspers' *General Psychopathology* (Chicago: University of Chicago Press, 1963, pp. 302, 364, 702). The sharp separation of art and science, so characteristic of much present-day thought too, invites correction by the example of the Renaissance. Leonardo, to use a perhaps unfair example, appears not to have worked scientifically *or* artistically but used the two methods inseparably. Such a phenomenon gives me courage to describe psychiatric methods as technology.

5. A thoughtful and detailed account appears in Novey's *The Second Look: The Reconstruction of Personal History in Psychiatry and Psychoanalysis* (Baltimore: John Hopkins Press, 1968).

6. For an excellent brief discussion and useful bibliography of the "working-through process," see Sandler, J., Dare, C., and Holder, A., Basic psychoanalytic concepts: IX. Working through, *Brit. J. Psychiat.* 117:617, 1970.

7. Here is Binswanger's tribute to Freud's methodological advances.

We may say that it was Freud who raised psychiatric techniques of examination to the level of a technique in the truly medical sense of the word. In the pre-Freudian era, the psychiatric "auscultation" and "percussion" of the neurotic patient was, as it were, performed through the patient's shirt, in that all direct contact with personally erotic and sexual themes was avoided. Only when the physician was able to make himself into a *complete* physician, to include within the sphere of the examination his total person and the sympathetic, antipathetic, and sexual forces directed toward him by the patient, only then could he create between patient and doctor an atmosphere of personal distance and, at the same time, of medical cleanliness, discipline, and correctness. It was this atmosphere that was able to raise psychiatric technique to the level of general medicine. This, too, was possible for Freud only because his total existence was that of a *researcher,* and because of the quality of his system of thought as I have just sketched it. He saw in the "attitude" of the patient to the doctor only the regressive repetition of psychobiologically earlier parental "object-cathexes" and eliminated what was *new* in the patient's *encounter* with him. Insofar as he did this he was able to keep the physician as a person in the background and allow him to pursue his technical role unencumbered by personal influences—as is the case with surgeons or radiologists.

(*Being-in-the-World* [New York: Basic Books, 1963, pp. 201–202].) The whole passage from which this is taken deserves study.

8. Psychoanalytic and behaviorist ideas can be translated back and forth. See French, T. M., *The Integration of Behavior* (Chicago: University of Chicago Press, 1952); also Sloane, R. B., The converging paths of behavior therapy and psychotherapy, *Amer. J. Psychiat.* 125:7, 1969.

9. Freud, S., *The Ego and the Id* (1923). (Standard Ed., vol. XIX [London: Hogarth, 1961].)

10. I believe, too, that existential psychiatry opens the *world of feeling* to an extent so far largely unexplored. It may be that existential work is still in its beginnings, still under the domination of the objective schools, and that the world of feeling is capable of as detailed a topography as has been discovered in the visual representation of the human body and the intellectual understandings of the psyche and society. These remarks are not meant to underrate the start that existentialists have made in describing the experiences of color, time, space, etc., in the various states.

11. For a brilliant recent example, see the work of David Reiss (Intimacy and problem solving: an automated procedure for testing a theory of consensual experience in families, *Arch. Gen. Psychiat.* [Chicago] 25:442, 1971). A fine critical review of recent observations has been provided by Mishler, E. G., and Waxler, N. E., Family interaction processes and schizophrenia: A review of current theories, *Merrill-Palmer Quart.* 11:269, 1965.

Chapter 11

1. Here is a simple example. The author, Vamick Volkan, is a teacher of psychiatrists.

To clarify further, I will cite as an example a supervisory session with an inexperienced resident. During the resident's interaction with a patient she correctly observed and diagnosed the patient's angry state. In the hour of supervision that followed, the supervisor showed her that the patient's anger was not directed at her but was part of the transference manifestation in which the patient expressed his anger at his mother. During the therapy that followed the explanation, the resident was less irritated with the patient and was able to pick up his references to his mother, but by now she had lost her ability to diagnose the angry state that was still present. I am sure that others who supervise beginning residents have had similar experiences. This is a case of the "learning" of psychodynamics at the expense of diagnostic awareness.

(Discussion of paper, *Amer. J. Psychiat.* 128:133, 1972.) Some avoid the dilemmas by developing personal amalgams that lie between the schools. Bion sees himself as a psychoanalyst, but there is much here of the phenomenological reduction.

To attain to the state of mind essential for the practice of psychoanalysis I avoid any exercise of memory; I make no notes. When I am tempted to remember the events of any particular session I resist the temptation. If I find myself wandering mentally into the domain of memory I desist. In this my practice is at variance with the view that notes should be kept or that psycho-analysts should find some method by which they can record their sessions mechanically or should train themselves to have a good memory. If I find that I am without any clue to what the patient is doing and am tempted to feel that the secret lies hidden in something I have forgotten, I resist any impulse to remember what happened or how I interpreted what happened on some previous occasion. If I find that some half-memory is beginning to obtrude I resist its recall no matter how pressing or desirable its recall may seem to be.

(Bion, W., *Attention and Interpretation* [New York: Basic Books, 1971].) Such a suspension of active mental work has often been recommended to psychoanalysts, although seldom so radically. The principal difficulty is to determine when to suspend the suspension; at that point the schools diverge and fresh dilemmas arise. (I am indebted to Harold Boris of Boston for the Bion quotation.)

Perhaps the most popular solution to the dilemmas is to recommend, or acknowledge the necessity of, a flexible stance. One must be prepared to be empathic *and* objective at different times; there is no single place to stand in psychotherapy. Dieter Wyss (*Depth Psychology* [New York: Norton, 1966, p. 560]) has written eloquently to this effect:

The difficulty facing psychotherapy here, the need to strike a balance between perceiving and loving, the need to see through the patient whilst yet lovingly accepting him, the need to regard him not only as an object of transference but also as a human being in his own right, should not be underestimated. This point of balance, it would seem, is no sooner established than it is lost again.

Something similar has been written by Hammer, E. F., in his *Use of Interpretation in Treatment: Technique and Art* (New York: Grune & Stratton, 1968). One must be able to be both "tough-minded" and "tender-minded," without getting stuck at either extreme. Also Chessick, R. D., *Why Psychotherapists Fail* (New York: Science House, 1971; see especially p. 184). This dilemma, objectivity versus empathy, is the one most often discussed, often the only one discussed.

2. Ferenczi, S., *Further Contributions to the Theory and Technique of Psychoanalysis* (London: Hogarth, 1950), and Alexander, F., and French, T. M., *Psychoanalytic Therapy; Principles and Applications* (New York: Ronald, 1946).

3. Here is a sequence of perhaps increasingly empathic remarks: "I guess most people would be sore under those circumstances." "It would be hard not to be sore under those circumstances." "God, how sore you must be!" "That would have made me mad!" "How can you stand it?"

4. This produces in many students' minds a strong conviction of understanding and the expectation that everything can be explained—that everything is not only determined but also determined in ways we can grasp. Of course, explanations are by definition mental acts *after* the event; there is a great deal less predictive power. Indeed, the explanatory and predictive powers of psychoanalysis are sharply different.

Existential interest, in contrast, falls as heavily on the unpredictable (and the absurd) as analytic interest falls on the explained. For the latter, *formulations* are critical; for the former, it's *the brick* that travels 14 stories to land on one's head.

5. See Boyer, L. B., and Giovacchini, P. L., *Psychoanalytic Treatment of Characterological and Schizophrenic Disorders* (New York: Science House, 1967). These authors emphasize the needs many patients have for their therapists' providing "real objects" and being "receptive to patients' projections." I do not believe much disagreement will be found with this pronouncement. The difficulties arise when the advice is extended to a larger group of patients and situations (Greenson, R., *Technique and Practise of Psychoanalysis* [New York: International Universities Press, 1967]), especially in regard to the development and resolution of the transference neurosis. Boyer and Giovacchini are willing to leave parts of themselves behind in the patient, à la existential therapy, as opposed to complete resolution of the transference.

6. See her book *The Capacity for Emotional Growth* (London: Hogarth, 1970).

7. Perhaps all the ideas and feelings set going in us during a clinical encounter are messages from the patient, what David Reiss has called reenactments of something going on in the patient. This must surely be a simplification of what happens—for example, it seems to set aside complicated transference-countertransference processes—but at least it provides an idea as to how we can form ideas about patients without reducing patients to being objects of knowledge.

8. Janet, P., *Psychological Healing* (New York: Macmillan, 1925), and Wolberg, L., *Technique of Psychotherapy* (New York: Grune & Stratton, 1967).

INDEX

INDEX

Abrahams, Karl, 354
Acting out, 121
Adaptation
  catatonia as, 213–214
  concern with adaptive behavior, 56–57
  defined, 160
  existential vs. psychoanalytic concepts of, 160
  symptoms as, 211–212
  use as term, 150
Adjustment, symptoms as, 211–212
Adler, Alfred, 342
Affect(s)
  clarification of nature of, 88–89
  conflict of, 105, 107, 108
  contagious nature of, 212
  in dementia praecox, 28
  existential methods with, 318, 329
  ideas and, 104
  need for discharge of, 92, 97
  in paranoia, 342
  as primary causes, 353
  reversal of, 107, 108
  symptom formation and, 97
Alexander, Franz, 360
Ambivalence
  dealing with, 320–321
  dissociation and, 226
Amnesia
  anesthesia and, 39
  in fugues, 42
  in hysteria, 38, 39–40, 53, 68–69
  in obsessional states, 53
Anaclitic therapy, 195
Anesthesia
  amnesia and, 39
  in anorexic patients, 48
  in hysteria, 39, 48, 69, 73

Anger
  dealing with, 315–321
    existential method, 317–319
    interpersonal method, 319–321
    objective methods, 315–317
  in paranoia, 342
Anna O., case of Breuer, 81–90, 91, 94, 97, 101, 151, 340
Anorexia nervosa, 45–50
  behavior in, 48–50
  case histories, 46–47, 96–97
  euphoria in, 49–50
  as psychosis vs. neurosis, 50
Anxiety
  communication of, 212
  as indicator of parataxic processes, 311
Association(s). See also Free association
  in dementia praecox, 28
  dissociation concept and, 17
  hypnosis and, 89, 90
  idea discharge in, 104
  memory emergence in, 89, 104
  reality in, 341
  symptom formation and, 102
  to symptoms, 95
  in therapy, 91, 95, 102, 117
Attention-seeking in interpersonal method, 307–309
Auerbach, Erich, 181–182, 351
Autism
  Bleuler on, 244, 336–337
  ego in, 336–337
  reality relations in, 244
  in schizophrenia, 178

Bateson, Gregory, 350
Behavior, 230. See also specific type, e.g., Adaptation; Anger
  in anorexia, 48–50
  counterprojective, interpersonal psychiatry and, 307–309
  in dementia praecox, 24–27
  evaluation against ideal, 355
  genetic vs. environmental factors and, 248
  grandiose, 50
  in mania, 50
  in neuroses, 54–57, 61, 116
  in paranoia, 125–128, 343
  projective. See Projection(s)
  Skinner on, 352
Behavioral school, 352
  on learning, 304
  methods of, 284, 295
Bernheim, H., 37, 71, 288
Binet, Alfred, 40
Binswanger, Ludwig, 147–156, 165, 170
  contributions, 159–161
  on Freud, 357
  on phobia, 248–249
  on present and past, 233
  technique of, 155, 164, 262, 298, 299
  understanding of, 300
Bion, Wilfred R., 359
Bleuler, Eugene, 17, 333–334, 338, 352
  on affective elements, 247, 253
  autism concept, 244, 336–337
  on clinical signs, 32
  contributions, 334–335
  on "deep feeling," 259
  on dementia praecox, 123, 178, 334–335, 353
  on dissociation, 140, 225, 226, 334
  Janet vs., 334–335
  Minkowski and, 343
  on paranoia, 342
  on patient-physician relations, 210, 343
  process concepts, 243
  on psychoses, 334
  on social factors, 168
Breuer, Joseph, 55

on affect, 88
Anna O. case, 81–90, 91, 94, 97, 101, 151, 340
contributions, 90–92
on hypnoid moment, 102
on hysteria, 194
method of, 85–90, 164
Burton, Richard, on melancholy, 235–238, 240–243

Carter, Robert, 68
Catalepsy induction, 75–76
Catatonia
as adaptation, 213–214
in dementia praecox, 27
Kraepelin's tests, 284–285, 315
significance of gestures in, 242
Catecholamines, psychological states and, 245
Cathartic method, 92
aim of, 101
Breuer and, 85–90
discovery of, 336
emotion and ideas in, 89–90
Gestalt movement and, 345
goals in, 256
hypnosis and, 89
in psychoanalysis, 102
traumatic moment in, 102
Charcot, Jean-Marie, 61, 62, 65–80, 352
on affect, 88
on anorexia, 48
Breuer as link between Freud and, 90–92
contributions, 79–81, 159, 161, 228, 243, 340
on dissociation, 101, 244
experimental hysteria produced by, 72–77
Freud and, 81
on hypnoid moment, 102
hypnosis, use of, 89, 288
on hysteria, 32, 37, 65–80, 226, 288, 352

method of, 90
pathogenic sequences of, 94, 99, 105
process hypothesis of, 241–244
on sleep and nightmares, 85
on subconscious, 39
teaching method of, 65–66
on tics, 58–59
on unconscious, 92
Chemical hypotheses of psychoses, 32, 245
Childhood, 227, 228–234, 350–351
character of adolescence, 234
development of child psychiatry, 350–351
existential school on, 232, 233, 242, 353
Freud's study of infancy, 118, 119
psychoanalytic school on, 228–229, 292, 293, 308
Coles, Robert, 345, 350
Complexes
development of concept of, 351
Oedipus. See Oedipus complex
Compulsion
motivation and, 246
obsessive-compulsive neuroses, 58
repetition compulsion, 226, 290–291
Condensation. See also Displacement
unconscious, 117
wishes and, 117
Conflict(s)
of affects, case of, 105, 107, 108
awareness and, 101, 102, 321
dissociation and, 97–104
factors in resolution of, 149–150
Freud on, 39
insight and, 161, 293

Conflict(s) (*Cont.*)
  personality and, 140
  use of term, 150
Confrontation
  in existential method, 133–137,
    143–145, 158–159, 163–
    164, 281–282, 298
  in objective-descriptive method,
    281–282
Consciousness
  change of, 90
  changes in fugues, 42
  of conflict, results of, 99, 100,
    101–102
  dissociation and, 103–104
  elevation of neuroses to, 301
  in hypnoid moment, 102
  in hysteria, 51–53, 55–56, 59–
    60, 68, 77, 78, 79, 90
  in obsessional neuroses, 51–53
  pathological forms of, 60
  research on, 337–338
  therapy and psychic elements
    in, 101
Conversion in hysteria, 114, 264–
  265, 339
Counterprojective method, 301,
  307–309, 311
Countertransference, use of, 285,
  298–299
Cretinism, 15
Crowds, sociology of, 212

Decision-making by therapists,
  321–328
  external influences on, 322–
    324
  patient and, 327–328, 329,
    360–361
  temperament and, 324–325
  training and, 324–327
Defense mechanisms, 60–61. *See
    also specific type, e.g.,*
    Projection(s)
  management of

  in interpersonal psychiatry,
    310
  in psychoanalysis, 211
Delirium tremens, 21
Delusions
  in dementia praecox, 24–27
  dissociation and, 140
  intellectual activity and, 137–
    138
  Kraepelin on, 27
  in monomania, 351
  nature of, in hysteria vs. schizo-
    phrenia, 202–203
  as reproductions of family ex-
    perience, 213
Dementia praecox. *See also* Schiz-
    ophrenia
  attention discontinuities in, 60
  behavioral aberrations in, 24–
    27, 29
  Bleuler on, 123, 178, 334–
    335, 353
  catatonia in, 27
  delusions in, 24–27
  deterioration in, 333
  diagnosis, 264
  dissociation in, 60
  endogenous vs. exogenous fac-
    tors in, 29
  Kraepelin on, 15, 23–30, 123–
    124, 224, 332–333, 334,
    349–50, 352, 355
  manic-depressive psychoses vs.,
    26–27
  paranoia vs., 124–130
  paranoidal forms of, 27
  paresis diagnosis as, 25, 28, 35,
    123–124
  prognosis, 30, 124, 332–333
  retention of faculties in, 29
Denial, 39, 108–109, 113
Depression, 324. *See also* Manic-
    depressive psychoses
  catecholamine brain processes
    and, 245

late-life, 23
mental deterioration and, 25
Deterioration, mental, 25, 333
Displacement, 108, 114
denial and, 108–109, 113
unconscious, 114–115, 117
wishes and, 117
Dissociation, 350
ambivalence and, 226
in anorexia, 49
associationism and concept of,
17
Bleuler on, 140, 225, 226, 334
Breuer on, 140
Charcot on, 101, 244
conflict and, 97–104
consciousness and, 103–104
critical nature of, 161
delusions and, 140
in dementias, 60
ego and, 140, 164–165
existential school on, 154
external vs. internal, 141
family and, 350
in hysteria, 58, 59–60, 225–
226
interpersonal school on, 200
introduction of concept of functional, 50
Janet on, 140
Kraepelin on, 140, 225, 226
Minkowski on, 140
in neuroses, 61
objective-descriptive school on,
140, 225, 226, 244, 334
in obsessional states, 53–54,
58, 60
psychic disorders classified by, 60
psychological contradictions
and, 223–226
secondary symptoms and primary, 140
symptom formation and, 101
Dora, case of Freud, 104–116,
119, 120, 340–341

Dreams
association to, 95
in hysteria, 68, 77, 78
in pathogenic sequence, 91
somnambulism and, 335
symptoms and, 89
use in psychoanalysis, 289
wishes in, 100–101

Ego
autism concept, 336–337. *See
also* Autism
change in therapy, 164
concentration on defects of,
324
defined, 56
development of, 203
dissociation and, 140
Freud on, 142
functions of, 347
in hysteria, 60, 194
individuality concepts, 271–
273
Janet on failure of, 60
mental illness vs. disorders of,
56
psychoanalytic method and,
162, 282, 283, 294, 304
reality testing and, 336–337
in schizophrenia, 60
Ego psychology, 203, 347
concept, described, 60, 62
term as hybrid, 310
Electricity, clinical use of, 282,
284, 352
Ellenberger, Henri, 340, 343
Emotion(s)
of analyst in psychoanalysis,
285
cathartic method and, 89–90
conflict of, 97–102
consciousness of, 101–102
euphoria in hysteria vs. mania,
49–50

Emotion(s) (*Cont.*)
in hysteria, 49–50, 68, 72–73, 77, 78, 90
identification and field of, 303
Oedipus complex resolution and, 301–303
role in existential school method, 156–165, 298, 301–303, 358
role in objective school methods, 358
symptoms and, 89
theories of, 54
trauma and, 97–100, 101–102
Empathy
defined, 298
in existential method, 138–140, 153–154, 156–157, 161, 162, 298, 307, 317–318, 360
objectivity vs., 359–360
therapy and, 260
Energy, psychic abnormalities and, 16, 44
Environmental factors. *See* Social reality
Epilepsy, 71, 72
Erikson, Erik, 229, 350
diffuse etiology concepts of, 246
on life periods, 231–233
Esquirol, J. E. D., 221–222
Etiology. *See also specific disease or disorder*
concepts of childhood, 228–234, 350–351
development of doctrines of, 235–250, 350–354
in disease classification, 13–16
First Cause theory, 247–248
objective-descriptive school on, 229–230
process concepts of, 241–247, 264–267, 352–353, 355
psychoanalytic school on, 230–232

record analysis in determining, 227–228
relationships and symptoms in, 257–262
Euphoria, 49–50
Evolution, as psychiatric concept, 226–227
Existential psychiatry, 123–165, 283, 296–305, 329, 342–344. *See also specific topic*
adaptation concept, 160
advances in, 218
anger management in, 317–319
approaches to technical matters, 152
attitudes and approaches to patient in, 133–147, 152–157, 161–164, 261–262, 300, 304–305, 343
"being-in-the-world" concept, 203
Binswanger and, 147–156. *See also* Binswanger, Ludwig
complexities of method, 158–159, 164
confrontation in, 133–137, 143–145, 158–159, 163–164, 281–282, 298
contributions of, 150, 229
counterprojective method in, 301
development of, 131–132, 297–299
on dissociation, 154
emotions in, 156–165, 298, 301–303, 305
empathy in, 138–140, 153–154, 156–157, 161–162, 298, 307, 317–318, 360
explanation and prediction in, 360
on flowing "life periods," 232, 233

freedom from expectations in, 155–156
functions of, 328
on human condition, 268
on hysteria, 203, 204
ideals of, 158–159, 164–165, 268, 269, 271, 299–300, 303–304, 343
interpersonal psychiatry vs., 310, 343
Jaspers and, 124–132, 141, 342–343. *See also* Jaspers, Karl
Minkowski and, 133–147, 343. *See also* Minkowski, E.
on neuroses, 131–132
neutrality in, 307
origin of, 296
on past in etiology, 232, 233, 242, 353
phenomenological reduction, 155–156
on phobias, 248–249
problem emphasis in, 150
psychoanalytic psychiatry vs., 295, 304–305, 358
on psychoses, 131–132
reality-testing in, 305
resistance analysis in, 298–299
social phenomena and, 174
strength of, 147
on subject-object distinctions, 261–262
on successive present, 232
technical literature on, 296–297, 299
therapeutic power of, 299–302
Ey, Henry, 61

Fairbairn, R., 347
Fantasy, 346
in hysteria, 202–203
ideas and images in, 177
interpersonal school on, 184, 308, 319–320, 321

participant observation and, 200
projective, in therapy, 299
psychoanalytic school on, 121, 242, 270, 308, 311, 346
reality and, 200, 341
role in society, 199
in schizophrenia, 202–203
wishes and, 100–101, 117–118
Fears, 54–55. *See also* Phobias
Federn, Paul, 194
Feedback, negative, 212–213, 245
Ferenczi, Sandor, 360
First Cause theories, 247–248
Formalism, psychiatric, 356
Foucault, Michel, 354
Free association, 227. *See also* Association(s)
goals of, 117, 227
in psychoanalysis, 103, 285, 289–290, 295, 296
resistance analysis vs., 297
symptom formation and, 102
technique of, 95, 103
French, Thomas M., 357, 360
Freud, Anna, 347
Freud, Sigmund, 35, 62, 92, 94–121, 338, 352
on affect reversal, 104–116
on ambivalence, 226
on analytic listening, 161–162
analytic solutions of, 293
on association, 104
Breuer as link between Charcot and, 90–92
case study methods, 16
Charcot and, 81
on conflict, 39, 95–104
contributions, 16, 79, 81, 103, 159, 170, 184, 229, 287–288, 289, 357
on dissociation, 95–104, 140, 161, 226

Freud, Sigmund (*Cont.*)
Dora, case of, 104–116, 117, 119, 120, 340–341
on ego and id, 142
emotional involvement of, 285
emphasis of, 61
on goals of therapy, 293, 294
hyperbole of, 107–108
on hypnosis, 288
on hysteria, 25, 32, 194–195, 200, 226
on infantile elements, 118, 119
insights on psychological development, 120–121
Kraepelin and, 33
on life forces, 233
metaphors on etiology, 352
methods of, 94–95, 164
on neurologic concepts, 32
on neuroses, 81, 247–248
on Oedipus complex resolution, 301–303
on paranoia, 131
phases of work, 341–342
physical contact with patients, 94–95
on primary and secondary thought processes, 353
process concepts and pathogenic sequences, 244–245
on psychoanalysis vs. psychiatry, 339
psychological nature of data, 243
on psychoses, 194–195
public opinions on, 267
realism of, 191
on reality, 118, 175–176, 177
relationship with patients, 255
restrictions of method of, 312
on sexuality, 100, 115, 118, 119, 226, 247–248
social factor theories and, 168–169, 175–176, 177

on social institutions, 271
on subconscious, 39
on transformation, 79
on wishes and fantasy, 116–118, 341
on withdrawal, 178, 194
Fugues
amnesia in, 42
critical features in, 42
Janet on, 41–45
personality contrasts in, 42–45, 225
Function disorders in neuroses, 54–57, 61, 116. *See also* Behavior

Game-playing in therapy, 307–308
Generalization in neuroses vs. psychoses, 160
Genetic factors, 229, 248
in hysteria, 66–67
in psychoses, 30–31
Genital factors. *See* Sexuality
Gestalt therapy movement, 345
Goals. *See* Ideals, psychiatric
Griesinger, Wilhelm, on paranoia, 342
Group therapy, 170–171, 344–345

Hallucinations
in hysteria, 37
in paranoia, 126, 127, 129, 343
as reproductions of family experience, 213
Hawthorne effect, 349
Homosexuality, 115, 323
Horney, Karen, 344
Hypnosis, 227
association and, 89, 90
Charcot on, 89, 288

in hysteria production, 72–77,
339
objective correlates of, 339
patient manipulation in, 254–
255, 283–284
psychoanalytic method and,
288
symptom reproduction and, 89
transference in, 74
trauma and, 102
Hypochondriasis, 25
Hysteria, 69, 70–71, 75
advances in knowledge of, 93–
94
affect in, 105, 107, 108
amnesia in, 34, 38, 39–40, 53,
68–69
anesthesia in, 39, 48, 69, 73
anorexy, 45–50
Breuer on, 194
Charcot on, 32, 37, 65–80, 90,
226, 288, 352
concept of oral or primitive,
204
consciousness in, 55–56, 59–
60, 68, 77, 78, 79, 90
conversion symptoms and, 114,
264–265, 339
development of concept of, 32
diagnosis of, 264–265
displacement and, 108, 114
dissociation in, 58, 59–60,
225–226
Dora, case of Freud, 104–116,
119, 120, 340–341
drama in, 203–206
dreams and, 68, 77–79, 90
ego in, 60, 194
emotion in, 68, 72–73, 77, 78,
90
empathy for patients in, 260
epilepsy vs., 71, 72
euphoria in, 49–50
experimental, 72–77
fantasy in, 202–203

Freud on, 25, 32, 194–195,
200, 226
fugues, 41–45, 225
genetic factors in, 66–67
hallucinations in, 37
hypnosis and, 72–77, 102,
288, 339
hysterogenous zones in, 69, 70
id and, 60
ideas in, 77, 78, 90
importance of knowledge of,
62–64
interpersonal school on, 203–
204
Janet on, 34, 35–45, 65, 90,
194, 335
knowledge of mental life in,
51–53
Kraepelin on, 66
malingering vs., 75, 77
narcissism in, 205
objective-descriptive school on,
204
obsessions vs., 51–56, 58
oedipal element in, 204
paralysis and, 45, 75–77
pathogenic sequences in, 226–
227
personality traits in, 60, 225
projection in, 194
"pseudo–living" in, 203–204,
206
psychic element in, 68
psychoanalytic school on, 203–
204
reality concept in, 202–203
social understanding of, 199–
206
somnambulisms, 34, 35–40,
45, 335
stigmata in, 69, 70
subconscious in, 55–56
suggestibility in, 37–40, 59,
71–72, 94
Sullivan on, 194–195, 200

Hysteria (*Cont.*)
symptom sequence and persistence in, 38–39, 88, 90–91, 335
systemic manifestations of, 45
transference in, 74, 329
traumata and, 67–68, 72–73, 76–79, 90, 91, 102
unconscious and, 59–60
uterine, hypothesis of, 64–65, 338–339

Id
Freud on, 142
in hysteria, 60
Ideals, psychiatric, 263–273, 355–356
changing, 264–269
divergent, 270–273
of existential school, 158–159, 164–165, 268, 269, 271, 299–300, 303–304, 343
of interpersonal school, 265–271, 273, 311
need for redefinition of, 266
norms and, 262–263
of psychoanalytic school, 288–289, 293–294
therapy and, 263
unity of, 269–270
Ideas
affects and wishes and, 103–104
in cathartic method, 89–90
conflict and consciousness of, 101–102
content of, in traumatic moments, 98–99
discharge
in association, 104
need for, 92
extension of concept of, 50
hysteria and, 72–78, 90, 339
Identification, 301, 303
Identity concepts, 271–273

Illusion, illness and, 264
Infancy. *See* Childhood
Infantile neuroses, 96, 299
Inhibition, 355
Insight(s)
conflict and, 161
development of
in interpersonal method, 310
in objective-descriptive method, 286
in psychoanalysis, 290–293
of Freud on psychological development, 120–121
need for, in therapy, 72
symptoms and, 113
Instincts
conflict and, 293
psychoanalytic method and, 294, 295
Skinner on, 352
Institutional psychiatry, 251–262
advances in, 210–214, 217–218
artificial conditions of, 252
authority relations in, 252
"coming into relationship" in, 257–262
democratization of mental hospitals, 209–210
early descriptions of, 208–209
exposing reality of, 267
follow-up records in, 227
Laing on, 161, 210, 246, 343, 350
manipulation of patient in, 354
Sullivan on, 207–211
Szasz on, 164–165, 265, 343
understanding growth in, 252–257, 354
Interpersonal (social) psychiatry, 57, 167–214, 305–312, 329, 344–350. *See also* *specific topic*

active nature of, 281
anger management in, 319–321
approach to patient in, 179–181
attention-seeking in, 307–309
chemical etiology models, 352
concern of, 343
contributions, 150
counterprojective nature of, 307–309
dealing with ambivalence in, 320–321
defined, 167
demands of, 164
on dissociation, 200
existential school and, 310, 343
facts vs. fantasies in, 184, 308, 319–320, 321, 346
function of, 328
game-playing in, 307
historical tradition of, 319
hysteria interpretation in, 199–206
ideals of, 265–271, 273, 311
insight development in, 310
interview situation in, 190–199, 306, 310–311, 321
intimacy in, 307–310
Johnson and, 344
Meyer and, 167–183. See also Meyer, Adolf
neutrality in, 306–307, 309–310
new social areas of, 345
objectivity in, 306–307
origins of, 167–171
participant observation in, 305–307
participation in sociol processes, 311
past and present in, 231, 232
patient manipulation in, 320
patient role in, 145, 164
on preadolescence, 206–207

problem emphasis in, 150
process theories in, 242, 245–246, 353
projections in, 309
psychoanalytic school and, 295, 311
reality exposure by, 267–268
resistance management in, 295, 296, 309–310
results of, 214, 349–350
role-playing in, 309, 310
social reality in, 174–179, 184–187, 267–268, 306–308, 310–312, 345
society as focus of, 306–307, 310–312
Sullivan and, 167–171, 183–199, 346–348. See also Sullivan, Harry Stack
transference in, 199–200, 308
unconscious in, 311
Interpersonal relationships, 256–257
Intimacy, therapy and, 307–309

Jackson, Hughlings, 32
Janet, Pierre, 13, 32, 34–62, 338
on anorexy, 45–50
Bleuler vs., 334–335
concepts of normal and ethical, 44–45
on contact with subconscious, 85
degradation process theory, 243
on fugues, 41–45
functionalism of, 270
on hypnoid moment, 102
on hysteria, 34–50, 65, 71, 72, 90, 194, 225, 226, 335
illness classification, 353
on neuroses, 15, 34, 50, 243–244, 334, 336
pathogenic sequences of, 105
physical contact with patients, 94–95

Janet, Pierre (*Cont.*)
  on psychasthenias, 50–57
  social functions concept, 168
  on somnambulisms, 34, 35–40,
    335
  on subconscious, 39, 85
  theoretical background of, 34–
    35
  on tics, 58
Jaspers, Karl, 124–132, 134,
    342–343
  contributions, 159, 338
  existential technique, 141
  on first moment of observation,
    328
  on formation of illness, 175
  on inner experience, 174
  Kraepelin and, 124
  on paranoia, 124–130
  on psychosis vs. neurosis, 131–
    132, 342–343
Johnson, Adelaide, 213, 344
Jones, Maxwell, 210
Jung, Carl, 313, 342, 344

Kahlbaum, Karl, 229
Kraepelin, Emil, 13–32, 222–
    224, 331, 338
  Bleuler and, 27, 28
  on catatonia, 284–285, 315
  clinical pictures, 17–30, 32–
    34, 65, 66, 81, 131, 141,
    146, 177, 222–224, 332–
    333
  contributions, 16, 33–34, 80,
    159, 170, 229, 333–334,
    338
  data collection, 285–286
  on dementia praecox, 15, 23–
    30, 123–124, 224, 332–
    333, 334, 349–350, 355
  diagnostic tests, 281, 284–285,
    315
  disease concept, 13–17
  on dissociation, 140, 225, 226

  on etiology, 13–17, 30–33,
    242, 243, 334
  formalism of, 356
  on genetic aspects, 30–32
  on hysteria, 66
  limitations of work, 124
  on manic-depressive psychoses,
    17–23, 224, 226, 332
  on mental deterioration, 25
  methods vs. thinking of, 177
  Meyer and, 323
  on neurologic factors, 30–32
  process concepts, 243
  on psychological contradictions,
    224
  revisions of diagnostic criteria,
    123
  on significance of symptoms,
    258
  on social factors, 169
  theorizing by, 352
  on verbal material, 185
  on volition, 16–17
  Wundt and, 13, 16–17, 331
Kris, A. O., 334

Laing, R. D., 161, 210, 246,
    343, 350
Lasègue, E. C., 47, 48
Learning, reinforcement and, 304
Leighton, A. H., 346–347
Lévi-Strauss, Claude, 262, 354–
    355
Libido. *See* Sexuality
Lidz, Theodore, 348
Life, charts of, 176–177, 345–
    346. *See also* Social real-
    ity
Lobotomy, use of, 282, 352
Love, educational component of,
    301–303

Mania. *See also* Manic-depressive
    psychoses
  affect disorder in, 342

behavior in, 50
catecholamine brain processes
    in, 245
classification, 23
euphoria and grandiosity in,
    50
mental deterioration and, 25
Manic-depressive psychoses
    case study by Kraepelin, 15,
        17–23, 332
    differential diagnosis, 26–27
    mania classification in, 23
    prognosis, 30
    psychological contradictions in,
        224
Melancholia
    affect disorder in, 342
    Burton on, 235–236, 238,
        240–241, 242
    development in oral-narcissistic
        personalities, 354
    Rush on, 239–241
Memories
    association of symptoms and,
        89, 104
    emergence in association, 104
    forgotten, hypnotic symptoms
        and, 89, 104
Mesmer, Franz Anton, 89–90, 94
Meyer, Adolf, 25, 35, 171–183,
    213, 332, 338
    approach to patient, 179–181
    case histories, 170, 171–173,
        280
    contributions, 167–170, 180–
        183, 228–229, 330
    goals of, 198–199
    interest in facts, 346
    on Kraepelin, 323
    life charts of, 176–177, 345–
        346
    limitations of, 170
    methods of, 169–170, 177,
        186
    on schizophrenia, 44

on social interventions, 178–
    179
on social reality, 174–175,
    177–179, 345
on successive present, 232
on systems and habits, 211
on understanding patients, 185
Minkowski, E., 133–147, 152,
    153, 158, 170, 343
    attitudes and approaches to pa-
        tients, 133–147, 174, 343
    Bleuler and, 343
    contributions, 159, 162
    existential school technique,
        141–142, 162–164, 296–
        298, 334
    on life periods, 233
    on schizophrenia, 298
Monomania, 342, 351
de Montaigne, Michel Eyquem,
    336
Mullahy, Patrick, 184, 346

Narcissism, 203, 205
    narcissistic transference, in psy-
        choanalysis, 304–305
    process in narcissistic neuroses,
        178
Negative feedback, 212–213,
    245
Neurologic concepts of psychic
    disorders, 31–32, 245,
    295
Neuroses, 15, 34, 50, 243–244,
    334, 336
    anorexia nervosa, 50
    classification of, 14, 15, 50
    development stage and predis-
        position to, 57
    dissociation in, 61
    as disturbances of relationships,
        344
    Dora, case of Freud, 104–116,
        117, 119, 340–341
    elevation to consciousness, 300

Neuroses (*Cont.*)
    existential school on, 131–132
    formation of, 96, 292
    Freud on, 247–248
    function disorders in, 54–57, 61, 116
    generalization in, 160
    hysteria vs., 51–56
    infantile, 118–121
        defined, 96
        transferences and resistances in, 299
    Janet on, 34, 35, 50–57, 334
    Kraepelin on, 14
    obsessional. *See* Obsession(s)
    patients' problems in understanding, 253
    process in narcissistic, 178
    psyche in, 61
    psychoses vs., 131–132. *See also* Psychoses
    reality concepts in, 54–55, 57, 336–337
    reality in overcoming, 116
    resistances in, 299, 310
    sexuality in, 116, 217, 247–248. *See also* Sexuality
    transference. *See* Transference
Neutrality in therapy, 307
Niederland, W., 346
Nightmares, 85

Object-relations theory, 347
    interpersonal school on, 269, 271
    object cathexes in psychoses, 190
Objective-descriptive psychiatry, 18–62. *See also specific topic*
    anger management in, 315, 317
    on anorexy, 45–50
    attitude about patient, 142, 145, 146
    on catatonia, 284–285, 315
    categorization technique in, 279–280, 283
    contributions and development of, 229–230
    dangers of theorizing in, 352
    data collection in, 278–279, 285–286, 356
    demands of, 306
    on dementia praecox, 15, 23–30, 123–124, 222, 332–333, 334, 349–350, 355
    on dissociation, 140, 225, 226, 244, 334
    on etiology, 242, 243–244, 352
    on fugues, 41–45
    function of, 326
    on hysteria, 34–50, 65, 71, 72, 90, 194, 225, 226, 335
    ideals of, 272
    on illness vs. person, 191
    insight development in, 286
    Janet and, 13, 32, 34–62, 338. *See also* Janet, Pierre
    Kraepelin and, 13–32, 222–224, 331, 338. *See also* Kraepelin, Emil
    on manic-depressive psychoses, 17–23, 224, 226, 332
    methods of, 131, 278–287, 329
    on neuroses, 15, 34, 50, 243–244, 334, 336
    objectivity of, 284–286
    patient in, 278–287
        cooperation of, 282–283, 286
        manipulation of, 283–284
    process theories in, 243–245
    psychiatric formalism in, 356
    recognition powers in, 339
    on somnambulisms, 34, 35–40, 335
    subject-object split in, 283
    symptom use in, 96

tension in, 278–281
testing in, 281–283
transition to psychoanalysis,
80–81
Objectivity
empathy vs., 359–360
in interpersonal psychiatry,
306–307
in psychoanalysis, 285–288,
290, 292–294, 306–307,
316
Obsession(s), 34, 35, 50–57, 58
amnesia in, 53
consciousness in, 60
dissociation in, 53–54, 58, 60
fears in, 54–55
function disturbances in, 54–
55, 61
hysteria vs., 51–56, 58
Janet on, 34, 35, 50–57
knowledge of mental life in,
51–53
Obsessive-compulsive neuroses, 58
Oedipus complex
element of, in hysteria, 204
Freud on, 226
resolution of, 301–303
Operationalism, psychiatric, 260
Orne, Martin T., 339
Osler, William, 356
Ovesey, Lionel, 347

Paralysis
hysterical, 45, 73, 75–77
idea-dependent, 72
nature of phobic, 54
Paranoia
anger disorder in, 342
behavior in, 22, 125–128, 343
in dementia praecox, 27
dementia praecox distinguished
from 124–130
as disease of "false ideas," 247
hallucinations in, 126, 127,
129, 343

interpersonal school in management of, 188–190, 318–
319, 329
Kraepelin on, 15
personality defect in, 124, 125,
128, 129
in psychosis exploration, 130–
131
Parataxis. See Projection(s)
Paresis
diagnosis of, 25, 28, 35, 123–
124
Kraepelin on, 15
mental deterioration in, 25
Parsons, Talcott, 245
Participant observation, 200
Patient(s), 251–262, 278–287.
See also Institutional psychiatry
acceptance of, 142, 145–146
approaches to
existential school, 133–147,
150, 152–156, 343
interpersonal school, 145,
150, 164, 179–181
objective-descriptive school,
142, 145, 146
psychoanalytic school, 161–
163
attention paid to, 161–164
attitudes on, in existential
school, 133–147, 154–
157, 161–162, 343
authority relationships of therapist with, 252, 255
cooperation of, 282–283, 286
decisions by therapist and,
327–328, 329, 360–361
empathy with, 138–140, 153–
154, 156–157, 161–162,
298, 307, 317–318, 360
expectations of, 155–156
factors in attitudes of, 190,
192–194
fear of, 253

Patient(s) (*Cont.*)
  growth of understanding of,
    252–257, 354
  manipulation of, 254–255,
    354
    hypnosis as, 254–255, 283–
      284
    in interpersonal method,
      320
    narcissistic transference as,
      304–305
    need for, 329
    in objective-descriptive
      method, 283–284
  moral treatment era, 254
  physical contact with, 94–95,
    288–289
  problems in interview situ-
    ation, 190–199, 306,
    310–311, 321
  relationships, 252, 255
    coming into relationship,
      257–262
    diagnosis-treatment relation-
      ship, 259–260
    emotional, 256–257
    existential school on, 156–
      157, 261–262, 304–305
    psychoanalytic school on,
      142, 146
  as sinners, 253
  socioeconomic factors in diag-
    nosis and treatment, 254–
    256
  therapeutic goal changes, 256–
    257
  understanding of, 300
Pavlov, Ivan, 48
Perls, Fritz, 345
Perry, Helen, 184, 346
Persecutory delusions. *See* Paranoia
Personality. *See also* Behavior;
  Dissociation
  appearance vs., 173–174

changes in psychic illness,
  224–226
classification of disorders of, 15
conflict and, 140
in dementia, 60
ego psychology in interpretation of, 347
in hysteria, 60, 225
normal vs. fugue, 42–45, 225
in paranoia, 124, 125, 128,
  129
schizophrenia as advancement
  of, 44
social experience and, 242,
  245–246
social roles and, 270–271
Phenomenological reduction, 156
Phobias
  existential vs. psychoanalytic
    schools on, 248–249
  paralysis in, 54
Piaget, Jean, 353
Pinel, Philippe, 208, 219–221,
  241, 251, 254, 351
Plato, 64–65, 168
Pluralism in psychiatry, 328–330
Process concepts
  of definition of disease, 264–
    267, 355
  of etiology of disease, 241–
    247, 352–353
Projection(s)
  counterprojective behavior,
    301, 307–309, 311
  of fantasies in therapy, 299
  in hysteria, 194
  interpersonal school on, 307–
    309, 311
  prevalence in daily life, 308–
    309
  psychoanalytic school on, 307
  in psychoses, 190
  systematic methods for dealing
    with, 195–199
  testing for, 311

unconscious nature of, 194, 195

Psychasthenias. *See also specific type, e.g.,* Obsession(s)
consciousness in, 60
dissociation in, 58
hysteria compared with, 51–56, 58
Janet on, 50–57

Psyche, integrated vs. disintegrated, 61

Psychoanalytic psychiatry, 63–121, 287–295. *See also specific topic*
acting out and, 121
adaptation concept in, 160
alternatives in, 341
anger management in, 315–317
application of technology of, 131, 266–267
approaches to patient in, 142, 146, 161–163, 304–305
art vs. science in, 287, 356–357
association techniques in, 94–95, 102, 103, 285, 289–290, 295, 296
Breuer and, 85, 90–92. *See also* Breuer, Joseph
cathartic method in, 85, 90, 102
Charcot and, 65–80. *See also* Charcot, Jean-Marie
compulsion repetition in, 226, 290–291
consciousness in, 301
contributions, 228–229
countertransference biases in, 285
data collection and reporting in, 118, 119, 285
on defense mechanisms, 211, 310
demands of, 164

dream use in, 289
ego psychology and, 347
ego use in, 162, 282, 283, 294, 304
existential school vs., 304–305, 358
explanation and prediction in, 360
fact use in, 346
fantasy interpretation in, 121, 242, 270, 308, 311, 346
free association use in, 103, 285, 289–290, 295, 296
Freud and, 94–121. *See also* Freud, Sigmund
function of, 328
historical tradition of, 319
hypnosis and, 288
on hysteria, 203–204
id, role of, 162
ideals of, 265–267, 269, 271–273, 288–289, 293–294
on illness vs. person, 191
on influence of past, 228–233, 292–294, 308
insight development in, 290–293
instinct use in, 294, 295
interpersonal school vs., 311
intervention in, 289–290
methods vs. thinking in, 177
narcissism concept in, 203
narcissistic transference in, 304–305
neutrality in, 293–294, 306–307, 309
objective-descriptive school and, 80–81
objectivity in, 285–288, 290, 292–294, 306–307, 316
opinions on, 267, 355–356
origins and development of, 63–121, 287–297
passivity of, 292–294
on phobias, 248–249

Psychoanalytic psychiatry (*Cont.*)
  physical contact with patients
    in, 94–95, 288–289
  problem location in, 150, 341
  process theories, 242, 244–
    245, 352–353
  progress in, 218
  projection management in,
    195–196, 309
  reality and, 341
  reconstructive methods in, 231
  resistance management in, 289,
    291–293, 296, 309–311
  role of patient in, 95, 142,
    146, 161–163, 304–305
  role of therapist in, 95, 120,
    142, 146, 161–163, 282,
    289–290, 304–305
  schools of, 342
  on secretiveness, 355
  of sexuality, 115, 145, 164,
    266, 269–270
  on social institutions, 271
  social reality and, 293–294
  strength of, 146–147
  structured situations in, 281
  symptom use in, 96
  tension in, 280, 290, 292
  testing in, 316
  transference in, 104–105, 195–
    196, 198–200, 231, 290–
    292, 295, 304–305, 311,
    316–317
  unconscious use in, 120
  untoward results of, 272–273
  verbal nature of, 295
Psychoses. *See also specific psy-*
    chosis, e.g., Manic-
    depressive psychoses
  anorexia nervosa as, 50
  Bleuler on, 194, 334
  classification of, 15, 333
  components of, 300
  dementia praecox as endoge-
    nous, 29

  dissociation nature and degree
    in, 60
  etiology of infectious, 334
  Freud on, 194–195
  generalization in, 160
  genetic vs. neurologic concepts,
    30–33
  modern concepts, 50
  neuroses vs., 131–132
  object cathexes in, 190
  paranoia in study of, 130–131
  patient-therapist relations in,
    191–192, 253
  problems in understanding psy-
    chotic patients, 253
  prognosis, 333
  resistance analysis in, 309–310
  Sullivan on, 194–195
  withdrawal in, 194
"Pseudo-living" in hysteria, 203–
    204, 206
Psychosomatic states, 45
Psychotherapy, defined, 56

Random procedures, use of, 33
Reaction, symptoms and, 211–
    212
Reality. *See also* Social reality
  in association, 341
  in autism, 244
  changes in literary representa-
    tion of, 351
  concept in hysteria vs. schizo-
    phrenia, 202–203
  concepts in neuroses, 54–55,
    57, 336–337
  existential school on, 305
  fantasy and, 200, 341
  Freud's methods and, 118
  function of, 244
  in hysteria, 202–203
  interest in, in psychiatry, 346
  in obsessions, 60
  in overcoming neuroses, 116
  in psychasthenias, 60

reality-testing, 305, 336–337
  in unconsciousness, 341
Regression, described, 121
Reich, Wilhelm, 203
Reiss, David, 358, 361
Relationship disturbances in neuroses, 344
Repetition compulsion, 226, 290–
  291
Repression, 39
Resistance(s)
  analysis of, 297
  existential school on, 298–299
  interpersonal school on, 295,
    296, 309–311
  in neuroses, 299, 310
  use, in psychoanalysis, 289,
    291, 292–293
Responsiveness, volition and, 16
Rogers, Carl, 344
Role-playing
  in interpersonal psychiatry,
    309, 310
  narcissistic transference and,
    304
Rush, Benjamin, 208–209, 254
  on etiology, 238–242, 351–352
  on personality change, 224–
    225

Schildkraut, Joseph J., 353
Schizophrenia, 217. *See also* De-
    mentia praecox
  autism vs. withdrawal in, 178
  diagnosis, 264, 334
  effects of schizophrenics on
    therapists, 260, 327, 343
  ego in, 60
  family interactions in, 259
  fantasy vs. reality in, 202–203
  importance of knowledge of,
    63–64
  Minkowski on, 298
  paresis, diagnosed as, 25, 28,
    124

as personality advance, 44
  prognosis, 332–333
  psychological contradictions in,
    224
  Sullivan on, 60, 184–188
  thinking defect in, 353
  time sense in, 140–141
Searles, Harold, 193
Secretiveness, 355
Senile dementia, 23
Sexuality
  displacement and denial of,
    108–109, 116
  factors in sexual responsive-
    ness, 16, 116
  Freud on, 100, 115, 118, 119,
    226, 247–248
  homosexuality, 115, 323
  hysteria and, 105, 107, 204
  infantile, 118, 119
  libido maturation, 164
  in neuroses, 116, 217, 246–
    248
  oedipal elements, 204, 226,
    301–303
  psychoanalytic school on, 100,
    115, 118, 119, 145, 146,
    226, 247–248, 269–270
  sexual implications of hystero-
    genous zones, 70
Skinner, B. F., 352
Sloane, R. B., 357
Social psychiatry. *See* Interper-
    sonal (social) psychiatry
Social reality, 190–191
  behavior and, 248
  Bleuler on, 168
  delusions and, 213
  dementia praecox and, 29
  existential school on, 232, 233,
    268
  Freud on, 175–177
  improvement of social interven-
    tions, 178–179
  instincts and, 293

Social reality (*Cont.*)
  interpersonal school on, 174–179, 184–187, 267–268, 306–308, 310–312, 345
  life chart use, 176–177, 345–346
  Meyer on, 174–179, 345
  present and past life forces, 228–234, 350–351
  psychoanalytic school on, 267–268
  responsiveness and, 16
  Sullivan on adaptation of to patient, 184–187
  symptoms and, 177–179, 183–184
  therapy adjustment to, 180–181
  widening representation of, 181–183
Somnambulism, 35–40, 355
  dreaming and, 335
  personality contrasts in, 225
Stanton-Schwartz phenomenon, 349
Statistical techniques, use of, 33
Subconscious, 39
  contact with, 85
  in hysteria, 55–56
  Janet on, 39, 85
Subjectivity, 33
Sublimations, role of, 293, 294
Suggestibility in hysteria, 37–40, 59, 71–72, 94
Sullivan, Harry Stack, 164, 183–199, 346, 347–348
  on attitudes of patients, 30, 192–194, 195
  contributions, 167–170, 183–184, 207–213
  on diagnosis related to treatment, 259
  on ego, 347
  emphases of, 344
  followers of, 345

Horney and, 344
  on human interests, 347
  on human transactions, 267–268
  on hysteria, 194–195, 200–206
  interest in facts vs. fantasies, 184, 346
  on interview situation, 190–199
  on intimacy vs. neutrality, 309
  limitations of, 170
  method of, 169, 170, 184–199, 312, 316, 347
  paranoia management, 188–190
  participant observation by, 305–307
  on patient-physician barriers, 30
  on personality, 270–271
  on preadolescent life, 206–207
  process theories, 245, 353
  projection management, 195–199, 229, 307
  restrictions of method, 312
  on schizophrenia, 311, 322–323
  social illness concept, 311–312
  style of, 184, 186, 346
  on successive present, 232
  understanding of, 300
  on verbal material, 185
Sutton, Thomas, 21
Syphilitic dementia. *See* Paresis
Szasz, Thomas, 164–165, 265, 343

Tension
  in objective-descriptive method, 278–281
  in psychoanalytic method, 280, 290, 292
Testing
  by objective-descriptive school, 281–283

for projection, 311
in psychoanalysis, 316
reality-testing, 305, 336–337
Tics, 57–59
Training of therapists
    decision-making and, 324–327
    problems in, 358–359
Transference, 159–161
    analysis by Freud, 341
    countertransference, 285, 298–299
    development of, 194
    distortions of, 195–196, 198
    in hypnosis, 74
    in hysteria, 74, 329
    infantile neuroses and, 299
    interpersonal psychiatry and, 199–200, 308, 311
    narcissistic, 304–305
    in psychoanalysis, 104–105, 195–196, 198, 199–200, 231, 290–292, 295, 304–305, 311, 316–317
    therapist and, 120
    working through, 328, 329, 360
Transformation in hysteria, 79
Traumata
    cathartic method and, 102
    extension of concept of, 50
    hypnosis and, 102
    hysteria and, 67–68, 72–73, 76–79, 90, 91, 102
    ideas and emotions in moments of, 98–99
    important facets of, 91
    intrusion into sleep, 85
    Kraepelin on, 20
    repetition in therapy of, 102
    symptom production and awareness of, 98–102

Unconscious, 39
    access to, 91
    Charcot on, 92

displacement in, 114–115, 117
in hysteria, 59–60
ideas and emotions in, 92
importance in psychoanalysis, 120
interpersonal school on, 311
order in, 117
projection and, 194, 195
reality in, 341
Uterine hypothesis of hysteria, 64–65, 338–339

Vaillant, George E., 333
Virchow, Rudolph, 14
Volition concept, 16–17. *See also* Wishes
Volkan, Vamick, 358

Wernicke, Carl, 211, 352, 356
    on dissociation, 225, 226
    process theory, 243
    on social factors, 168
Will, volition and, 16–17
Winnicott, D. W., 344
Wishes
    displacement and, 117
    dreams and, 100–101
    fantasy and, 100–101, 117–118
    Freud on, 116–118, 341
    ideas and, 103–104
    prohibitions and, 100–101
    strength of, 117
    symptoms and, 114
Withdrawal
    Freud on, 178, 194
    in psychoses, 190, 191, 194
    in schizophrenia, 178
Wölfflin, Heinrich, 80
Wundt, Wilhelm, 1, 13, 331
    Kraepelin and, 13, 16–17, 331
Wyss, Dieter, 359

Zetzel, Elizabeth, 329
Ziehen, Theodor, 15–16